Ramzi Ajjan • Stephen M. Orme

Editors

Endocrinology and Diabetes

Case Studies, Questions and Commentaries

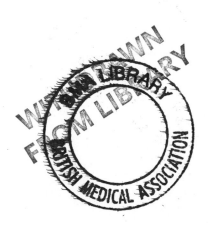

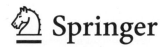 Springer

Editors
Ramzi Ajjan
Cardiovascular and Diabetes Research
University of Leeds
Leeds, UK

Stephen M. Orme
Department of Endocrinology
St. James's Hospital
Leeds, UK

ISBN 978-1-4471-2788-8   ISBN 978-1-4471-2789-5   (eBook)
DOI 10.1007/978-1-4471-2789-5

Library of Congress Control Number: 2015936752

Springer London Heidelberg New York Dordrecht

Printed on acid-free paper

Springer-Verlag London Ltd. is part of Springer Science+Business Media (www.springer.com)

This book is dedicated to our mentors, trainees, students and patients, and our wives and daughters.

Preface

The practice of diabetes and endocrinology is a clinical discipline, which relies on structured detective work in order to make the correct diagnosis. This in turn requires a combination of good observational skills and an ability to interpret complex results within the clinical context. Presentation of patients with the same endocrine condition can be variable, which adds to the complexity making this field of medicine both challenging and enjoyable.

In this book, we assembled a number of real-life clinical cases that illustrate aspects of both diabetes and endocrinology. The clinical vignettes presented have been written by practising physicians and surgeons who encountered these patients in their day-to-day practice. Some represent common presentations of relatively rare conditions, whilst others describe uncommon presentations of more familiar disorders.

The cases are described as they may present to the clinician, followed by a series of questions that illustrate the clinical problem and provide background information.

The list is not intended to be exhaustive, and a systematic approach is deliberately avoided. The main aim of this book is to whet the appetite of trainees in diabetes and endocrinology and provide an alternative approach to cover a wide variety of clinical scenarios for the more experienced practitioner.

Leeds, West Yorkshire, UK   Ramzi Ajjan, FRCP, MMed. Sci, PhD
Stephen M. Orme, MBChB, MD, FRCP

Contents

Contributors

Afroze Abbas BSc (Hons), MBChB, MRCP, PhD Leeds Centre for Diabetes & Endocrinology, Leeds Teaching Hospitals NHS Trust, Leeds, West Yorkshire, UK

Sabah Alvi MBChB, MD Department of Paediatric Endocrinology, Leeds Children's Hospital, Leeds, West Yorkshire, UK

Ramzi Ajjan FRCP, MMed. Sci, PhD Cardiovascular and Diabetes Research, University of Leeds, Leeds, Yorkshire, UK

Akwasi A. Amoako BSc, MBChB, PhD, MRCOG Leeds Centre for Reproductive Medicine, Department of Obstetrics and Gynaecology, Leeds Teaching Hospitals, Leeds, West Yorkshire, UK

Adam H. Balen MBBS, MD, DSc, FRCOG Leeds Centre for Reproductive Medicine, Department of Obstetrics and Gynaecology, Leeds Teaching Hospitals, Leeds, West Yorkshire, UK

Julian H. Barth FRCP, FRCPath, MD Chemical Pathology/Metabolic Medicine, Department of Blood Sciences, Leeds Teaching Hospitals NHS Trust, Leeds, West Yorkshire, UK

William M. Bennet MD, MBChB Department of Endocrinology, Royal Hallamshire Hospital, Sheffield, Yorkshire, UK

John S. Bevan BSc, MBChB, MD, FRCP Department of Endocrinology, J.J.R. Macleod Centre for Diabetes, Endocrinology and Metabolism (Mac-DEM) Aberdeen Royal Infirmary, Aberdeen, UK

Aberdeen University, Aberdeen, Grampian, UK

Deepak Chandrajay MBBS, MRCP, FRCPath Metabolic Medicine and Chemical Pathology, Leeds Teaching Hospitals NHS Trust, Leeds, West Yorkshire, UK

Bernard Y. P. Chang BSc, MBChB, FRCSEd, FRCOphth Department of Ophthalmology, Leeds Teaching Hospitals NHS Trust, Leeds, West Yorkshire, UK

Fiona M. Fairlie MD, FRCOG Department of Obstetrics and Gynaecology, The Royal Hallamshire Hospital, Sheffield, Yorkshire, UK

Brian M. Frier BSc (Hons), MD, FRCPE, FRCPG BHF Centre for Cardiovascular Science, The Queen's Medical Research Institute, University of Edinburgh, Edinburgh, Lothian, Scotland, UK

Earn H. Gan MBChB, MRCP Institute of Genetic Medicine, Newcastle University, Newcastle upon Tyne, UK

Endocrine Unit, Royal Victoria Infirmary, Newcastle upon Tyne, UK

Nigel G. L. Glynn MB, BCh, BAO Department of Endocrinology, Barts and The London School of Medicine, Queen Mary University of London, London, UK

Alex J. Graveling MBChB, MRCP (UK) Department of Diabetes and Endocrinology, Aberdeen Royal Infirmary, Aberdeen, Aberdeenshire, UK

Jubbin J. Jacob MD, DNB Endocrinology and Metabolism (Mac-DEM), J.J.R. Macleod Centre for Diabetes, Aberdeen Royal Infirmary, Aberdeen, UK

Endocrine and Diabetes Unit, Department of Medicine, Christian Medical College and Hospital, Ludhiana, Punjab, India

Haqeel A. Jamil MbChB, MRCP Department of Cardiology, Leeds Institute of Genetics, Health and Therapeutics, University of Leeds, Leeds, UK

Rhodri J. King MD Division of Cardiovascular and Diabetes Research, The University of Leeds, Leeds, UK

Márta Korbonits MD, PhD Department of Endocrinology, William Harvey Research Institute, Barts and the London School of Medicine, Queen Mary University of London, London, UK

Katarina Kos MD, PhD Diabetes and Obesity Research, University of Exeter, Exeter, Devon, UK

Ioannis Kyrou MD, PhD Endocrinology and Metabolism (WISDEM), Warwickshire Institute for the Study of Diabetes, University Hospitals Coventry and Warwickshire NHS Trust, Coventry, UK

Division of Metabolic and Vascular Health, Warwick Medical School, University of Warwick, UHCW, Coventry, UK

Wycliffe Mbagaya MBChB, MRCP (UK), FRCPath Laboratory Medicine, Leeds Teaching Hospitals NHS Trust, Leeds, West Yorkshire, UK

Robert D. Murray BSc, MD, FRCP Department of Endocrinology, Leeds Teaching Hospitals NHS Trust St. James's University Hospital, Leeds, West Yorkshire, UK

Deepa Narayanan MBBS, MRCP Chemical Pathology/Metabolic Medicine, Department of Blood Sciences, Leeds Teaching Hospitals NHS Trust, Leeds, West Yorkshire, UK

Stephen M. Orme MBChB, MD, FRCP Department of Endocrinology, St. James's Hospital, Leeds, West Yorkshire, UK

Katharine R. Owen MD, MRCP Endocrinology and Metabolism (OCDEM), Oxford Centre for Diabetes, University of Oxford, Churchill Hospital, Oxford, Oxon, UK

Simon H. S. Pearce MD, FRCP Institute of Genetic Medicine, Newcastle University, Newcastle upon Tyne, UK

Endocrine Unit, Royal Victoria Infirmary, Newcastle upon Tyne, UK

Nick Phillips MBChB, FRCS, FRCS (SN) PhD Department of Neurosurgery, Leeds General Infirmary, Leeds, West Yorkshire, UK

Chinnadorai Rajeswaran MBBS, FRCP(UK), MSc Department of Diabetes, Endocrinology and Obesity, Dewsbury District Hospital, Dewsbury, West Yorkshire, UK

Mohan Ramasamy MScPT Weight Management Service, The Mid Yorkshire Hospitals NHS Trust, Dewsbury, West Yorkshire, UK

Harpal Singh Randeva MBChB, PhD, FRCP Endocrinology and Metabolism (WISDEM), Warwickshire Institute for the Study of Diabetes, University Hospitals Coventry and Warwickshire NHS Trust, Coventry, UK

Division of Metabolic and Vascular Health, Warwick Medical School, University of Warwick, UHCW, Coventry, UK

Arelis Rodriguez-Farradas RD Diabetes Centre, Adult Weight Management Services, Mid Yorkshire Hospitals NHS Trust, Dewsbury, West Yorkshire, UK

Eleanor M. Scott BM, BS, BMedSci, MD, FRCP Leeds Institute of Genetics Health and Therapeutics, University of Leeds, Leeds, West Yorkshire, UK

Tolulope Shonibare Bsc, MBChB, MRCP Department of Diabetes, Endocrinology and Obesity, Dewsbury District Hospital, Dewsbury, West Yorkshire, UK

Roly Squire MBBS, FRCS (Paed) Paediatric Surgery, Leeds Children's Hospital, Leeds General Infirmary, Leeds, West Yorkshire, UK

Mark W. J. Strachan BSc, MBChB, MD, FRCP Metabolic Unit, Western General Hospital, Edinburgh, Midlothian, UK

Eberta J. H. Tan MBBS, MRCP (UK) Endocrinology, Changi General Hospital, Singapore, Singapore

Martin O. Weickert MD, FRCP Endocrinology and Metabolism
(WISDEM), Warwickshire Institute for the Study of Diabetes,
University Hospitals Coventry and Warwickshire NHS Trust, Coventry, UK

Division of Metabolic and Vascular HealthWarwick Medical School,
University of Warwick, UHCW, Coventry, UK

Klaus K. Witte MD, FRCP Division of Cardiovascular
and Diabetes Research, University of Leeds, Leeds, UK

Nicola N. Zammitt BSc (Med Sci), MBChB, MD, FRCPE Department
of Diabetes, Royal Infirmary of Edinburgh, Edinburgh, Lothian,
Scotland, UK

Difficult-to-Treat Hyperthyroidism

Case 1

Earn H. Gan and Simon H.S. Pearce

Abstract

This case illustrates a 31-year-old female who presented with thyrotoxicosis and mild thyroid eye disease. Questions relating to this common thyroid condition are addressed in a systematic fashion, including a summary of the clinical signs and symptoms, the appropriate biochemical and radiological investigations, management and follow-up. This case nicely demonstrates the spectrum and heterogeneity of hyperthyroidism in terms of disease severity and response to medication. Although most patients respond well to anti-thyroid drugs, this patient was refractory to this treatment, as shown by her growing goitre and worsening biochemical results despite high dosages of carbimazole. Her condition was eventually treated with total thyroidectomy. The management options for more aggressive Graves' disease are discussed along with other questions about the case study.

Keywords

Hyperthyroidism • Thyrotoxicosis • Thyroid autoantibody • Antithyroid medication • Radioiodine therapy

Case Presentation

A 31-year-old lady with a 6-month history of dizziness, heat intolerance and shakiness was referred to the endocrine unit. Her primary care practitioner reported the following results: TSH <0.05 mU/l, free T4 29.2 pmol/l.

> What are the questions to be asked?

The brief history from the patient suggested symptoms of hyperthyroidism. Other symptoms associated with thyrotoxicosis were explored systematically as shown in Table 1.1. The symptoms reported by the patient include intermittent palpitation, excessive sweating and increased irritability with short attention span. She had also lost 5 kg in 6 months despite having a good

E.H. Gan, MBChB, MRCP (✉)
S.H.S. Pearce, MD, FRCP
Institute of Genetic Medicine, Newcastle University, Centre Parkway, Newcastle upon Tyne NE1 3BZ, UK

Endocrine Unit, Royal Victoria Infirmary, Centre Parkway, Newcastle upon Tyne NE1 3BZ, UK
e-mail: earn.gan123@gmail.com

R. Ajjan, S.M. Orme (eds.), *Endocrinology and Diabetes: Case Studies, Questions and Commentaries*,
DOI 10.1007/978-1-4471-2789-5_1, © Springer-Verlag London 2015

Table 1.1 Symptoms of hyperthyroidism

Systems	Symptoms of hyperthyroidism
Skin	Heat intolerance, hair loss, hyperhidrosis, urticaria, pruritis, eczema
Cardiopulmonary	Palpitation, exercise intolerance, dyspnoea on exertion, angina pectoris, orthopnoea, obstructive symptoms from enlarged thyroid (dysphagia or breathing difficulty).
Gastrointestinal	Increased bowel frequency from rapid intestinal transit, weight loss from increased caloric requirement, nausea or vomiting (may suggest concurrent pregnancy)
Renal and electrolytes	Polydipsia and polyuria
Reproductive system	Amenorrhea, oligomenorrhea, hypomenorrhea and anovulation, infertility
Neuromuscular system	Tremor, muscle weakness, especially proximal muscle involvement. Less commonly, patients might have bulbar and oesophagolaryngeal muscle weakness presenting with dysphonia, dysphagia and dysarthria. Reversible diaphragmatic weakness has occasionally being reported and presented with dyspnoea [1]
Mental and cognition	Anxiety, irritability, emotional liability, apprehension and difficulty concentrating, shortened attention span, distractibility and impaired short-term memory. Apathetic symptoms are common in the older group such as depression and pseudodementia

appetite. Patients with hyperthyroid Graves' disease or nodular thyrotoxicosis (solitary toxic nodule or multinodular goitre) generally have symptoms for several months with no clear day of onset. The onset of symptoms over 1 or 2 days would raise the possibility of thyroiditis.

It is important to elicit symptoms of thyroid eye disease in patients suffering from thyrotoxicosis as this condition is clinically apparent in 50 % of patients with Graves' disease [2]. Indeed, this patient admitted that her father noticed her eyes appear to be more prominent but she denied having pain or grittiness in her eyes. Questions addressing the risk factors and potential causes of hyperthyroidism were also explored, as summarized in Box 1.1.

Box 1.1: Risk Factors for Hyperthyroidism
A. Past medical history of autoimmune diseases (pernicious anaemia, vitiligo, etc.)
B. Past history of postpartum thyroiditis
C. Family history of thyroid disease or autoimmune conditions
D. Medication: Amiodarone, lithium, radiology imaging with iodine contrast, excessive thyroxine replacement
E. Diet: Excessive consumption of high-iodine content food such as kelp or seaweed

---

F. Recent hepatitis B vaccination, recent treatment for chronic hepatitis C (interferon and ribavirin), HIV or with alemtuzumab. This group of patients is at risk of both self-limiting thyroiditis or autoimmune hyperthyroidism (Graves' disease)
G. Demographic factors such as age (range 20–50 years), female sex and previous pregnancy [5]

There was no relevant past medical history in this patient. She did not have any previous thyroid disorders or other associated autoimmune diseases. She is a non-smoker with two healthy children aged 6 and 11 years old. Smoking history is particularly important as Graves' ophthalmopathy is more common among smokers and they seem to respond poorly to treatment compared to non-smokers [3, 4]. Her mother has hypothyroidism and her great grandmother suffered from hyperthyroidism and pernicious anaemia. Her current medication includes Dianette for contraception and oxytetracycline as required for acne treatment.

What signs to look for?

Table 1.2 Signs of thyrotoxicosis

Systems	Signs of hyperthyroidism
Cardiovascular	Sinus tachycardia or atrial fibrillation, systolic hypertension with widened pulse pressure, cardiac flow murmur and third heart sounds from high-output congestive heart failure
Respiratory	Stridor or facial plethora as a result of compression of trachea or vena cava from enlarged thyroid
Bone	Osteoporosis, osteopenia, occasionally hypercalcaemia
Skin	Warm, smooth and moist hands, fine hair, alopecia, shiny, soft and friable nails (onycholysis), thyroid acropachy, facial or palmar erythema, hyperpigmentation, telangiectasia, pretibial myxoedema
Renal and electrolyte metabolism	Hypertension, pedal oedema, nephrocalcinosis, thyrotoxic periodic paralysis (associated with hypokalaemia), distal renal tubular acidosis, proteinuria in patients with autoimmune thyroid disease [6]
Haematology	Microcytosis, pernicious anaemia, lymphoid enlargement and splenomegaly, and rarely thymic enlargement; thrombocytopenia [7]
Mental/central nervous system	Tremor, agitation, fidgetiness or hyperactivity, muscle weakness and wasting, hyperactive deep tendon reflex with shortening of relaxation phase
Eyes	Lid retraction, proptosis, chemosis, plica and conjunctival redness
Gastrointestinal	Elevated transaminase enzymes, protein-calorie malnutrition and hypoalbuminaemia from severe thyrotoxicosis

The clinical manifestations of hyperthyroidism are multi-system, mainly caused by the acceleration of various physiological processes in all organs. Nevertheless, most of these signs are non-specific. The frequency and severity of these features vary widely among affected patients, and in rare cases the first presentation may be with life-threatening thyroid storm. The signs to look out for in hyperthyroidism are summarized in Table 1.2.

Summarise Key Symptoms and Provide a List of Differential Diagnoses

This case illustrates a 31-year-old lady presented with a 6-month history of significant weight loss, palpitation, hyperhidrosis, agitation and short attention span. Physical examination revealed a diffusely enlarged goitre with bruit, palmar erythema and tremors in both hands. Her pulse was regular at 88 beats per minute and her reflexes were normal. Her eyes appeared to be proptotic, without any dysmotility or redness. All these features are in keeping with thyrotoxicosis and the differential diagnosis include:

- Graves' hyperthyroidism (most likely diagnosis as patient has a diffuse goitre with eye symptoms)
- Silent or subacute thyroiditis
- Toxic nodular thyroid disease
- Factitious thyrotoxicosis

> What biochemical and radiological tests are needed to reach a diagnosis?

A comprehensive clinical history and physical examination should be sufficient to confirm thyrotoxicosis in most cases. Nevertheless, it is necessary to make an aetiological diagnosis in all cases in order to plan treatment and assess prognosis.

Thyroid status is determined biochemically by the measurement of serum free thyroxine (FT4), free triiodothyronine (FT3) and thyroid stimulating hormone (TSH) concentration. Serum TSH secretion is very sensitive to inhibition by excess circulating thyroid hormones and hence is a remarkably sensitive test for thyrotoxicosis. Importantly, in all cases of true primary hyperthyroidism, the TSH is fully suppressed (i.e., <0.05 mU/l), as non-thyroidal illness and several drugs may commonly lead to low but not suppressed TSH concentrations (0.1–0.4 mU/l) [8].

However, one also has to bear in mind that normal or raised serum TSH levels are found in the rare instances of thyrotoxicosis caused by a TSH-secreting pituitary adenoma or resistance to thyroid hormone. Serum FT3 is the next most sensitive test for hyperthyroidism, and a state of "T3 thyrotoxicosis" is defined by a suppressed TSH with an elevation of serum FT3 but with normal FT4. In evolving hyperthyroidism, serum FT4 is the last to become elevated. Use of modern free thyroid hormone assays has virtually eliminated interpretation problems caused by changes in serum binding protein levels that bedevilled total thyroid hormones assay.

The relative elevation of serum T3 and T4 concentrations can suggest the cause of thyrotoxicosis. For instance, excessive free T3 production is commonly found in Graves' hyperthyroidism and toxic nodular goitre, whereas T4-predominant thyrotoxicosis usually suggests thyroiditis, iodine-induced thyrotoxicosis or exogenous T4 ingestion. A free T4/free T3 ratio (pmol/l:pmol/l) of 3 or less being typical of Graves' hyperthyroidism [9].

The measurement of thyroid autoantibodies, such as TSH receptor-binding inhibitory immunoglobulin (TBII) and thyroid peroxidise antibody (TPO) are necessary to confirm the diagnosis of Graves' disease in the absence of eye signs. TBII test is positive in more than 95 % of Graves' disease patients and measurement is particularly useful in euthyroid individuals who present with features of thyroid eye disease, or differentiating toxic nodular goitre from Graves' disease, as well as assessing the risk of foetal or neonatal thyroid dysfunction in pregnant women with autoimmune thyroid disorders. TPO antibodies are less helpful as elevated levels are found in only 80 % of patients with Graves' disease.

In the event of negative thyroid auto-antibodies, measurement of radioactive iodine or pertechnetate uptake in the thyroid gland is useful for differentiating thyrotoxicosis caused by excessive thyroid hormone production (increased uptake) from various conditions resulting in low thyroid uptake, as stated in Table 1.3. In addition, elevated ESR and CRP are found in patients suffering from subacute thyroiditis. Hypercalcaemia, elevated liver transaminases or alkaline phosphatase, ferritin and sex hormone binding globulin may also be found.

Table 1.3 Pattern of thyroidal uptake in radionuclide imaging

Causes of thyrotoxicosis	Radionuclide uptake pattern
Graves' disease	Increased uptake homogenously
TSH-induced thyrotoxicosis	Increased uptake homogenously
Toxic nodular goitre	Increased uptake in regions of autonomy only (uni or multiple)
Subacute thyroiditis[a]	Little or no uptake
Silent thyroiditis[a]	Little or no uptake
Iodine or radiographic contrast induced	Little or no uptake
Factitious or iatrogenic thyrotoxicosis	Little or no uptake

[a]In thyroiditis, thyroid uptake mirrors serum TSH, so scans need to be performed during the suppressed TSH phase to see low uptake

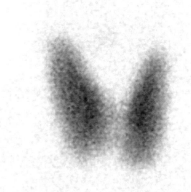

Uptake 6.6 % (N < 3.5)

Fig. 1.1 Pertechnetate scan showed an increased uptake at 6.6 % (normal <3.5 %) in homogenous pattern

Discuss the Results and Provide a Final Diagnosis

Thyroid function tests were carried out by the referring general practitioner and showed a fully suppressed serum TSH with a raised FT4 (29.2 pmol/l). This was then repeated at the endocrine clinic which showed a further increase in FT4 (72 pmol/l) and FT3 (35 pmol/l). Her TBII antibody was positive at 13.4 u/ml (normal <1.5). A pertechnetate thyroid scan showed an increased homogenous uptake at 6.6 % (normal <3.5 %), in keeping with Graves' disease (Fig. 1.1). Given the strongly positive TBII result and clinical evidence of eye disease, the nuclide scan was not strictly necessary to confirm the final diagnosis of Graves' hyperthyroidism complicated by mild thyroid eye disease.

Management of the Case and Follow-Up

There are three options currently available to alleviate hyperthyroidism: antithyroid drugs, radioactive iodine therapy and total thyroidectomy. Each of these treatments has certain drawbacks and the optimal treatment depends on patient preference, disease presentation and severity. Because of her severe thyrotoxicosis at presentation, it was mandatory to try and improve her thyroid state before definitive treatments (radioiodine or surgery) could be considered. The patient was therefore started on anti-thyroid medication, carbimazole 40 mg once a day. The patient was warned about the rare side effect of agranulocytosis with this medication. Nevertheless, a TBII level of over 5 u/ml predicts a low probability of medical remission [10], particularly with severe hyperthyroidism, and so definitive therapy was planned from the start. In general, however, relapse prediction using TBII is not that practical in daily practice as a large proportion of patients have antibody levels in the "inconclusive range."

Six weeks after being started on carbimazole, levothyroxine 100 mcg daily was added in block and replace regimen, as her FT4 had dropped significantly (Fig. 1.2). She also reported increased grittiness in her eyes with significant bilateral eyelid swelling and retro-orbital tightness. Examination revealed minimal right-sided proptosis, bilateral upper lid retraction and equivocal injection of the conjunctiva. She was reviewed in a combined ophthalmologist/endocrinologist thyroid eye clinic and was found to have inactive thyroid eye disease, with discomfort on up-gaze as the only sign of disease activity. She had lid retraction of 3 and 4 mm in the right and left eye, respectively; whereas proptosis was symmetrical and borderline at 19.5 mm. Her eye symptoms improved with topical lubricants.

At review, a further 12 weeks later she reported increased tiredness and had lost a further 2 kg in weight. Examination showed that she was still thyrotoxic with mild tremor and regular heart rate at 100 beats per minute. Her thyroid function had rebounded and was consistent with her worsening symptoms; showing a raised FT3 of 13.7 pmol/l and FT4 of 89.9 pmol/l. The importance of drug compliance was reinforced but the patient claimed to have good concordance with the treatment. She denied having recent radiological imaging (this was confirmed through the hospital radiology system) and she reported only occasional consumption of seafood and no vitamin or iodine supplements.

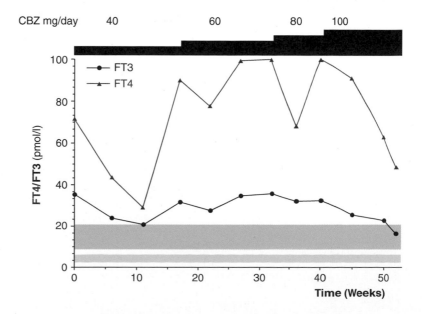

Fig. 1.2 The time course of free T4/free T3 profile and carbimazole (CBZ) dosage from diagnosis until just before total thyroidectomy

The carbimazole dose was increased to 60 mg once a day and the 'block and replace' regimen was carried on. This resulted in some improvement in her symptoms and biochemical results (see Fig. 1.2).

Unfortunately, over the next few months the patient developed intolerance to 60 mg of carbimazole owing to nausea and vomiting every morning after taking medication. This led to worsening thyrotoxicosis, with increased sweatiness and palpitation. She was advised to split up her carbimazole doses to 20 mg three times a day, which she tolerated much better, but despite this her goitre continued to enlarge with persistent loud bruit. The more concerning issue was she started to report difficulty in swallowing, indicating obstructive symptoms from an enlarged thyroid. She was referred urgently to a surgeon for total thyroidectomy and carbimazole dosage was increased further to 40 mg twice a day. Thyroxine was stopped at this point.

The patient continued to respond poorly to antithyroid medication. She remained symptomatic with palpitation, heat intolerance and tiredness. Her FT3 and FT4 remained elevated at 32.7 pmol/l and 100 pmol/l respectively, with fully suppressed TSH. Carbimazole dose was further increased to 100 mcg daily and propanolol LA 80 mg was added while waiting for total thyroidectomy. Her thyroid function improved slightly 4 weeks later but she remained thyrotoxic with FT4 of 63.2 pmol/l and FT3 of 22.8 pmol/l. In light of her poorly controlled

thyrotoxicosis, she was admitted 10 days before the surgery for thyroid blockade with iopanoic acid therapy (Fig. 1.3).

An Update on the Condition

The patient was rendered euthyroid prior to the operation and underwent total thyroidectomy uneventfully. Histology showed a 34-g thyroid gland with toxic hyperplastic cells in keeping with treated Graves' disease. Postoperatively, she had transient hypocalcaemia, necessitating therapy with calcium supplements (Sandocal 1 g 4 times per day) for 1 month, followed by a phased reduction over the next 2 months. She was also started on 150 mcg levothyroxine daily after the operation. Her FT3 normalised following total thyroidectomy (see Fig. 1.3) and her quality of life has also improved significantly. Her thyroid eye disease steadily improved, with improvement in eyelid retraction and mild proptosis over the next 6 months. She was discharged back to her GP for thyroid function monitoring while on lifelong thyroxine replacement.

Learning Points

Failure to achieve control of hyperthyroidism with antithyroid drugs can be problematic to manage. In many cases it is due to poor patient

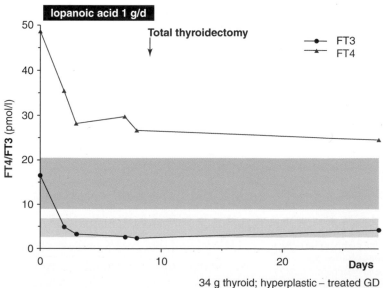

Fig. 1.3 Free T$_3$ (FT$_3$) normalized after total thyroidectomy, but free T4 (FT4) remains marginally elevated. Iopanoic acid 1 g od was administered for 10 days prior to surgery

concordance with therapy. However, it seems likely that aggressive Graves' disease with high titres of stimulating antibodies was the culprit in this case. Other causes including administration of iodinated contrast media during CT scanning or a high iodine diet/iodine supplements should also be excluded. The thionamide antithyroid drugs act as a competitive substrate for iodination by thyroid peroxidase, and there is no established "upper dose limit" for either carbimazole or propylthiouracil, although adverse reactions (agranulocytosis) appear more frequent on doses of carbimazole of 100 mg daily or above [11]. While the patient was being treated with high dose carbimazole, she was being seen every 2 weeks with blood count monitoring and strict instructions about what to do in the event of sore throat or fever. In the end, she did not achieve sufficient improvement in her thyrotoxicosis with carbimazole to make surgery a safe option, so a rapid blockade regimen using iopanoic acid (1 g daily) was used. An alternative would have been to administer Lugol's iodine or saturated solution of potassium iodide. In the overwhelming majority of patients, any of these three methods results in normalisation of serum FT3 within 7 days, at which point the patient would be suitable for immediate surgery, such as in this case (see Fig. 1.3). Serum FT4 may stay the same or even go up during iopanoic acid treatment due to inhibition of deiodination, and this should not delay surgery if FT3 is normal. An alternative treatment might have been to give her radioiodine 6 or 8 weeks after carbimazole had been started. Of concern is that radioiodine may precipitate or cause exacerbation of existing thyroid eye disease [12]. Nevertheless, administration of radioiodine under prednisolone cover (e.g., prednisolone 20 mg daily for a month, starting on the day of radioiodine) might have been an equally satisfactory and safe treatment option [13].

References

1. Mier A, Brophy C, Wass JA, Besser GM, Green M. Reversible respiratory muscle weakness in hyperthyroidism. Am Rev Respir Dis. 1989;139(2):529–33.

2. Kendall-Taylor P, Perros P. Clinical presentation of thyroid associated orbitopathy. Thyroid. 1998;8(5): 427–8.
3. Bartalena L, Marcocci C, Tanda ML, Manetti L, Dell'Unto E, Bartolomei MP, et al. Cigarette smoking and treatment outcome in Graves' ophthalmopathy. Ann Intern Med. 1998;129:633–5.
4. Vestergaard P. Smoking and thyroid disorders – a meta-analysis. Eur J Endocrinol. 2002;146(2):153–61.
5. Strieder TG, Tijssen JG, Wenzel BE, Endert E, Wiersinga WM. Prediction of progression to overt hypothyroidism or hyperthyroidism in female relatives of patients with autoimmune thyroid disease using the Thyroid Events Amsterdam (THEA) score. Arch Intern Med. 2008;168(15):1657–63.
6. Weetman AP, Tomlinson K, Amos N, Lazarus JH, Hall R, McGregor AM. Proteinuria in autoimmune thyroid disease. Acta Endocrinol (Copenh). 1985;109(3):341–7.
7. Androuny A, Sandler RM, Carmel R. Variable presentation of thrombocytopenia in Graves' disease. Arch Intern Med. 1982;142(8):1460–4.
8. Mitchell AL, Pearce SH. How should we treat patients with low serum thyrotropin concentrations? Clin Endocrinol. 2010;72(3):292–6.
9. Yoshimura Noh J, Momotani N, Fukada S, Ito K, Miyauchi A, Amino N. Ratio of serum free triiodothyronine to free thyroxine in Graves' hyperthyroidism and thyrotoxicosis caused by painless thyroiditis. Endocr J. 2005;52(5):537–42.
10. Eckstein AK, Plicht M, Lax H, Neuhauser M, Mann K, Lederbogen S, et al. Thyrotropin receptor autoantibodies are independent risk factors for Graves' ophthalmopathy and help to predict severity and outcome of the disease. J Cin Endocrinol Metab. 2006;91(9): 3464–70.
11. Grebe SK, Feel CM, Ford HC, Fagerstrom JN, Cordwell DP, Delahunt JW, et al. A randomized trial of short-term treatment of Graves' disease with high-dose carbimazole plus thyroxine versus low-dose carbimazole. Clin Endocrinol (Oxf). 1998;48(5):585–92.
12. Bartalena L, Marcocci C, Bogazzi F, Manetti L, Tanda ML, Dell'Untol E, et al. Relation between therapy for hyperthyroidism and the course of Graves' ophthalmopathy. N Engl J Med. 1998;338(2):73–8.
13. Lai A, Sassi L, Compri E, Marino F, Sivelli P, Piantanida E, et al. Lower dose prednisolone prevents radioiodine-associated exacerbation of initially mild or absent graves' orbitopathy: a retrospective cohort study. J Clin Endocrinol Metab. 2010;95(3):1333–7.

Suggested Reading

Braverman LE, Cooper D. Werner & Ingbar's the thyroid: a fundamental and clinical text. 10th ed. Philadelphia: Lippincott, Williams & Wilkins; 2012.

Hypothyroidism Complicated by Hypothyroid Coma

Case 2

Ramzi Ajjan

Abstract

A 68-year-old lady is admitted to hospital after being found unconscious by her neighbour with little clues in the history to make a firm diagnosis. The case turns out to be a typical example of a common medical condition with a rare and serious clinical presentation.

The various symptoms and signs at presentation are discussed in order to aid in the diagnosis. This is followed by making a list of the possible diagnoses and the appropriate tests are subsequently requested. The importance of understanding the unusual, and potentially misleading, laboratory results associated with this condition are discussed. Finally, treatment options and controversies in the management of this condition are reviewed.

Keywords

Hypothyroidism • Hypothyroid coma

Case

A 68-year-old lady with a history of mild chronic obstructive airway disease (COAD) was admitted to accident and emergency after being found unconscious by her neighbour. In addition to COAD, she has a history of osteoarthritis (OA), treated with both regular and as required pain killers. She lives alone, fully independent and does not keep in touch with any members of her family. The neighbour mentioned that the patient has been acting strangely recently, becoming withdrawn and having issues with her memory, raising the possibility of dementia. However, the patient refused to see her GP with her symptoms. Family history includes a niece with type 1 diabetes and a daughter with eczema. Her list of medications comprised of ibuprofen 400 mg tds, salbutamol and fluticasone inhalers, bendrofluazide 2.5 mg od and paracetamol as required. She stopped smoking 22 years ago (20/day for 19 years prior) and drinks up to 5 units of alcohol/week.

R. Ajjan, FRCP, MMed.Sci, PhD
Cardiovascular and Diabetes Research,
University of Leeds, Clarendon Way, Leeds,
Yorkshire LS2 9JT, UK
e-mail: r.ajjan@leeds.ac.uk

R. Ajjan, S.M. Orme (eds.), *Endocrinology and Diabetes: Case Studies, Questions and Commentaries*,
DOI 10.1007/978-1-4471-2789-5_2, © Springer-Verlag London 2015

> Comment on the history. What would you like to do next?

The patient, admitted to hospital with a collapse, is an ex-smoker with a history of COAD and OA. She has been having behavioural issues and problems with her memory, suggesting that she may have developed dementia. There is a family history of autoimmunity. More details should be obtained on the behavioural changes from the neighbour. Also, it is worth ringing her GP to obtain an up-to-date list of medications and discuss her medical history. We should now proceed to a full examination.

On examination she had:

Temperature: 36.1 °C

Blood pressure: 155/72 mmHg, pulse 52/min (regular), respiratory rate 14/min

Oxygen saturation: 88 %

Her GCS was 12/15 (E3, V4 and M5) with normal pupils and no clear neurological signs. Her JVP was raised at 4.5 cm, and she had a faint mitral regurgitation (MR) murmur with mild pedal oedema.

> What are the three most striking abnormalities in her examination?

Low GCS, reduced oxygen saturation, and relatively low respiratory rate.

Raised JVP may be due to right heart failure secondary to her COAD, whereas MR is quite common and pedal oedema may also be due to her right heart failure.

Her preliminary investigations showed the following:

FBC: Hb 10.5 g/dl, MCV 104 fL, WBC 9.1×10^9/L (normal differential), platelets 350×10^{12}/L

U&Es: sodium 130 mmol/L, potassium 3.8 mmol/L, Urea 16.1 mmol/L, creatinine 120 µmol/L, bicarbonate 31 mEq/L and eGFR 49 ml/kg/m².

Arterial blood gas analysis: pO2: 7.1 kPa, pCO2: 8.8 kPa, pH: 7.24

Chest x-ray (CXR): see Fig. 2.1.

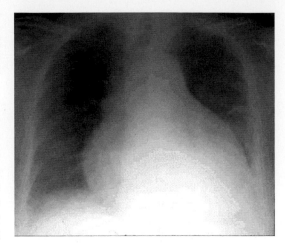

Fig. 2.1 Chest x-ray on admission to accident and emergency

ECG: rate 50/min regular, flat T waves in III, AVF, V4–6.

Urgent CT-head, no abnormality detected.

Comment on Her FBC

This lady has anaemia with normal WBC and platelet counts She has raised MCV and therefore the differential diagnosis for her anaemia includes:

- Alcohol
- Vitamin B12 or folate deficiency
- Myelodysplasia
- Hypothyroidism
- Haemolytic anaemia
- Drugs: particularly those interfering with DNA synthesis such as Azathioprine, methotrexate, Zidovudine
- Aplastic anaemia
- Acquired sideroblastic anaemia

However, the mild abnormality in her FBC is unlikely to have contributed to the clinical presentation.

Comment on Her U&Es

This lady has hyponatraemia and raised bicarbonate. The commonest cause of low sodium is the use diuretics, some of which can also cause metabolic alkalosis. This patient is on bendrofluazide, which may have caused this abnormality although there are other possibilities (for full review of hyponatraemia, please see Case 10). The modest drop in her sodium is unlikely to be the cause for her presentation.

Comment on the CXR

The heart shows significant enlargement and there is a mild degree of pleural effusion, more evident on the left. There are no clear signs of heart failure in the lung fields and therefore the enlarged globular heart does not necessarily represent dilated cardiac chambers and more likely to be due to pericardial effusion.

> How would you proceed in this patient?

There are few clues in the history to point towards a clear diagnosis. In a situation like this, it is helpful to make a list of the main abnormalities to try to reach the right diagnosis.
Admission: collapse and drop in GCS.
History: memory problems and behavioural issues with a family history of autoimmunity.
Investigations: decompensated respiratory acidosis (raised bicarbonate may be a marker of chronic metabolic alkalosis). Large heart on CXR and non-specific ECG abnormalities.
Focussing further on one serious abnormality likely to be the cause of her clinical presentation, respiratory acidosis is a clear culprit.

> What is the differential diagnosis of respiratory acidosis?

This includes:
Lung pathology: COAD is a potential cause in our patient but normal chest auscultation and clear lung fields argue against this being the main cause of the symptoms.
Central nervous system pathology: The failure to detect neurological signs and normal CT head makes this an unlikely diagnosis. Central

hypoventilation may occur secondary to opioid use. Our patient has osteoarthritis and may have been prescribed additional pain killers. Therefore, a careful drug history from the GP is mandatory. Normal pupils that are reactive to light effectively rules out this possibility but checking with the GP is still recommended. In cases of doubt, naloxone can be administered to reverse the action of any opioid. Finally, endocrine disorders such as hypothyroidism may cause hypoventilation but there is no history of a thyroid disorder in our patient.
Neuromuscular disease: This includes myasthenia gravis, Guillain-Barré and amyotrophic lateral sclerosis. These conditions are not consistent with the history of the presentation or patient examination.
Obesity-hypoventilation: this can occur in individuals with significant weight problems (see Case 10), but our patient had a weight of 69 kg with a BMI of 25.7 kg/m^2, making this an unlikely diagnosis.

> The patient deteriorates over the next few hours and her GCS drops to 9/15. Repeat blood gas analysis shows a rise in $pCO2$ to 9.1 kPas and a drop in pH to 7.19. What would you do?

Summarising the major abnormalities, the patient has a central hypoventilation disorder together with an enlarged heart on CXR and a small pleural effusion. The GP cannot be reached and therefore a trial with naloxone is not unreasonable.

> The patient is given naloxone, but no change in her condition is noted. Would you request thyroid function tests at this stage?

Thyroid tests should NOT be generally requested in patients who are ill and the only exception is when it is thought the illness is directly related to thyroid dysfunction. Therefore, it is important to undertake an examination of the thyroid status and palpate the neck followed by requesting thyroid function tests.

On examination, the patient is noted to have a dry skin but there are no other convincing signs of hypothyroidism. One doctor reports slow relaxation of ankle reflexes, whereas another, who is more senior, disagrees. Neck palpation is unremarkable. Her TFTs show:

FT4: 1.1 pmol/L (normal 10–20)
TSH: 97 mIU/L (normal 0.2–4.5 mIU/L)

> Does this patient have hypothyroidism, or are these abnormal TFTs related to euthyroid sick syndrome (ESS)?

In ESS, T3 levels are typically low and in more advanced cases T4 levels can fall, whereas TSH is normal or low normal [1, 2]. TSH levels can marginally rise, particularly as the acute illness is brought under control, but these never reach the levels seen in our patient. Therefore, our diagnosis fits with primary hypothyroidism [3, 4]. Positive thyroid peroxidase antibodies will confirm the autoimmune nature of hypothyroidism and it is a test worth requesting.

> Does primary hypothyroidism offer a unifying diagnosis for the symptoms and signs in our patient?

Primary hypothyroidism can cause memory loss and alter behaviour. Dry skin and bradycardia are classical signs of hypothyroidism [5, 6]. Low thyroid hormones can result in hyponatraemia and non-specific ST-T segment changes on ECG. Mild anaemia with raised MCV is seen with hypothyroidism whereas pericardial and pleural effusions are known to occur, particularly in severe thyroid hormone deficiency. Respiratory acidosis is one of the criteria to diagnose myxoedema coma and therefore the likely unifying diagnosis in our patient is hypothyroidism causing myxoedema coma.

The criteria used to diagnose myxoedema coma can vary greatly and recent work attempted to diagnose this condition using a scoring system that includes alteration in thermoregulation, central nervous, cardiovascular, gastrointestinal and metabolic systems with and without a precipitating event [7]. Even using this system, some cases can be missed and therefore the diagnosis requires a high degree of suspicion and appropriate expertise.

> What would you do in this patient?

This patient, with a diagnosis of myxoedema coma, should be managed in intensive care setting as she can deteriorate quickly (mortality is up to 50 %, although this is now on the decrease) [8].

Given the rarity of this condition and the potentially serious consequences, there are no randomised controlled trials investigating the best management strategy. In general these patients need: thyroid hormone replacement, glucocorticoid replacement, treatment with broad spectrum antibiotics and general supportive measures [9, 10].

Thyroid hormone replacement: T4 is the main thyroid hormone used for replacement and can be given IV or via nasogastric tube in doses between 100 and 500 μg/day. The intravenous route is preferred due to compromised GI absorption in these patients. Frequently a loading dose of 200–500 μg is used followed by maintenance dose of 100–200 μg/day. Doses higher than 500 μg/day are thought to be associated with increased mortality and should be avoided. Some advocate the use of T3, given it is the active hormone, but evidence for superiority of such an approach has not been proven [11–14].

Glucocorticoid replacement: Adrenal insufficiency commonly occurs in patients with severe hypothyroidism and therefore glucocorticoid replacement in mandatory in these patients. A baseline cortisol check is recommended before starting therapy, although this is not strictly necessary. Dose of hydrocortisone used is between 50 and 100 mg every 6–8 h. The length of treatment should be guided by the physical condition of the patient and improvement in thyroid hormone levels.

Broad-spectrum antibiotics: The precipitating cause of myxoedema coma is frequently an infection; therefore, these patients should have appropriate cultures followed by a course of broad-spectrum antibiotics. It is unclear whether our patients had a concomitant infection but cover with antibiotics is necessary given the high risk involved.

General supportive measures:

- Intubation in case respiratory acidosis cannot be corrected medically
- IV fluid with strict input/output balance
- Correction of electrolyte imbalance: in particular hyponatraemia. This should be corrected gradually and according to the fluid status of the patient
- Oxygen supplementation as necessary
- Vasopressors in case of hypotension not corrected with IV fluid
- Passive external rewarming as a management of hypothermia aiming for a slow rise of temperature of around 0.5 °C/h. Hypothermia is common in hypothyroid coma, although core temperature was normal in our patient.
- General monitoring, including cardiac monitoring (risk of arrhythmias)
- An experienced endocrinologist with daily input into care of the patient should be involved in the management.

This patient had raised temperature at 38.5 °C less than 2 days after her admission and her urine cultures were positive for E coli. Is the rise in temperature a poor prognostic sign?

Patients with myxoedema coma are usually hypothermic and the rise in temperature in our patient may simply be related to the presence of infection and normalisation of body responses following thyroid hormone therapy. Therefore, this may be a good rather than a poor prognostic sign. Naturally, we should ensure that the she is on appropriate antibiotics to cover her urinary infection.

What are the three commonest predisposing factors to myxoedema coma?

Infection, administration of central nervous system depressants and cold exposure.

This lady had a number of routine additional tests that showed:

Creatine kinase (CK): 4,423 U/L (normal <300)

Troponin <50 pg/ml

CA125: Five-fold increase in levels (requested due to recent diagnosis of ovarian cancer in the patient's sister)

What do these tests mean and would you ask a cardiologist to review the patient given the abnormal ECG?

Elevated CK can be found in hypothyroidism, particularly severe disease. Moreover, this patient was found collapsed, which may have contributed to her raised CK.

Normal troponin is reassuring but perhaps it is worth repeating this test to be absolutely sure (given the ECG abnormalities). If repeat troponin is normal then there is no need to ask for a cardiology review as non-specific ST-T segment changes can occur in individuals with severe hypothyroidism, which normalise after therapy.

Raised CA-125 levels are a marker of ovarian cancer. However, levels can be raised in individuals with ascites due to any cause and raised tumour markers have been documented in patients with hypothyroidism, particularly in the presence of ascites [15]. Imaging is mandatory here to exclude an ovarian pathology and clarify the nature of raised CA-125.

CT scan of the abdomen/pelvis is performed, which showed the presence of moderate amounts of ascetic fluid with no other abnormality detected.

The patient makes an uneventful recovery and her TSH 3 weeks later drops to 15 mIU/l on 100 mcg of thyroxine/day. She is feeling much better in herself, and the previous issues with her memory resolve. However, she is very concerned about raised CA-125 levels. Would you advocate repeating these, or would you simply reassure the patient that these were related to her hypothyroidism and ascites and will normalise?

Given her normal imaging, it is almost certain that raised CA-125 levels are related to this patient's hypothyroidism, complicated by ascites. However, it is important to monitor levels to make sure these are normalising.

What else would you like to do?

Repeat CXR and ECG should be performed. Also, a cardiac ultrasound should have been requested on admission (after her CXR results) to assess cardiac function and confirm pericardial effusion.

Four weeks after the initial presentation, her CXR shows major improvement with smaller heart shadow and disappearance of her pleural effusion, whereas her ECG normalises. Cardiac ultrasound on admission showed a trivial MR with a significant pericardial effusion and no evidence of tamponade. Her repeat cardiac ultrasound one month later showed a very small amount of fluid in the pericardium. Does the patient require any further cardiac investigations?

No, as the pericardial effusion is resolving and she has no major cardiac structural abnormalities. It should be noted that severe hypothyroidism can lead to cardiac muscle dysfunction leading to congestive cardiac failure, which was not the case in our patient.

What is the frequency of ascites, pleural and pericardial effusions in hypothyroidism?

Ascites and pleural effusion occur in less than 10 % of cases. A small amount of pericardial effusion may be evident in up to 30 % of patients with hypothyroidism, but this is not usually clinically significant [16].

References

1. McIver B, Gorman CA. Euthyroid sick syndrome: an overview. Thyroid. 1997;7:125–32.
2. De Groot LJ. Dangerous dogmas in medicine: the nonthyroidal illness syndrome. J Clin Endocrinol Metab. 1999;84:151–64.
3. Adler SM, Wartofsky L. The nonthyroidal illness syndrome. Endocrinol Metab Clin North Am. 2007;36:657–72.
4. Warner MH, Beckett GJ. Mechanisms behind the nonthyroidal illness syndrome: an update. J Endocrinol. 2010;205:1–13.
5. Vaidya B, Pearce SH. Management of hypothyroidism in adults. BMJ. 2008;337:a801.
6. Almandoz JP, Gharib H. Hypothyroidism: etiology, diagnosis, and management. Med Clin North Am. 2012;96:203–21.
7. Popoveniuc G, Chandra T, Sud A, Sharma M, Blackman MR, Burman KD, et al. A diagnostic scoring system for myxedema coma. Endocr Pract. 2014;20:808–17.
8. Wartofsky L. Myxedema coma. Endocrinol Metab Clin North Am. 2006;35:687-viii.
9. Hampton J. Thyroid gland disorder emergencies: thyroid storm and myxedema coma. AACN Adv Crit Care. 2013;24:325–32.
10. Mathew V, Misgar RA, Ghosh S, Mukhopadhyay P, Roychowdhury P, Pandit K, et al. Myxedema coma: a new look into an old crisis. J Thyroid Res. 2011;2011:493462.
11. Chernow B, Burman KD, Johnson DL, McGuire RA, O'Brian JT, Wartofsky L, et al. T3 may be a better agent than T4 in the critically ill hypothyroid patient: evaluation of transport across the blood–brain barrier in a primate model. Crit Care Med. 1983;11:99–104.
12. McCulloch W, Price P, Hinds CJ, Wass JA. Effects of low dose oral triiodothyronine in myxoedema coma. Intensive Care Med. 1985;11:259–62.
13. Yamamoto T, Fukuyama J, Fujiyoshi A. Factors associated with mortality of myxedema coma: report of eight cases and literature survey. Thyroid. 1999;9:1167–74.

14. Rodriguez I, Fluiters E, Perez-Mendez LF, Luna R, Páramo C, García-Mayor RV. Factors associated with mortality of patients with myxoedema coma: prospective study in 11 cases treated in a single institution. J Endocrinol. 2004;180:347–50.

15. Krishnan ST, Philipose Z, Rayman G. Lesson of the week: hypothyroidism mimicking intra-abdominal malignancy. BMJ. 2002;325:946–7.

16. Roberts CG, Ladenson PW. Hypothyroidism. Lancet. 2004;363:793–803.

Hyperthyroidism in Pregnancy

Case 3

William M. Bennet and Fiona M. Fairlie

Abstract

Graves' disease presents frequently in females of reproductive age and is the most common cause of thyrotoxicosis in pregnancy, occurring in 0.15 %. In addition transient gestational hyperthyroidism occurs in 2–3 % of pregnancies in Europe. Thyrotoxicosis may adversely impact on the outcome of pregnancy. Where hyperthyroidism complicates pregnancy it is important to correctly diagnose the condition so as to guide appropriate management. In this chapter, the presentation of the three common causes of thyrotoxicosis in pregnancy and the puerperium are described using clinical scenarios. Pregnancy complications are considered and management options discussed.

Keywords

Pregnancy • Thyrotoxicosis • Hyperthyroidism • Thyroiditis • Maternal • Gestational • Graves' disease

Introduction

Hyperthyroidism is present where there is an overactive thyroid gland with elevated thyroid hormones, free thyroxine (free T4) and free tri-iodothyronine (free T3), and thyrotoxicosis is where symptoms are also present. Thyrotoxicosis may adversely impact on the outcome of pregnancy. Graves' disease is common in females of reproductive age and is the most frequent cause of thyrotoxicosis in pregnancy, occurring in 0.15 %. Transient gestational hyperthyroidism occurs in 2–3 % of pregnancies in Europe. Where hyperthyroidism arises during pregnancy it is important to correctly diagnose the condition so as to guide appropriate management.

In this chapter, the presentation of the three common causes of thyrotoxicosis in pregnancy and the puerperium are described using clinical scenarios. Pregnancy complications are considered and management options discussed.

W.M. Bennet, MD, MBChB (✉)
Department of Endocrinology,
Royal Hallamshire Hospital,
Glossop Road, Sheffield, Yorkshire S10 2JF, UK
e-mail: William.bennet@sth.nhs.uk

F.M. Fairlie, MD, FRCOG
Department of Obstetrics and Gynaecology, The
Royal Hallamshire Hospital, Sheffield, Yorkshire UK

R. Ajjan, S.M. Orme (eds.), *Endocrinology and Diabetes: Case Studies, Questions and Commentaries*,
DOI 10.1007/978-1-4471-2789-5_3, © Springer-Verlag London 2015

Case 1: Overt Thyrotoxicosis – Pre-pregnancy

A 34-year-old woman is referred to you by her general practitioner because she has abnormal thyroid function test (TFT) results. She has recently miscarried at 11 weeks gestation. This was her first pregnancy. She has a history of primary infertility for which no cause has been found and she is keen to conceive again soon. Her general practitioner has investigated thyroid function because she complained of palpitations and weight loss after her miscarriage.

> What symptoms would you ask about?

As well as querying about the duration and of her extent of her weight loss and palpitations, you should probe for additional symptoms of thyrotoxicosis including increased appetite, heat intolerance, tremor, sweating, anxiety, insomnia and poor concentration (full details can be found in Case 10).

You should establish if she has a personal or family history of thyroid disease or other autoimmune condition.

A spectrum of typical symptoms would support a diagnosis of continuing thyrotoxicosis. Some of these symptoms, especially palpitations, occur in normal pregnancy. A short duration of symptoms, lasting only days, would be suggestive of subacute or postnatal thyroiditis whereas a longer time course would be typical of Graves' toxicosis.

> What signs would you look for?

You should examine her for signs of thyrotoxicosis including tachycardia, warm peripheries, sweating and tremor. You look for a thyroid goitre and thyroid eye disease, which would indicate Graves' disease.

Summarise the Symptoms/Signs and Provide a List of Differential Diagnoses

She has had typical symptoms of thyrotoxicosis for 6 months and you have identified subtle signs of thyrotoxicosis including pulse 88 beats per minute, a minor tremor and warm hands. There is a bilateral fullness in the neck but no discrete goitre and she has minor chemosis with periorbital oedema. Differential diagnoses include:

- Graves' disease
- Toxic multinodular goitre
- Single toxic adenoma
- Subacute thyroiditis
- Iodine-induced hyperthyroidism
- Struma ovarii
- Thyrotropin receptor activation

The most likely diagnosis is therefore Graves' thyrotoxicosis and this may explain her infertility. Transient gestational hyperthyroidism would not cause overt thyrotoxicosis and would have resolved on fetal loss.

> What biochemical and immunological tests are needed to reach a diagnosis?

You should request TFT, including thyrotropin (TSH), free T4 and free T3, which confirm thyrotoxicosis (Table 3.1). Also, request anti-TSH receptor antibody (TRAb); the result is elevated consistent with Graves' disease (see Table 3.1). The final diagnosis is therefore Graves' disease. Her thyrotoxicosis might explain her infertility as she has lost weight which may result in weight-related anovulation.

> How would you manage this case?

She wants to conceive again soon but this poses risks from uncontrolled thyroid disease in pregnancy. There may be infertility due to anovulation and there is an increased miscarriage rate. She may develop uncontrolled thyrotoxicosis and is at risk of cardiac failure. Very rarely retrosternal extension of a goitre may cause dysphagia or

Table 3.1 TFT and antibody results

Test, units	Result	Reference range
TSH, mIU/l	<0.02	0.27–4.2
FreeT4, pmol/l	48	12–22
FreeT3, pmol/l	12.6	3.1–6.8
TRAb, IU/l	7.2	≤0.9

tracheal obstruction, which can be a problem if the patient requires to be intubated.

There are risks to the fetus or neonate from uncontrolled maternal thyrotoxicosis. Miscarriage rates are increased in thyrotoxicosis. Premature delivery may occur, either due to preterm labour if thyrotoxicosis is uncontrolled or there may be iatrogenic prematurity due to concerns about fetal growth and wellbeing or secondary to thyroidectomy in pregnancy. Fetal and neonatal thyrotoxicosis may develop due to TRAb.

Despite her desire to become pregnant you should explain that she must use contraception until she is euthyroid. You need to outline the risks, both to her and to her fetus, of uncontrolled thyroid disease. She should be treated with propylthiouracil (PTU). Once the patient has been rendered euthyroid by a high dose for 4–6 weeks the PTU should be titrated to the minim dose which will maintain her free T4 at the upper limit of the reference range. She could then attempt to conceive again.

She was commenced on PTU using an initial dose of 200 mg twice daily which has been reduced to 50 mg twice daily. She is now 8-weeks pregnant. Her free T4 is 22.1 pmol/l (first-trimester reference range 12.1–19.6). You should adjust the PTU to the minimum dose that will keep her free T4 at or just above the *non-pregnant* reference range [1]. You could continue to treat her with PTU 50 mg twice daily but you should anticipate that the PTU dose will need to be reduced; therefore you should monitor her TFT closely, every month. PTU infrequently causes severe hepatitic reactions so consider changing to carbimazole or methimazole (CBZ/MMI) after the first trimester when organogenesis is complete; the equivalent dose of carbimazole is 10–15 times less than for PTU. In a patient receiving only a small dose of PTU you could anticipate reducing and stopping it within 2 months. In addition to TFT, liver function tests should be monitored in patients receiving PTU.

Fetal anatomy ultrasound is usually undertaken at 18–20 weeks. In the event that antithyroid medication is continued after 20 weeks gestation or the TRAb is elevated over 4 IU/l (or two to three times the reference range) when rechecked at this stage, then additional growth scans should be arranged every 4–6 weeks or as indicated

clinically. Evidence of fetal thyroid dysfunction includes goitre, tachycardia, growth retardation, hydrops and cardiac failure. An alert should be sent to the paediatrician to assess the newborn baby for transient neonatal Graves' disease.

Whereas Graves' toxicosis ameliorates during pregnancy you should anticipate a rebound after delivery. You will need to arrange ongoing close endocrine monitoring and should expect to restart or increase antithyroid drugs. Both CBZ/MMI and PTU are secreted in breast milk and borderline elevation of TSH can occur in breastfed infants. CBZ/MMI in doses up to 30 mg daily are preferred to PTU, used in doses up to 300 mg daily, in view of the risk of hepatitis with PTU [2]. Treatment should be taken in divided doses immediately after breastfeeding.

Update of Graves' Disease Before and During Pregnancy

Antithyroid drugs are the mainstay of treatment. CBZ/MMI would normally be the drugs of first choice to treat Graves' thyrotoxicosis in the non-pregnant situation. However, in a patient trying to conceive PTU is more appropriate than CBZ/MMI which are teratogenic [1, 3]. Treatment with CBZ/MMI in the first trimester is associated with the congenital skin defect aplasia cutis, and infrequently choanal atresia (posterior nasal passage), oesophageal atresia, omphatocele and omphalo-mesenteric duct abnormalities. The incidence of aplasia cutis combined with the latter two congenital defects is 1.6 % of patients treated with CBZ/MMI in the first trimester [4]. However CBZ/MMI should be used after 13 weeks gestation for patients requiring continued antithyroid medication or presenting de novo with thyrotoxicosis. Indications for thyroidectomy in pregnancy include severe adverse reactions to antithyroid drugs, ongoing high doses of these medications, for example CBZ/MMI >30 mg per day or PTU >450 mg per day, or inability to control thyrotoxicosis due to compliance issues. If surgery is required, the optimum time is the second trimester. Radioiodine treatment is not used in pregnancy.

It is important to measure TRAb in pregnant women who are hypothyroid following prior radioiodine treatment or in those who had thyroidectomy. Elevated levels may persist and these immunoglobulin G (IgG) antibodies freely cross the placenta and may render the fetus toxic. Conversely in patients who have had prior Graves' disease in remission, not requiring anti-thyroid drugs, then fetal growth is not likely to be compromised.

Compared to pre-pregnancy levels *total* T4 and *total* T3 are increased in pregnancy, secondary to a rise in thyroid-binding globulin which is caused by an elevation in oestradiol. Conversely free T4 and free T3 show small progressive decreases during the course of pregnancy. These changes depend on the assay used and trimester-specific ranges should be obtained from your local laboratory. TSH falls transiently during the first trimester, mirroring the rise seen for human chorionic gonadotropin (hCG).

Case 2: First-Trimester Hyperthyroidism

A 21-year-old Asian woman presents with frequent vomiting. It is 8 weeks since her last menstrual period and a pregnancy test is positive. This is her first pregnancy. She is unable to tolerate any oral food or fluid and she has been admitted to the local gynaecology unit for hydration and administration of antiemetic. Investigation of thyroid function has shown abnormal results with TSH fully suppressed and free T4 raised 40 % above the first trimester reference range.

What questions should be asked?

Has she had symptoms suggestive of thyrotoxicosis, e.g., heat intolerance, palpitations, emotional lability, weight loss and tremor? If these symptoms have been present did they precede the pregnancy or develop only recently?

Has she previously had thyrotoxicosis and is there a family history of thyroid disease?

Is there a personal or family history of other autoimmune disease?

What are the signs to look for?

Look for evidence of weight loss and examine for the presence of tremor, tachycardia, lid lag, exophthalmos and goitre.

What differential diagnosis would you consider?

Transient gestational hyperthyroidism is the most likely diagnosis.

Graves' disease can present for the first time in early pregnancy: thyroid eye disease and goitre are signs of this condition.

Consider other causes of vomiting in early pregnancy, notably urinary tract infection, peptic ulceration, pancreatitis (both usually associated with abdominal pain) and Addisonian crisis (very rare).

What biochemical and immunological tests are needed to reach a diagnosis?

Request TRAb and repeat the TFT (free T4 and free T3) every 4–6 weeks until 18–22 weeks gestation. In transient gestational hyperthyroidism overt thyrotoxicosis is uncommon, spontaneous resolution occurs by mid-gestation and TRAb is not significantly elevated. Conversely in Graves' disease TRAb is normally elevated and antithyroid medication is often required. Measure thyroid peroxidase (TPO) antibody if there is a significant goitre.

Request mid steam urine for microscopy and culture.

Monitor her urea and electrolytes.

Table 3.2 Changes in TFT results as gestation advances

	8 weeks	13 weeks	19 weeks
TSH, mIU/l	<0.02	<0.1	2.4
Free T4, pmol/l	28.1	24.6	15.7
Free T3, pmol/l	6.2	5.9	5.1

Results of Investigations

Thyroid function normalised by 19 weeks gestation (Table 3.2).

Urine culture was negative.

The initial urea and electrolyte profile was indicative of dehydration with hyponatraemia, hypokalaemia and hypochloraemic alkalosis. These abnormalities resolved once she was rehydrated and her vomiting was controlled with antiemetics (see management).

> What is the final diagnosis?

She had transient gestational hyperthyroidism associated with hyperemesis gravidarum.

> How would you manage this patient?

The woman should be admitted to hospital and given intravenous fluids to correct her dehydration and electrolyte imbalance. Normal saline (0.9 % sodium chloride) is appropriate with the addition of potassium chloride to correct the hypokalaemia.

Antiemetics are helpful to control nausea and vomiting in this situation. Any of the following agents can be prescribed orally or parentally. To date there is no evidence that these drugs are teratogenic.

- Antihistamines, e.g., promethazine and cyclizine
- Phenothiazines, e.g., chlorpromazine
- Dopamine antagonists, e.g., metoclopramide and domperidone
- Ondansetron

Hyperemesis may cause vitamin deficiencies, notably of the B vitamins B1, B6 and B12. Oral (25–50 mg three times daily) or intravenous (100 mg weekly) thiamine should be given to any woman with prolonged vomiting.

The woman's risk of thrombosis should be assessed (pregnancy itself is a risk factor in addition to bed test and dehydration). In most cases thromboprophylaxis with low molecular weight heparin is indicated during hospital admission.

Excessive vomiting in pregnancy may be due to multiple pregnancy or hydatidiform mole. The woman should have an early pelvic ultrasound scan to exclude these conditions and to confirm viable pregnancy.

Update on Transient Gestational Hyperthyroidism

In this condition there is a self-limiting hyperthyroidism occurring in early pregnancy. It usually resolves by 20 weeks gestation and is not due to intrinsic thyroid disease [5]. It is often but not always associated with nausea and vomiting of varying severity. Overt thyrotoxicosis is rarely seen when there is a pre-existing multinodular goitre. The condition is more common among south Asian women compared with Caucasian women and it tends to recur in subsequent pregnancies.

Whereas free T3 and T4 are raised and/or TSH is suppressed, affected women are clinically euthyroid and TRAb is not significantly elevated.

hCG levels peak in early pregnancy. The hCG alpha subunit is closely homologous with that of TSH and is thought to stimulate the thyrotropin receptor in gestational thyrotoxicosis, similarly to stimulation of the receptor by TRAb in Graves' disease. The level of hCG directly correlates with the severity of vomiting and free thyroxine concentrations.

Transient gestational hyperthyroidism is more likely if the pregnancy is complicated multiple pregnancy or hydatidiform mole, conditions associated with high levels of hCG.

The diagnosis of transient gestational hyperthyroidism is one of exclusion. TRAb should be absent and the woman should be clinically euthyroid. TSH, free T3 and T4 levels should return to normal in the second trimester as nausea and vomiting resolves. Antithyroid drugs should only be considered where the patient is clinically toxic and both free T3 and free T4 are elevated, following rehydration if appropriate, as Graves' disease or toxic nodular goitre are the likely diagnoses.

The majority of women with vomiting in early pregnancy respond to rehydration and antiemetics. Corticosteroids (oral prednisolone 50 mg daily or intravenous hydrocortisone 100 mg twice daily) have been shown in randomised trials to be beneficial in severe cases resistant to antiemetics and rehydration.

Case 3: Postpartum Thyroiditis (PPT)

A woman presents with a history of fatigue and palpitations since the birth of her daughter 3 months ago. Since the birth she has never felt well but thought her symptoms were due to lack of sleep and anxiety. Her symptoms are suggestive of thyrotoxicosis.

What questions should you ask?

Has she previous pregnancies and if so, did she experience similar symptoms in the postpartum period?

Is there a family history of thyroid disease or other autoimmune conditions?

Has she experienced postpartum depression?

What signs do you look for?

You should look for signs of thyrotoxicosis (tachycardia, warm peripheries, tremor) and examine for a goitre.

Summarise the Symptoms/Signs and Provide a List of Differential Diagnoses

PPT may present with signs and symptoms attributable to either hyperthyroidism or hypothyroidism depending on the phase of the condition (see update below).

Differential diagnoses include:
- Postpartum Graves' disease
- Postpartum thyroiditis
- Hashimoto's thyroiditis
- Toxic multinodular goitre
- Postpartum depression

What biochemical and immunological tests are needed to reach the diagnosis?

You should request TSH, free T3 and T4, which in her case confirms thyrotoxicosis, with values approximately two times the upper limit of the reference range. In addition, request TRAb and TPO antibodies.

TRAb is usually absent in self-limiting postpartum thyroiditis but present in Graves' disease. An elevated TPO antibody titre is usually seen in PPT.

How would you manage this patient?

If she finds thyrotoxic symptoms debilitating, she can be offered treatment with beta blockers. However, she is at risk of entering a hypothyroid phase so her thyroid function and symptoms should be closely monitored, every 4–6 weeks.

If she becomes hypothyroid then levothyroxine replacement will be necessary. She should be advised that the condition commonly resolves after 6–8 months so levothyroxine can be stopped when she is 12 months postpartum and TFT checked after 4 weeks off the medication. If levothyroxine is discontinued there is a 10 % annual risk of developing hypothyroidism so ongoing thyroid monitoring is appropriate. PPT may recur in future pregnancies.

Update on PPT

PPT is defined as thyroid dysfunction occurring within the 12 months of delivery (whether live birth, stillbirth or miscarriage). There is disagreement over the incidence but most reviews quote a range from 5 to 10 % [6]. The condition usually presents 3–4 months postpartum. It may be monophasic (either transient hypothyroidism or hyperthyroidism) or biphasic with initial hyperthyroidism followed by hypothyroidism. The common symptoms (fatigue, insomnia, anxiety, palpitations) are often overlooked by the woman as she regards them as normal postpartum changes. It may interfere with lactation.

It is an autoimmune disorder, more common in women with type 1 diabetes, or a family history of thyroid disease or with thyroid peroxidise antibodies. Histological features are similar to Hashimoto's thyroiditis.

In the biphasic form there is an initial destructive phase with release of thyroxine resulting in hyperthyroidism. This lasts about 2–3 months and is followed by hypothyroidism as the stores of thyroxine are depleted.

Differentiating postpartum Graves' disease from PPT is usually achieved by testing for TRAb. If uncertainty remains then a radioactive technetium scan can be performed but breast-feeding needs to be deferred for 30 h. Uptake will be low in PPT but high in Graves' disease.

Most cases resolve spontaneously by 12 months postpartum. The need for treatment depends on the severity of the woman's symptoms rather than the biochemical abnormalities

There is a 70 % risk of recurrence in future pregnancies [6]. Up to 60 % of women with PPT will develop permanent hypothyroidism in later life, especially if TPO antibody positive, and an annual check of thyroid function is advisable.

References

1. De Groot L, Abalovich M, Alexander EK, Amino N, Barbour L, Cobin RH, et al. Management of thyroid dysfunction during pregnancy and parturition: an Endocrine Society clinical practice guideline. J Clin Endocrinol Metab. 2012;97:2543–65. PubMed PMID: 22869843.
2. Stagnaro-Green A, Abalovich M, Alexander E, Azizi F, Mestman J, Negro R, et al. Guidelines of the American Thyroid Association for the diagnosis and management of thyroid disease during pregnancy and postpartum. Thyroid. 2011;21:1081–125. PubMed PMID: 21787128.
3. Lazarus JH. Antithyroid drug treatment in pregnancy. J Clin Endocrinol Metab. 2012;97:2289–91. PubMed PMID: 22774211.
4. Yoshihara A, Noh JY, Yamaguchi T, Ohye H, Sato S, Seyika K, et al. Treatment of Graves' disease with antithyroid drugs in the first trimester of pregnancy and the prevalence of congenital malformations. J Clin Endocrinol Metab. 2012;97:2396–403. PubMed PMID: 22547422.
5. Rodien P, Jordan N, Lefèvre A, Royer J, Vasseur C, Savagner F, et al. Abnormal stimulation of the thyrotrophin receptor during gestation. Hum Reprod Update. 2004;10:95–105. PubMed PMID: 15073140.
6. Lazarus JH. The continuing saga of postpartum thyroiditis. J Clin Endocrinol Metab. 2011;96:614–6. PubMed PMID: 21378224.

Rhodri J. King

Abstract

Patients with Graves' disease are common to all general endocrine outpatient clinics and management options for these individuals are generally straight forward. Thyroid nodules are also frequently encountered and can present more of a clinical challenge. Less common is the finding of thyroid nodules associated with Graves' and these individuals may require greater consideration. This case addresses the treatment options available for Graves' disease along with the management and investigation of thyroid nodules.

Keywords

Graves' disease • Hyperthyroidism • Thyroid nodule • Cold nodule • Thyroid cancer

Case

A 65-year-old lady is referred as an outpatient following the discovery of a neck lump. A thyroid ultrasound arranged by the GP is reported:

> Both lobes of the thyroid are diffusely enlarged. Within the right lobe of the thyroid there lies a 15×26 mm hypoechogenic nodule with some areas of calcification. No other worrying features are identified. The remainder of the thyroid tissue appears normal. There is no local lymphadenopathy

Her thyroid function tests prior to clinic are as follows:

FreeT4 35 pmol / l, TSH < 0.05 miu / l

What are the salient points to obtain from the history and examination?

History

What (if any) thyrotoxic symptoms are present?
History and amount of weight loss.
When was the lump first noticed? Has it increased in size and if so how quickly? Is it painful?
Any difficulties with swallowing or change in quality of voice?
Is there a past medical history (PMH) of thyroid disease or autoimmune disease?

R.J. King, MD
Division of Cardiovascular
and Diabetes Research, The University of Leeds,
Clarendon Way, Leeds LS2 9JT, UK
e-mail: R.J.KING@LEEDS.AC.UK

Any history of radiation exposure?

Is there a family history of thyroid disease or head and neck cancer?

Examination

Is she thyrotoxic?

Any evidence of cardiac compromise? This includes atrial fibrillation and/or signs of heart failure.

Are signs of thyroid eye disease present?

Goitre? Is it tender/diffusely enlarged?

Is the nodule palpable? Is it mobile/fluctuant/hard?

Is lymphadenopathy present?

Does the patient have pre-tibial myxoedema?

What are the factors associated with an increased likelihood malignancy in a thyroid nodule?
- History of neck irradiation in childhood
- FH of hereditary thyroid carcinoma (MTC, PTC, MEN 2)
- Male
- Age (<20 or >70)
- Firm, hard and fixed nodule or rapidly growing nodule
- Cervical lymphadenopathy
- Persisting dysphonia, dysphagia or dyspnoea
- Other: Hashimoto's thyroiditis (lymphoma), polyposis coli

What are the features of malignancy in a thyroid nodule on ultrasound examination?
- Hypoechoic and solid nodule
- Irregular margins
- Microcalcification
- Increased and/or chaotic vascularity
- Presence of cervical lymphadenopathy or extra-capsular growth

The patient tells you that she has had classical thyrotoxic symptoms for 8–10 weeks and had lost approximately two stone in weight over 4 months. She first noticed the lump in her neck about 6 months ago and does feel that it has become more noticeable. She has a PMH of post-menopausal osteoporosis for which she takes alendronate weekly. She has no relevant family history.

On examination you note that she is tremulous with moist palms. She has a regular tachycardia (120 bpm) with no evidence of heart failure. She has no signs of active thyroid eye disease. The thyroid is moderately and diffusely enlarged with a palpable nodule within the right lobe of the thyroid which is non-tender and mobile. There is no cervical lymphadenopathy.

What are the differential diagnoses and how would you proceed at this stage?
1. Toxic adenoma
2. Graves' disease with a simple nodule
3. Toxic multinodular goitre
4. Graves' disease with a cold nodule, which may be malignant

How would you manage this patient?

The overriding issue at this stage is to treat this patient's hyperthyroidism and the symptoms related to this. Anti-thyroid medication such as carbimazole 40 mg od along with a beta-blocker (propranolol 80–160 mg bd) would be the initial treatment option. Longer term management will vary significantly depending on the final diagnosis and so further investigation is warranted at this stage. A thyroid radionuclide uptake scan will indicate if the nodule is "hot" or "cold" and provide useful information to aid the diagnosis. Thyroid function tests (TFTs) should be repeated 4–6 weeks after commencing treatment and reviewed in clinic with the results of the uptake scan.

In her follow up visit, the patient reports an improvement in her symptoms and her weight loss has plateaued. Her repeat TFTs are as follows:

FT4 10 pmol / l, TSH 0.04 miu / l

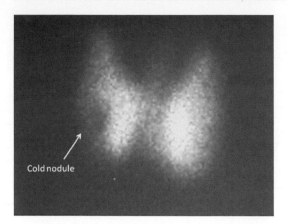

Fig. 4.1 Thyroid uptake scan demonstrating increased uptake within most of the thyroid tissue, with an area of reduced uptake within the right lobe indicating a "cold" nodule

The thyroid radionuclide uptake scan is reported:

> The nodule within the right lobe of the thyroid does not take up the radio-isotope, whereas within the remainder of the thyroid tissue there is increased uptake.

The picture is consistent with Graves' disease with a non-functioning nodule within the right lobe of the thyroid (Fig. 4.1).

The diagnosis is now suggestive of Graves' disease with an indeterminate thyroid nodule that requires further investigation.

> How common are thyroid nodules? What is the significance of the combination of Graves' disease and thyroid nodules?

The presence of thyroid nodules in the general population is common, with a prevalence of around 5 %, which can increase to 30–40 % when ultrasound is used to visualise the thyroid, and which is consistent with autopsy studies [1]. The causes of thyroid nodules are shown in Table 4.1. Thyroid cancer is rarer than nodules and accounts for 1–2 % of all cancers. The link between Graves' disease, thyroid nodules and thyroid cancer has been the subject of much debate. Palpable nodules are present in 10–15 % of Graves' disease patients, two to three times higher than in the general population [1], and nodules may also develop de novo

Table 4.1 Causes of thyroid nodules

Benign (90 % of nodules)	Malignant (10 % of nodules)
Benign nodular goitre	Papillary carcinoma
Follicular adenomas	Follicular carcinoma
Simple or haemorrhagic cysts	Hurthle cell carcinoma
Chronic lymphocytic thyroiditis	Poorly differentiated carcinoma
	Medullary carcinoma
	Anaplastic carcinoma
	Primary thyroid lymphoma
	Sarcoma, teratoma and miscellaneous tumours
	Metastatic tumours

during the course of the disease [2]. In terms of malignancy and Graves' disease, the overall risk is approximately 5 % [3–5]; however, this risk is greatly increased in the presence of cold, palpable nodules, ranging from 15 to 48 % [3, 4, 6]. The malignancy rate of palpable nodules within the general population is around 5 %, suggesting that thyroid nodules associated with Graves' are at increased risk of developing differentiated thyroid carcinoma than nodules within euthyroid individuals. Malignant nodules also appear more aggressive in Graves' disease, presenting at a more advanced staged and associated with a worse outcome than tumours in matched euthyroid individuals [7, 8].

The co-existence of Graves' disease and toxic thyroid nodule(s) is known as the Marine Lenhart syndrome. It is a very rare condition, with autonomously functioning nodules occurring in approximately 3 % of Graves' disease patients. Thyroidectomy or radioactive iodine (RAI) is typically the treatment of choice, with reports suggesting that an increased dose of radioactivity is required compared to conventional RAI treatment [9].

> What now?

In terms of the thyroid medication, there are two options
1. Reduce the carbimazole to 20 mg od
2. Continue with carbimazole 40 mg od and add levothyroxine 100 µg od

The thyroid nodule requires further characterisation through ultrasound-guided fine-needle

Fig. 4.2 Flowchart for the diagnosis and management of palpable thyroid nodules (Adapted from AATA guidelines [10])

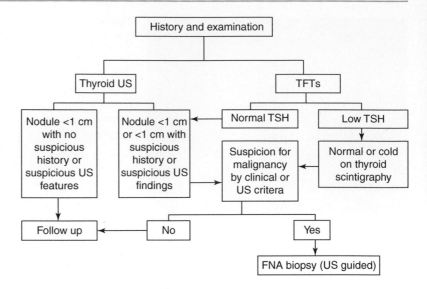

aspiration (FNA) as illustrated in Fig. 4.2. To treat the Graves' disease there are three options:

1. A course of anti-thyroid medication (6–18 months)
2. Primary radioactive iodine (RAI) *if* the nodule is deemed to be benign
3. Thyroidectomy – which would also allow characterisation of the nodule.

The patient favours a titrating regime of anti-thyroid medication. She tells you that she has several friends who have had "thyroid operations" and have experienced problems with stabilising their thyroid afterwards. She is therefore put off the idea of surgery and RAI at this stage and would like to undergo a course of medication as this would give her a chance at least of staying off extra tablets altogether. She is happy to undergo FNA of the lump. It is worth noting that "hot" nodules on a thyroid uptake scan do not usually require FNA as the risk of malignancy within a hyperfunctioning nodule is very small, providing there are no suspicious features.

Follow Up 6-Week OP Review

FT4 14 pmol/l, TSH 2.4 miu/l on CMZ 20 mg od

The cytology of the USS guided FNA is reported as thy1. This is repeated and a better sample is obtained and reported as thy2.

Are you re-assured by this result and what are your plans for follow-up?

It seems reasonable at this stage to continue with her current dose of CMZ and repeat TFTs every 6 weeks. A second benign cytology result of the nodule is required (Table 4.2) which is arranged at 6 months.

Repeat USS FNA

There is a slight increase in the size of the nodule which appears to have slightly more irregular margins. No lymphadenopathy seen.

The cytology of the FNA is reported as thy3.

What are the options now?

There is no value in repeating the FNA given the latest cytology result and the increased risk of malignant nodule associated with Graves' disease. Surgery, typically a lobectomy, is usually required with all Thy3 cytology as it is not possible to distinguish between a benign or malignant follicular lesion with FNA cytology. The patient agrees to proceed with total thyroidec-

Table 4.2 Cytological classification of thyroid nodules and action required

Cytological result of FNA	Description	Action
Thy1	**Non-diagnostic**[a] Inadequate sample or artefacts do not allow interpretation	Repeat FNA Use ultrasound guidance if not used initially
Thy2	**Non- neoplastic**[a]	Repeat 3–6 months Two thy2 results are generally required to exclude neoplasia
Thy3	**Follicular lesion/suspected follicular neoplasm**	Most patients require thyroid lobectomy and should be discussed at an MDT meeting
Thy4	**Suspicious of malignancy** Suspicious but not diagnostic of papillary, medullary or anaplastic carcinoma or lymphoma	Surgery is usually indicated All cases to be discussed by MDT
Thy5	**Diagnostic of malignancy**	Surgery is indicated Further management, investigation, radiotherapy, chemotherapy to be discussed by MDT

Adapted from Perros [11]
[a]Cysts may be described as thy1 in the absence of epithelial cells and presence of colloid and histiocytes (and clearly described as cysts) or thy2 if benign epithelial cells are also present

tomy, following which she is commenced on levothyroxine 100 μg.

The histology confirms benign follicular thyroid tissue.

What may have caused this?
1. Poor compliance
2. Reduced absorption

Follow Up 8 Weeks Post-surgery

The patient is now taking levothyroxine 125 μg and most recent TFTs are as follows:

FT4 13 pmol / l TSH 2.6 miu / l

She is discharged from endocrine follow-up, and the GP is advised to repeat her TFTs annually or sooner should she develop symptoms of thyroid dysfunction.

Longer-term Follow-up

After 6 months, she visits her GP complaining of increasing lethargy and constipation. She remains on levothyroxine 125 μg, and her TFTs are now as follows:

FT4 8.4 pmol / l, TSH 8 miu / l

The patient is adamant that she does not miss any of her medication, taking them altogether with her breakfast. On further questioning it transpires that she has been commenced on calcium and vitamin D supplements which is likely to have reduced the absorption of her thyroxine. It is important that any medications that are known to interfere with the absorption of thyroxine are taken at least 4 h after the thyroxine itself. Numerous medications can alter thyroid function tests, as indicated in Table 4.3, and highlights the importance of an accurate drug history.

Summary

Patients with Graves' disease are frequently encountered in endocrinology outpatient clinics and it is important to be vigilant for the presence

Table 4.3 The effect of different medication on thyroid hormones

Decrease in TSH Secretion	Increased hepatic Metabolism of T4	Impaired absorption of thyroxine	Impaired T4 to T3 Conversion	Decreased thyroid Hormone secretion	Increased thyroid Hormone secretion
Dopamine Dopaminergic Agents	Phenytoin	Cholestyramine	Beta antagonists	Lithium	Iodide
Glucocorticoids	Carbamazepine	Cholestapol	Glucocorticoids	Iodide	Amiodarone
Cytokines	Barbiturates	Aluminium	Amiodarone	Amiodarone	Lithium (rare)
Octreotide	Rifampicin	hydroxide	Propylthiouracil		
Metformin		Ferrous sulphate	Iopanoic acid		
		Sucralfate	Radiocontrast		
		Calcium carbonate	dyes		
		Soy protein			
		Proton pump inhibitors			

Adapted from Association for Clinical Biochemistry and British Thyroid Association [12]

of thyroid nodules in these individuals given that a higher proportion of cold nodules will be malignant compared to euthyroid individuals. A thorough history and examination, as outlined above, will help identify those at high risk of malignancy. All cold nodules in Graves' disease require FNA at the very least, with surgery indicated in high risk individuals with suspicious features on ultrasound (see Table 4.2).

References

1. Belfiore A, Russo D, Vigneri R, Filetti S. Graves' disease, thyroid nodules and thyroid cancer. Clin Endocrinol (Oxf). 2001;55(6):711–8.
2. Cantalamessa L, Baldini M, Orsatti A, Meroni L, Amodei V, Castagnone D. Thyroid nodules in Graves disease and the risk of thyroid carcinoma. Arch Intern Med. 1999;159(15):1705–8.
3. Cappelli C, Pirola I, De ME, Agosti B, Delbarba A, Castellano M, et al. The role of imaging in Graves' disease: a cost-effectiveness analysis. Eur J Radiol. 2008;65(1):99–103.
4. Kraimps JL, Bouin-Pineau MH, Mathonnet M, De CL, Ronceray J, Visset J, et al. Multicentre study of thyroid nodules in patients with Graves' disease. Br J Surg. 2000;87(8):1111–3.
5. Mishra A, Mishra SK. Thyroid nodules in Graves' disease: implications in an endemically iodine deficient area. J Postgrad Med. 2001;47(4):244–7.
6. Carnell NE, Valente WA. Thyroid nodules in Graves' disease: classification, characterization, and response to treatment. Thyroid. 1998;8(8):647–52.
7. Belfiore A, Garofalo MR, Giuffrida D, Runello F, Filetti S, Fiumara A, et al. Increased aggressiveness of thyroid cancer in patients with Graves' disease. J Clin Endocrinol Metab. 1990;70(4):830–5.
8. Pellegriti G, Belfiore A, Giuffrida D, Lupo L, Vigneri R. Outcome of differentiated thyroid cancer in Graves' patients. J Clin Endocrinol Metab. 1998;83(8):2805–9.
9. Braga-Basaria M, Basaria S. Marine-Lenhart syndrome. Thyroid. 2003;13(10):991.
10. Gharib H, Papini E, Paschke R, Duick DS, Valcavi R, Hegedus L, et al. American Association of Clinical Endocrinologists, Associazione Medici Endocrinologi, and European Thyroid Association Medical guidelines for clinical practice for the diagnosis and management of thyroid nodules: executive summary of recommendations. Endocr Pract. 2010;16(3):468–75.
11. Perros P (ed), British Thyroid Association, Royal College of Physicians. Guidelines for the management of thyroid cancer. 2nd edn. Report of the Thyroid Cancer Guidelines Update Group. London: Royal College of Physicians; 2007.
12. Association for Clinical Biochemistry and British Thyroid Association. UK guidelines for the use of thyroid function tests; 2006. Available from: http://www.britishthyroidassociation.org/infoforpatients/Docs/TFT_guideline_final_version_July_2006.pdf

A Complicated Case of Thyroid Eye Disease

Case 5

Bernard Y.P. Chang and Ramzi Ajjan

Abstract

Clinical thyroid eye disease (TED) is found in up to 50 % of patients with Graves' disease. Fortunately, the majority of cases are mild requiring topical treatment or no intervention at all. However, some cases can be severe and in extreme cases may threaten vision.

The current chapter addresses the management of a patient with type 1 diabetes who develops Graves' disease complicated by severe TED. This case illustrates the difficulties encountered in the management of patients with complicated TED.

Keywords

Thyroid eye disease • Clinical activity score • Proptosis • Optic nerve compression • Pulsed iv methylprednisolone • Orbital decompression

Case

A 54-year-old with type I diabetes for 30 years is referred by her general practitioner to the endocrine clinic with newly diagnosed thyrotoxicosis. The patient has had a number of symptoms suggestive of hyperthyroidism including heat intolerance, weight loss, anxiety and palpitations for at least 3 months prior to the referral. She is seen in the endocrine clinic and found to have clear signs of hyperthyroidism (tachycardia at 104/min/regular, hand tremor, lid lag and sweaty palms). Neck palpation reveals a smooth uniform goitre, and mild thyroid eye disease is noted with a clinical activity score of 1/7 (conjunctival redness). Her thyroid function tests (TFTs) confirm hyperthyroidism (FT4 64 pmol/l with TSH <0.05 mIU/L) and her thyroid stimulating hormone receptor antibodies are positive. Her diabetes is complicated by retinopathy that needed laser treatment 5 years earlier. She had no other diabetes complications or other medical conditions.

> What is the differential diagnosis of thyroid eye disease (TED) and does this lady need treatment for her eye symptoms?

B.Y.P. Chang, BSc, MBChB, FRCSEd, FRCOphth
Department of Ophthalmology, Leeds Teaching Hospitals NHS Trust, Leeds, West Yorkshire, UK

R. Ajjan, FRCP, MMed.Sci, PhD (✉)
Cardiovascular and Diabetes Research,
University of Leeds, Clarendon Way, Leeds,
Yorkshire LS2 9JT, UK
e-mail: r.ajjan@leeds.ac.uk

TED is commonly misdiagnosed as allergic conjunctivitis, which may delay appropriate management of this condition. Other differential diagnoses to consider include:

- Myasthenia gravis: In case diplopia is the presenting complaint. It should be noted that ocular myasthenia and TED may co-exist.
- Orbital tumour/pseudotumour: Whilst these conditions are relatively rare, they should be considered in individuals with unilateral disease.
- Carotid-cavernous fistula: A "pulsating" eye ball should raise suspicion of this condition.
- Orbital myositis: This is usually unilateral, has a severe inflammatory component and develops quickly.

Given that this lady has mild TED with a clinical activity score of 1/7 (secondary to conjunctival injection) no systematic treatment is necessary. She can be offered artificial tears in case her eyes feel uncomfortable (itchy, dry, etc.).

> What is the natural history of TED and how are disease activity and severity assessed?

TED is a self-limiting condition, and it should be explained to the patient that the condition "burns itself out." However, the period taken for the condition to stabilise varies from one patient to another, and the role of the attending physician is to control the active phase in order to reduce disease severity and avoid long-term complications. Rundle's curve demonstrates the clinical course of TED as shown in Fig. 5.1 [1].

It is important to assess disease activity and severity. Full guidelines can be found on the European Group for Graves' Opthalmopathy (EUGOGO) website (http://www.eugogo.eu). These can be summarised as follows:

Disease Activity
- Spontaneous retrobulbar pain
- Pain on eye movement
- Redness of conjunctiva
- Redness of eye lids
- Swelling of eyelids
- Swelling of caruncle
- Conjunctival oedema (chemosis)

Each gets one point and usually a score of 3 or more suggests that systematic therapy is required.

Disease Severity
- Assessment of disease severity is summarised in Table 5.1.

This patient was treated with block and replace regimen for her Graves' disease. When reviewed in clinic 3 months later, she was complaining of pain around her eyes that becomes worse on eye movement. She has also noticed intermittent diplopia. Visual acuity was normal and her colour vision was intact. Figure 5.2 represents a picture of this lady.

> Describe what you see?

The patient has periorbital odema, swollen and red eyelids, conjunctival injection and early chemosis on the left and swelling of the caruncle. She has full eye closure and therefore no risk of exposure keratitis.

> What would you do at this stage?

Fig. 5.1 Rundle's curve depicting the clinical course of TED demonstrating disease activity (*dotted line*) and severity (*solid line*) against time (Reproduced from Perros et al. [1] © 2009 with permission from BMJ Publishing Group Ltd)

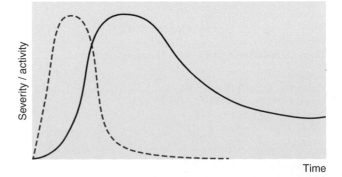

Severity / activity

Time

Table 5.1 Assessment of disease severity

Sign	Mild	Moderate/severe
Eyelid retraction	<2 mm	≥2 mm
Exophthalmus	<3 mm	≥3 mm
Orbital muscle pathology	Diplopia: none/intermittent	Constant diplopia
Soft tissue pathology	Mild	Moderate/severe
Corneal pathology	Absent or mild	Significant/severe

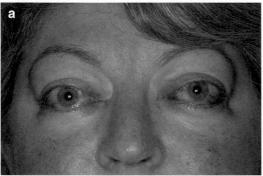

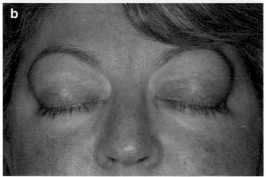

Fig. 5.2 The patient 3 months after the initial presentation. (**a**) Conjunctival and eyelid abnormalities are clearly evident (see text). (**b**) Full eye closure rules out the possibility of exposure keratitis

This lady's TED is showing clear signs of progression with a clinical activity score of 7/7. She has pain on eye movements, together with eyelid redness and swelling. She also has swelling of the caruncle, conjunctival redness and chemosis. Therefore, systemic treatment with steroid is advised. The lady was started on intravenous methylprednisolone using a EUGOGO-approved regimen. Alternatively, she can be treated with oral steroids, but these are generally less effective and associated with more systemic side effects [2, 3].

It should be noted that steroid use is a relative contraindication in our patient due to the diagnosis of diabetes. However, given the severity of the condition, methylprednisolone can be used with close monitoring of the blood glucose and adjustments in therapy as appropriate.

> What would you need to monitor whilst on methylprednisolone therapy?

The patient should have baseline tests like any other patient starting on steroids (full blood count, U&Es, glucose, HbA1c and LFTs). Particular emphasis should be placed on liver function tests as methylprednisolone therapy can cause hepatitis and should be avoided in patients with a history of significant liver disease [4]. However, severe cases of hepatitis were generally related to the use of a particular regimen (1 g methylprednisolone daily for 3 days), which is perhaps best avoided. The authors prefer to use methylprednisolone at 500 mg doses weekly for 6 weeks, followed by 250 mg weekly for 6 weeks (cumulative dose of 4.5 g). Maximum dose of methylprednisolone used should not exceed 6.5 g, as per EUOGOGO guidelines.

> What the best treatment strategy for the management of hyperthyroidism in TED?

There are no randomised controlled trials on this, which remains an area guided by personal experience rather than hard evidence. It is generally accepted that fluctuation of thyroid function should be avoided (particularly hypothyroidism), as this may exacerbate TED; therefore, the majority of these patients are treated with block and replace regimen during the active phase of TED [5].

> The patient improves significantly after the second dose of methylprednisolone, and she completes a full course of 4.5 g with clinical activity score dropping to 2/7. However, 5 weeks after stopping treatment she presents with impaired colour vision,

> severe diplopia and a clinical activity score of 7/7. On examination there is a sharp drop in visual acuity both eyes, particularly the left (6/12 on Snellen chart). Moreover, examination using Ishihara chart confirms impairment in colour vision, and there was a loss of peripheral vision on Humphrey visual field testing. What would you do now?

This patient is developing symptoms/signs consistent with optic nerve compression. An urgent MRI of the orbit will help to confirm this suspicion, and the patient should be started on treatment immediately.

> Given her previous response to methylprednisolone, this treatment is restarted and MRI of the orbit confirms optic nerve compression, which is particularly severe on the left. The patient is placed on regular follow-up, but her condition fails to improve after 2 weeks of therapy. What would you advise at this stage?

Given the sight-threatening nature of her TED, emergency decompression surgery is the safest option. Orbital surgery to deal with consequences of TED (proptosis, diplopia) is usually delayed until the acute phase is over. The only exception is individuals with sight-threatening disease, in whom emergency orbital decompression is the best way forward.

> Her surgical decompression was a success but her eye disease remained active. What are the options now?

It is clear that steroid therapy is becoming less effective and longer-term use will be associated with side effects, giving an unfavourable benefit/ risk ratio. Therefore, steroid-sparing immuno-suppressants should be considered and ciclosporin has been used in TED patients with reasonable success. Azathioprine has been used in a limited number of patients, but its efficacy appears to be inferior to ciclosporin. There are no large RCTs on the use of either of these agents in TED; therefore, our knowledge is more experience- than evidence-based. Radiotherapy is another option, but it is contraindicated in this patient owing to her long-standing diabetes and retinopathy.

More advanced immunosuppressive agents such as rituximab (anti-CD20 monoclonal antibody modulating B-cell responses) and etaner-cept (anti-tumour necrosis factor-α) have been successfully used to treat TED, but these were case reports rather than randomised controlled trials; therefore, our experience with these agents remains limited [6–8].

Once the disease is inactive, cosmetic surgery can be undertaken to improve appearance (Fig. 5.3) or squint surgery can be performed to correct diplopia.

> Following decompression, and after discussion with the patient, it was decided to start oral steroids together with ciclosporin therapy. Is there any monitoring that needs to be undertaken in this patient?

Ciclosporin has renal toxic effects and may also affect the liver. Therefore, close monitoring of U&Es (every 2 weeks initially and whenever the dose is increased) is essential with regular checks of LFT. Blood pressure should also be regularly monitored, as ciclosporin can cause raised blood pressure, which is of particular importance in or patient who has diabetes.

> How long would you continue on ciclosporin therapy?

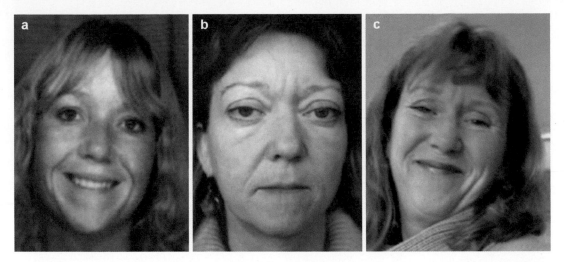

Fig. 5.3 A patient with thyroid eye disease (TED). (**a**) Before TED. (**b**) After the acute phase of TED. (**c**) Following cosmetic surgery (Reproduced from Perros et al. [1] © 2009 with permission from BMJ Publishing Group Ltd)

There are no RCT investigating this area; length of treatment, therefore, differs between centres. A pragmatic approach is to treat for around 6 months after bringing clinical activity of the condition under control. It should be noted that topical ciclosporin has been trialed as a treatment for TED with disappointing results [9].

What are the criteria for urgent referrals for specialised TED clinics?

Urgent referrals should be made in the presence of the following symptoms and signs:

Symptoms
- Sudden deterioration in vision
- Issues with colour vision
- Sudden proptosis

Signs
- Failure of full lid closure
- Corneal opacity
- Abnormal discs

Summarise Main Treatment Options for TED

Treatment options according to severity of TED are summarised in Fig. 5.4.

Summary

Although the incidence of TED is on the decrease, diagnosis is often delayed, which may affect clinical outcome of these patients. A high degree of suspicion is needed to make the diagnosis, and management of these individuals should take place in specialised joint clinics. The condition should be brought under control in the acute stage to avoid long-term complications. Glucocorticoids remain the main therapeutic agents to be used, and the intravenous route using methylprednisolone is preferred to oral steroids. The risk of hepatitis with methylprednisolone is relatively low, provided daily regimens are avoided. In chronic conditions, steroid-sparing immunosuppressive agents or radiotherapy offer alternative options. Decompression surgery

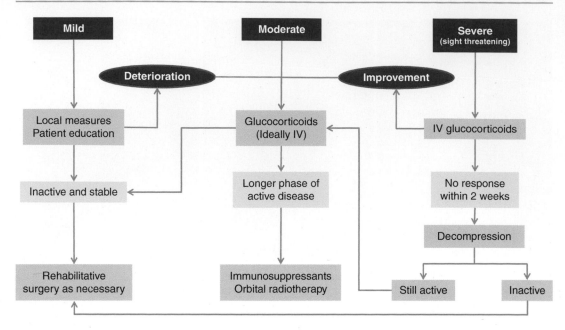

Fig. 5.4 Management of thyroid eye disease

for the acute management of this condition is becoming rare, and surgical intervention is usually reversed for cosmetic reasons or for improving the disabling diplopia.

References

1. Perros P, Neoh C, Dickinson J. Thyroid eye disease. BMJ. 2009;338:b560.
2. Bartalena L, Marcocci C, Tanda ML, Piantanida E, Lai A, Marinò M, et al. An update on medical management of Graves' ophthalmopathy. J Endocrinol Invest. 2005;28:469–78.
3. Stiebel-Kalish H, Robenshtok E, Hasanreisoglu M, Ezrachi D, Shimon I, Leibovici L. Treatment modalities for Graves' ophthalmopathy: systematic review and metaanalysis. J Clin Endocrinol Metab. 2009;94: 2708–16.
4. Verity DH, Rose GE. Acute thyroid eye disease (TED): principles of medical and surgical management. Eye (Lond). 2013;27:308–19.
5. Bartalena L. The dilemma of how to manage Graves' hyperthyroidism in patients with associated orbitopathy. J Clin Endocrinol Metab. 2011;96:592–9.
6. Shen S, Chan A, Sfikakis PP, Hsiu Ling AL, Detorakis ET, Boboridis KG, et al. B-cell targeted therapy with rituximab for thyroid eye disease: closer to the clinic. Surv Ophthalmol. 2013;58:252–65.
7. Bhatt R, Nelson CC, Douglas RS. Thyroid-associated orbitopathy: current insights into the pathophysiology, immunology and management. Saudi J Ophthalmol. 2011;25:15–20.
8. Bartalena L, Fatourechi V. Extrathyroidal manifestations of Graves' disease: a 2014 update. J Endocrinol Invest. 2014;37:691–700.
9. Altiparmak UE, Acar DE, Ozer PA, Emec SD, Kasim R, Ustun H, et al. Topical cyclosporine A for the dry eye findings of thyroid orbitopathy patients. Eye (Lond). 2010;24:1044–50.

Cushing's Syndrome

Case 6

Robert D. Murray

Abstract

Cushing's syndrome is the resultant clinical phenotype consequent on chronic glucocorticoid excess. The most common cause of Cushing's syndrome is exposure to exogenous glucocorticoids in the treatment of chronic inflammatory and malignant conditions. In contrast, endogenous Cushing's syndrome is rare, occurring in around one to two individuals per million population a year. Untreated Cushing's syndrome is associated with significant complications, and a 5-year mortality rate in the region of 50 %. The excess mortality relates primarily to vascular and infective causes. Early identification and appropriate diagnosis is essential to providing the patient an optimal outcome. Treatment of endogenous Cushing's syndrome is dependent on identification of the aetiology, which may be pituitary, adrenal or ectopic. A number of tests are available for diagnosis, and identifying the aetiology, but all are subject to false positive and false negative results, placing weight upon clinical suspicion of the disease. Cushing's syndrome should therefore be managed exclusively by individuals with extensive experience with this condition. Treatment is generally surgical and directed at the cause. Although surgery is highly successful, medical therapy where remission is not achieved can leave the physician wanting.

Keywords

Cushing's syndrome • Cushing's disease • Pseudo-Cushing's • Dexamethasone suppression test • Inferior petrosal sinus sampling • Corticotropin releasing hormone (CRH) • Adrenocorticotrophin hormone (ACTH)

R.D. Murray, BSc, MD, FRCP
Department of Endocrinology, Leeds Teaching
Hospitals NHS Trust St. James's University Hospital,
Beckett Street, Leeds, West Yorkshire LS14 3AR, UK
e-mail: robertmurray@nhs.net

Case

Presenting History

A 34-year-old woman presents complaining of a 12-month history of facial swelling, general lethargy, low mood, irritability, poor concentration, increased appetite, and weight gain of 6 kg. On direct questioning she admits she has noted some redness of her face, an increase in facial hair, a number of bruises on her legs and arms, shortness of breath, and difficulties climbing the stairs. Her menses had become irregular, with cycle lengths of 32–45 days.

The putative diagnosis in this woman is of Cushing's syndrome. Additional characteristic features of Cushing's syndrome include reduced libido, impaired memory, insomnia; and in children a reduced growth rate. The probability of a diagnosis of Cushing's syndrome is increased with the number of concurrent features at presentation, and progression of those features [1]. The woman in question has a collection of symptoms in keeping with the suggested diagnosis that have worsened over the last 12 months and therefore would be at high clinical suspicion of Cushing's syndrome.

What are the additional questions to be asked?

Once the possibility of Cushing's syndrome has been raised questions should be asked to elucidate relevant history relating to the following:

1. Exogenous Cushing's syndrome: Before any tests for Cushing's syndrome are performed an in depth history needs to be taken to exclude exogenous glucocorticoids (i.e., topical, local or systemic glucocorticoid therapy) as the aetiological factor. Medroxyprogesterone acetate, a synthetic progestogen, has glucocorticoid activity at high doses [2, 3] and can lead to Cushing's syndrome.
2. Pseudo-Cushing's: Consideration needs to be given to the possibility of pseudo-Cushing's.

These patients have a mild Cushingoid phenotype, and false positive tests for Cushing's syndrome (i.e., pregnancy, depression, anxiety disorders, alcohol excess, morbid obesity, poorly controlled diabetes mellitus, and glucocorticoid resistance) [4].
3. The aetiology of the syndrome: After exclusion of exogenous Cushing's syndrome questions should be asked to elucidate whether the aetiology is Cushing's disease, ectopic ACTH, or adrenal (i.e., rapid onset and progression of symptoms in keeping with an ectopic source; headaches or visual field defects consistent with a pituitary adenoma, etc.).
4. Complications of Cushing's syndrome (proximal myopathy, diabetes mellitus, hypertension, osteoporosis, vascular disease, carpal tunnel syndrome, nephrolithiasis) [5].
5. Differential diagnoses (i.e., hypothyroidism).

The patient denied any further symptoms, though notably previously complained of some difficulties climbing stairs and carrying her shopping consistent with the presence of a proximal myopathy. There were no symptoms suggestive of aetiology, alternative diagnosis, pseudo-Cushing's, or further complications.

What signs to look for?

On examination the patient showed a rounded facies with facial plethora, BMI 28.4 kg/m², and an intrascapular fat pad. Her skin was thin for her age, with two small areas of purpura on her forearms. She could not recall any significant trauma to this arm. Although there was moderate hirsutism, no acne was present. No striae were present on her abdomen, axilla or proximal thighs. Her BP was 138/92 mmHg. She was unable to rise from sitting without using her hands and showed power 4/5 in the shoulder abductors. There was no glycosuria on urinalysis.

The signs of Cushing's syndrome vary between the classical "apple on sticks" phenotype to relatively subtle signs that may be hard to discern [6]. At their most fulminant, signs include

1. Central, intra-scapular (buffalo hump), and facial (moon face) fat deposition
2. Muscle wasting*, greatest in the proximal limb muscles
3. Skin thinning with poor healing
4. Purpura* in the absence of injury
5. Violaceous striae*, most commonly on the lower abdomen, and proximal aspects of the limbs
6. Facial telangiectasia*/plethora
7. Acne
8. Hirsutism and male pattern baldness in women
9. Peripheral oedema
10. Hypertension
11. Glycosuria
12. In children; reduced growth velocity, pseudo-precocious or delayed puberty

Most of the signs of Cushing's syndrome are not unique to this pathology. The most discerning (*) are proximal muscle wasting, purpura in the absence of trauma, facial telangiectasia, and violaceous striae [7].

> What tests are needed to reach a diagnosis?

The results of investigations of our case are presented in Table 6.1.

Table 6.1 Investigation results from a patient with a putative diagnosis of Cushing's syndrome

	Results	Normal range
24 h urinary free cortisol	564 nmol/day (vol 1.62 L)	<147 nmol/day
24 h urinary free cortisol	489 nmol/day (vol 1.93 L)	<147 nmol/day
1 mg overnight DST	256 nmol/l	<50 nmol/l
Midnight cortisol	206 nmol/l	<50 nmol/l
ACTH	42 pmol/l	<47 ng/l
IPSS (central: peripheral ratio)	Baseline 1.6	Baseline >2[a]
	Post CRH 3.5	Post CRH >3[a]
MRI pituitary	No abnormality observed	–

Abbreviations: *ACTH* adrenocorticotropin hormone, *IPSS* inferior petrosal sinus sampling
[a]Results consistent with a diagnosis of Cushing's disease in contrast to ectopic Cushing's syndrome

The frequency of incidental pituitary and adrenal incidentalomas on imaging is reported to be up to 10 and 4 %, respectively [8–10]. It is therefore mandatory that before considering imaging a biochemical diagnosis of Cushing's syndrome is established. This ideally encompasses demonstration of excess cortisol secretion, failure of suppression to exogenous glucocorticoids and loss of the normal diurnal secretion. Excess cortisol secretion is usually demonstrated by measurement of 24-h urinary free cortisol (UFC) levels, which reflect daily integrated cortisol secretion. Normative ranges depend on the assay methodology used in the local laboratory. At least two measurements should be undertaken as the hypercortisolism of Cushing's syndrome can vary significantly day to day.

In normal individuals supraphysiological doses of exogenous glucocorticoids suppress both ACTH and cortisol. Failure of suppression of ACTH and cortisol by exogenous glucocorticoids occurs in Cushing's syndrome, and can be investigated either using an overnight dexamethasone suppression test (DST) or low-dose DST. Both show a sensitivity and specificity of more than 90 %. The overnight DST entails the taking of 1 mg dexamethasone at midnight with measurement of serum cortisol level at 09.00 h the following morning. The low dose DST involves ingestion of dexamethasone 0.5 mg 6 hourly for 2 days, commencing at 09.00 and the final dose at 03.00 h. Following the final dose of dexamethasone the serum cortisol level is measured at 9 am. In both DSTs a cortisol level of <50 nmol/l effectively excludes active Cushing's syndrome. The dexamethasone-CRH test has been proposed as an alternative to the low-dose DST. Theoretically the normal individual will not respond to CRH under dexamethasone suppression; however, patients with Cushing's disease do respond. The dexamethasone-CRH test thus aims to exaggerate the difference in responses between patients with and without Cushing's disease to increase sensitivity and specificity. The test involves administration of CRH 1 µg/kg intravenously two hours after the last dose of dexamethasone of a low-dose DST. The serum cortisol is measured every 15 minutes for one hour following injection of the CRH. A further diagnostic option in Cushing's disease is the desmopressin stimulation test. This test involves measurement of ACTH before, 10, 20 and 30 min after 10 g arginine vasopressin. Patients with Cushing's disease generally show an increased ACTH, where as normal individuals and those with Cushing's syndrome of a non-pituitary source do not respond. This test requires further study, however, before becoming accepted in to routine clinical practice.

Cortisol shows a clear diurnal rhythm with highest levels around 06.00–07.00 h, following which levels fall progressively throughout the day [11]. Lowest levels occur at around 24.00 h, and in normal individuals who are asleep cortisol levels are <50 nmol/l. Autonomous cortisol secretion in Cushing's syndrome leads to loss of circadian rhythm, and resultant elevation of midnight cortisol levels. Obtaining an accurate measurement of midnight cortisol is difficult logistically as the blood should be taken with the patient asleep, or within 5–10 min of waking. As a consequence this investigation is frequently not performed. More recently, the use of a late-night (23.00–24.00 h) salivary free cortisol measurement has become an alternative to a midnight serum cortisol, though availability of this test is not yet widespread. Salivary free cortisol levels reflect serum free cortisol levels, and reach equilibrium with serum values within several minutes. The value of this test is dependent on establishing an appropriate "late evening" reference range for salivary cortisol, but has the advantage that the test can be performed at home and the sample sent in to the investigating unit for analysis.

In interpreting the results of urinary free cortisol measurements and the DST a diagnosis of pseudo-Cushing's needs to be considered due to the high incidence of false positive results in these individuals [4]. Additionally, false positive results for the 24-h UFC and overnight/ low-dose DST can occur in patients under physical stress (hospitalisation, surgery, pain), malnutrition, anorexia nervosa, intense chronic exercise, hypothalamic amenorrhoea, and in the presence of excess cortisol binding globulin (i.e., oestrogen therapy) [7]. Twenty-four hour UFCs are unreliable where there is significant renal dysfunction (false negative) and increased with excess fluid intake (false positive) [7]. A number of concomitant drugs (i.e., phenytoin, carbamezapine, rifampicin, pioglitazone) can result in false positive results during the DST by induction of CYP 3A4, which increases metabolism of dexamethasone [7]. The diurnal rhythm of cortisol is affected by shift work, depression, and critical illness making midnight serum cortisol and salivary free cortisol measures unreliable in these circumstances [7]. Clinical suspicion is imperative to establishing a diagnosis of Cushing's syndrome, and thus the importance of involvement of an Endocrinologist familiar with managing this condition. This is particularly important where test results are normal, but symptoms progress or the suspicion of Cushing's syndrome is high.

Once a diagnosis of Cushing's syndrome is proven biochemically the aetiology needs to be established. The first step is to determine if the Cushing's syndrome is ACTH-dependent or independent by measurement of plasma ACTH. Notably ACTH is a relatively unstable hormone so the sample needs to reach the laboratory for processing within 30 min. A suppressed ACTH is indicative of an adrenal aetiology and imaging of the adrenal gland should be performed. Both CT or MRI can be used to image the adrenal gland, however, CT imaging provides a measure of attenuation (Houndsfield units) to determine if an observed nodule has a high fat content. An attenuation of <10 Houndsfield units is highly likely to be a benign adenoma.

Where ACTH is measurable the diagnosis lies between that of Cushing's disease and ectopic ACTH. Approximately 80–90 % of ACTH-dependent Cushing's syndrome relates to Cushing's disease. Traditionally the high dose DST has been used to determine whether ACTH-dependent Cushing's syndrome is the consequence of pituitary disease or ectopic ACTH. This test involves measurement of serum cortisol, followed by ingestion of dexamethasone 2 mg 6 hourly for 2 days, commencing at 09.00 and the final dose at 03.00 h. Following the final dose of dexamethasone the serum cortisol level is measured at 9 am. If the 9 am cortisol is less than

50 % of the basal value after 48 h of dexamethasone this is classified as showing suppression, and indicative of Cushing's disease. The sensitivity and specificity of the high-dose DST is around 70–80 %, such that the test positive prediction rate fails to exceed that of the pre-test likelihood of Cushing's disease. Because of the low sensitivity and specificity of this test many Units have stopped using the high-dose DST. The gold standard for differentiating ectopic Cushing's syndrome from Cushing's disease is inferior petrosal sinus sampling (IPSS). This test involves insertion of a catheter in to the petrosal sinus bilaterally. ACTH levels are measured simultaneously in both petrosal sinuses and in the peripheral circulation prior to and following an injection of CRH 100 μg. Measurements of ACTH are performed at −5, 0, 2, 5, and 10 min. A central to peripheral ACTH ratio of greater than two basally, or three following CRH, is highly suggestive of Cushing's disease. Sensitivity and specificity of this test approaches 100 %. The test is less sensitive, however, in lateralising the lesion within the pituitary gland. Once a diagnosis of Cushing's disease is made a dedicated MRI scan of the pituitary gland should be performed.

Although initial investigation is aimed towards establishing a diagnosis of Cushing's syndrome and the aetiology of this, it is important not to forget to investigate the potential complications of Cushing's syndrome. This should include investigation of carbohydrate handling and assessment of bone mass by dual energy X-ray absorptiometry (DXA). Co-existent hypertension should be managed aggressively before any surgical intervention is undertaken.

> What are the key results that help to reach the final diagnosis?

The results obtained in our patient (see Table 6.1) show grossly elevated 24-h urinary free cortisol levels in keeping with excess cortisol secretion; failure of cortisol levels to suppress during the overnight DST in keeping with autonomous cortisol secretion; and an elevated midnight cortisol representing loss of the normal diurnal rhythm of cortisol. Together these results support a diagnosis of Cushing's syndrome in this patient.

The measurable ACTH suggests the aetiology is either pituitary driven or ectopic ACTH. To investigate this further the patient underwent IPSS. Although the central: peripheral ratio at baseline was not suggestive of pituitary disease the elevated ratio following CRH confirms the diagnosis to be Cushing's disease. The dedicated pituitary MRI scan performed following biochemical confirmation of Cushing's disease showed no abnormality. This is seen in up to 30 % of cases of Cushing's disease. There is a suggestion from the differential in ratios from the right and left side that the lesion is on the left.

> How would you manage this patient?

The case in question ideally requires pituitary surgery as definitive treatment. Consideration should be given to medical therapy prior to surgery, as in the presented case the clinical features suggest her to be catabolic (muscle wasting, skin thinning and bruising etc.). Given the absence of a discreet MRI abnormality surgery will initially entail exploration of the left side of the gland, as a putative adenoma is often visualised at surgery. Where this is not the case a left hemihypophysectomy can be performed. Peri- and post-operatively the patient should have hydrocortisone cover as the normal corticotroph cells are likely suppressed from the high circulating cortisol levels. Thus should the corticotroph adenoma be successfully removed at surgery the patient would be rendered cortisol deficient. The hydrocortisone dose is generally weaned to physiological within 3–4 days. A serum cortisol level <50 nmol/l on post-operative day 4 or 5, prior to receiving the morning hydrocortisone dosage is indicative of successful surgery. Levels greater than 50 nmol/l suggest some residual adenoma tissue. If levels remain significantly elevated further early surgery can be considered. Low levels, though >50 nmol/l, are consistent with remission and patients can potentially be observed clinically and biochemically for the possibility of relapse.

Where surgery fails to induce remission, repeat surgery is usually considered in the week following initial surgery. If further pituitary surgery is not considered to be an option, medical therapy can be instituted whilst alternate definitive therapy is considered. Alternative therapy to pituitary surgery includes conformal (conventional) radiotherapy, stereotactic radiotherapy, and bilateral adrenalectomy. Conformal radiotherapy to the pituitary takes at least 2 years to control ACTH secretion. There are few data concerning the effects of stereotactic radiotherapy in Cushing's disease, and whether control of excess ACTH secretion occurs more rapidly than with conformal radiotherapy. Following radiotherapy the patient should be observed regularly for evolving hypopituitarism. Bilateral adrenalectomy performed laproscopically is a significantly smaller undertaking than previous open operations, however, leaves the patient adrenal insufficient with all the associated risks. Medical therapy for Cushing's disease primarily entails use of metyrapone or ketoconazole. Both drugs act by inhibition of adrenal steroidogenesis; metyrapone is a 11-hydroxylase inhibitor whereas ketoconazole acts on several P450 enzymes, including the first step in cortisol synthesis, cholesterol side-chain cleavage, and conversion of 11-deoxycortisol to cortisol. Titration of the drug dosage is monitored by the use of regular cortisol day curves. It is not uncommon to combine the use of metyrapone with ketoconazole where excess cortisol secretion is difficult to control, or where use of higher doses of either drug is limited by side-effects. Additionally, many Physicians employ a combination of a physiological replacement dose of hydrocortisone with inhibitors of adrenal steroidogenesis in the form of a "block and replace" regimen to prevent over suppression of the endogenous glucocorticoids. There have been recent concerns over abnormalities of liver function when ketoconazole has been used as an antifungal agent, leading to withdrawal of use for this indication. As a consequence availability of ketoconazole for use in Cushing's syndrome is presenting difficulties.

Follow-up of Patients and Further Management/Complications of Original Condition or Treatment as Appropriate

Post-pituitary surgery, where remission has been suggested by the day 4/5 "9 am cortisol" level a cortisol stimulation test (SST, GST, ITT) should be performed at 6 weeks post-operatively to assess the endogenous axis. If an acceptable cortisol level is achieved the hydrocortisone can be discontinued. If a subnormal cortisol level is achieved physiological hydrocortisone replacement (15–20 mg/day) can be continued and the stimulation test repeated in 3–6 months. In patients defined as panhypopituitary during the initial stimulation test and basal pituitary bloods the likelihood of recovery of the cortisol axis is small and therefore repeated testing is probably unnecessary. In patients with suboptimal stimulated cortisol levels, but a peak cortisol of >300 nmol/l it may be possible to manage these individuals with hydrocortisone only during periods of intercurrent stress until a repeat stimulation test is performed.

Long-term follow-up of patients with Cushing's disease is essential to manage excess cortisol secretion where surgical cure has not been achieved; for surveillance of symptoms and signs of recurrence following successful surgery; for optimisation of any pituitary hormone replacement therapies; and management of any residual sequelea (osteoporosis, hypertension, diabetes, etc.).

An Update on the Condition

Cushing's syndrome is the clinical syndrome resulting from chronic excessive cortisol secretion. Most commonly this results from the use of exogenous glucocorticoid therapy as an anti-inflammatory agent. Endogenous Cushing's syndrome is however rare, with an incidence of two to three cases per million per year [12] and occurs as a consequence of autonomous cortisol production from the adrenal or hyperstimulation of the adrenal from excessive ACTH production. An early study of untreated Cushing's syndrome reported mortality to be 50 % at 5 years due to vascular and infective complications [13]. More recent reports though have shown an SMR of at least two-fold, and suggested normalisation of mortality after successful treatment [14, 15]. Where cortisol levels are not adequately controlled an excess mortality persists (SMR 3.8–5.5) [12, 14].

Diagnosis and treatment of Cushing's disease have been covered in the described case. Recently described novel aspects of Cushing's disease requiring further reading include:

1. The phenotype of long-term survivors of Cushing's disease. Treatment of patients with Cushing's disease reduces both morbidity and mortality. With the consequent fall in cortisol levels resolution of the characteristic clinical phenotype and improvements in well-being are observed. The generally held belief has been that with resolution of the hypercortisolaemia, in addition to the clinical manifestations, carbohydrate, protein, lipid and vascular anomalies are normalised. More recent studies have shown that despite "cure" of Cushing's syndrome, these patients may be left with features reminiscent of their original diagnosis, though not usually to a level that is appreciable clinically [16]. Bone mass improves over several years, but remains suboptimal in a proportion of patients [17]. Although quality of life improves it frequently remains lower than expected [18]. Body composition, blood pressure, carbohydrate handling, coagulation and inflammatory markers improve markedly with treatment but do not fully normalise [16, 19] suggesting these individuals may remain at risk of excess vascular morbidity and mortality. Direct evidence for continued vascular damage is exemplified by increases in carotid intima-medial thickness and plaque formation. A recent meta-analysis has also concluded that patients in remission from Cushing's disease retain an excess mortality, at least in the first 5 years [20].

2. Thromboembolic risk in Cushing's disease. There are increasing data to suggest an increase in both spontaneous and post-operative venous thromboembolism in patients with Cushing's disease [21, 22]. A recent systematic review has confirmed an enhanced risk of spontaneous and post-operative venous thrombosis [21], though highlighted the lack of high-quality studies. The risk of spontaneous VTE was estimated to be up to ten fold that of an age-matched normal population; and that of post-operative VTE to be equivalent to a total knee/hip replacement when both are under conditions of thromboprophylaxis [21, 23]. The risk of VTE is higher with rapid lowering of cortisol levels independent of the treatment leading to this [23]. Most VTE events and deaths from VTE in Cushing's syndrome are reported to occur within 3 months of surgery [21, 23, 24], with higher rates of events in those patients with persistent hypercortisolaemia [24]. Prophylactic anticoagulation post-operatively reduces thromboembolic events and fatalities from this [24]. Pathophysiologically patients with Cushing's syndrome have anomalies within both the coagulation and fibrinolytic pathways [21, 22, 24, 25]. In keeping with the increased risk of VTE within the first 3 months after surgery, the described coagulation and fibrinolytic anomalies fail to correct within 80 days of biochemical control of Cushing's disease induced by medical therapy [25]. Several Units now recommend the use of VTE prophylaxis therapy in Cushing's disease perioperatively and for 3 months post-operatively [21].

3. New drug therapies for Cushing's disease. A number of novel medical therapies have recently been investigated to determine their utility in Cushing's disease. Although none of these therapies are likely to become the default therapy for Cushing's disease they do add to the therapeutic armamentarium available to manage this condition. Cabergoline is a dopaminergic agonist which has long been used in the management of both prolactinomas and acromegaly to control hormonal hypersecretion. Data using bromocriptine in Cushing's disease have shown some success in the short-term control of cortisol levels and in long-term

management of sporadic cases [26, 27]. Studies of cabergoline, a more potent dopaminergic agonist, in Cushing's disease has shown control of cortisol secretion in up to 40 % of patients and tumour shrinkage of >25 % in 20 % of patients. Clinical improvement in body composition, blood pressure, and carbohydrate handling paralleled changes in UFC levels [28, 29]. Mifepristone is a progesterone receptor antagonist with glucocorticoid receptor antagonist activity at higher doses, but no significant action at the mineralocorticoid receptor. Several case reports and small series have suggested a role for mifepristone in the medical therapy of Cushing's syndrome [30–32]. In a prospective study of the effects of mifepristone in patients with Cushing's syndrome significant clinical improvement was observed in 87 % of individuals [33] with improvements in body composition, carbohydrate handling, quality of life, well-being and cognition. Mean blood pressure remained unchanged, however, 40 % showed a lowering of diastolic BP of more than 5 mmHg, and 28 % decreased their antihypertensive agents [33]. Levels of both ACTH and cortisol increased in treated Cushing's disease patients. Adverse effects including nausea, fatigue, headache, hypokalaemia, arthralgia, oedema, dizziness, and endometrial thickening were common [33]. An increase in BP was observed in a subset of patients. The elevated BP, oedema, and hypokalaemia likely reflect the action of the elevated cortisol levels via the mineralocorticoid receptor. Corticotrophomas responsible for Cushing's disease express somatostatin receptors (SSTR), with the highest density being SSTR subtype 5 (SSTR5). Until recently the only two commercially available somatostatin analogues (lanreotide and octreotide) showed high affinity at SSTR2, but limited binding at the additional SSTRs. Pasireotide (SOM230), a novel somatostatin analogue that binds SSTR1, 2, 3, and 5 with high affinity, displays ~40 fold greater affinity for SSTR5 than either octreotide or lanreotide. Following pre-clinical [34] and phase II studies [35], a definitive phase III study was performed in 162 patients with Cushing's disease [36]. Patients were randomised to pasireotide 600 or 900 g bd for 6 months, followed by 6 months open treatment. A greater than 50 % reduction in urinary free cortisol occurred in 60 % of patients, although only 15 and 26 % in the low- and high-dose groups showed normalisation of UFCs [36]. Patients who were responders could be identified within the first 2 months. Clinical improvement paralleled the biochemical changes with reductions in blood pressure, LDL cholesterol and weight. Quality of life improved, and a reduction in facial rugor and supraclavicular and dorsal fat pads was observed [36]. The incidence of GI side effects and gallstones was similar to other somatostatin analogues, however, hyperglycaemia-related side effects were much more frequent occurring in 73 % of patients [36].

References

1. Ross EJ, Linch DC. Cushing's syndrome–killing disease: discriminatory value of signs and symptoms aiding early diagnosis. Lancet. 1982;2(8299):646–9.
2. Malik KJ, Wakelin K, Dean S, Cove DH, Wood PJ. Cushing's syndrome and hypothalamic-pituitary adrenal axis suppression induced by medroxyprogesterone acetate. Ann Clin Biochem. 1996;33(Pt 3): 187–9.
3. Learoyd D, McElduff A. Medroxyprogesterone induced Cushing's syndrome. Aust N Z J Med. 1990; 20(6):824–5.
4. Newell-Price J, Trainer P, Besser M, Grossman A. The diagnosis and differential diagnosis of Cushing's syndrome and pseudo-Cushing's states. Endocr Rev. 1998;19(5):647–72.
5. Arnaldi G, Mancini T, Tirabassi G, Trementino L, Boscaro M. Advances in the epidemiology, pathogenesis, and management of Cushing's syndrome complications. J Endocrinol Invest. 2012;35(4):434–48.
6. Valassi E, Santos A, Yaneva M, Tóth M, Strasburger CJ, Chanson P, et al. The European registry on Cushing's syndrome: 2-year experience. Baseline demographic and clinical characteristics. Eur J Endocrinol. 2011;165(3):383–92.
7. Nieman LK, Biller BM, Findling JW, Newell-Price J, Savage MO, Stewart PM, et al. The diagnosis of Cushing's syndrome: an Endocrine Society clinical practice guideline. J Clin Endocrinol Metab. 2008; 93(5):1526–40.
8. Freda PU, Beckers AM, Katznelson L, Molitch ME, Montori VM, Post KD, et al. Pituitary incidentaloma: an endocrine society clinical practice guideline. J Clin Endocrinol Metab. 2011;96(4):894–904.

9. Molitch ME. Nonfunctioning pituitary tumors and pituitary incidentalomas. Endocrinol Metab Clin North Am. 2008;37(1):151–71, xi.

10. Davenport C, Liew A, Doherty B, Win HH, Misran H, Hanna S, Kealy D, et al. The prevalence of adrenal incidentaloma in routine clinical practice. Endocrine. 2011;40(1):80–3.

11. Debono M, Ghobadi C, Rostami-Hodjegan A, Huatan H, Campbell MJ, Newell-Price J, et al. Modified-release hydrocortisone to provide circadian cortisol profiles. J Clin Endocrinol Metab. 2009;94(5): 1548–54.

12. Lindholm J, Juul S, Jørgensen JO, Astrup J, Bjerre P, Feldt-Rasmussen U, et al. Incidence and late prognosis of Cushing's syndrome: a population-based study. J Clin Endocrinol Metab. 2001;86(1):117–23.

13. Plotz CM, Knowlton AI, Ragan C. The natural history of Cushing's syndrome. Am J Med. 1952;13(5): 597–614.

14. Clayton RN, Raskauskiene D, Reulen RC, Jones PW. Mortality and morbidity in Cushing's disease over 50 years in Stoke-on-Trent, UK: audit and meta-analysis of literature. J Clin Endocrinol Metab. 2011;96(3):632–42.

15. Swearingen B, Biller BM, Barker 2nd FG, Katznelson L, Grinspoon S, Klibanski A, et al. Long-term mortality after transsphenoidal surgery for Cushing disease. Ann Intern Med. 1999;130(10):821–4.

16. Barahona MJ, Sucunza N, Resmini E, Fernández-Real JM, Ricart W, Moreno-Navarrete JM, et al. Persistent body fat mass and inflammatory marker increases after long-term cure of Cushing's syndrome. J Clin Endocrinol Metab. 2009;94(9):3365–71.

17. Hermus AR, Smals AG, Swinkels LM, Huysmans DA, Pieters GF, Sweep CF, et al. Bone mineral density and bone turnover before and after surgical cure of Cushing's syndrome. J Clin Endocrinol Metab. 1995;80(10):2859–65.

18. Lindsay JR, Nansel T, Baid S, Gumowski J, Nieman LK. Long-term impaired quality of life in Cushing's syndrome despite initial improvement after surgical remission. J Clin Endocrinol Metab. 2006;91(2): 447–53.

19. Colao A, Pivonello R, Spiezia S, Faggiano A, Ferone D, Filippella M, et al. Persistence of increased cardiovascular risk in patients with Cushing's disease after five years of successful cure. J Clin Endocrinol Metab. 1999;84(8):2664–72.

20. Ntali G, Asimakopoulou A, Siamatras T, Komninos J, Vassiliadi D, Tzanela M, et al. Mortality in Cushing's syndrome: systematic analysis of a large series with prolonged follow-up. Eur J Endocrinol. 2013;169(5): 715–23.

21. Van Zaane B, Nur E, Squizzato A, Dekkers OM, Twickler MT, Fliers E, et al. Hypercoagulable state in Cushing's syndrome: a systematic review. J Clin Endocrinol Metab. 2009;94(8):2743–50.

22. Manetti L, Bogazzi F, Giovannetti C, Raffaelli V, Genovesi M, Pellegrini G, et al. Changes in coagula-

tion indexes and occurrence of venous thromboembolism in patients with Cushing's syndrome: results from a prospective study before and after surgery. Eur J Endocrinol. 2010;163(5):783–91.

23. Stuijver DJ, van Zaane B, Feelders RA, Debeij J, Cannegieter SC, Hermus AR, et al. Incidence of venous thromboembolism in patients with Cushing's syndrome: a multicenter cohort study. J Clin Endocrinol Metab. 2011;96(11):3525–32.

24. Boscaro M, Sonino N, Scarda A, Barzon L, Fallo F, Sartori MT, et al. Anticoagulant prophylaxis markedly reduces thromboembolic complications in Cushing's syndrome. J Clin Endocrinol Metab. 2002; 87(8):3662–6.

25. van der Pas R, de Bruin C, Leebeek FW, de Maat MP, Rijken DC, Pereira AM, et al. The hypercoagulable state in Cushing's disease is associated with increased levels of procoagulant factors and impaired fibrinolysis, but is not reversible after short-term biochemical remission induced by medical therapy. J Clin Endocrinol Metab. 2012;97(4):1303–10.

26. Lamberts SW, Klijn JG, de Quijada M, Timmermans HA, Uitterlinden P, de Jong FH, et al. The mechanism of the suppressive action of bromocriptine on adrenocorticotropin secretion in patients with Cushing's disease and Nelson's syndrome. J Clin Endocrinol Metab. 1980;51(2):307–11.

27. Invitti C, De Martin M, Danesi L, Cavagnini F. Effect of injectable bromocriptine in patients with Cushing's disease. Exp Clin Endocrinol Diabetes. 1995;103(4): 266–71.

28. Pivonello R, De Martino MC, Cappabianca P, De Leo M, Faggiano A, Lombardi G, et al. The medical treatment of Cushing's disease: effectiveness of chronic treatment with the dopamine agonist cabergoline in patients unsuccessfully treated by surgery. J Clin Endocrinol Metab. 2009;94(1):223–30.

29. Pivonello R, Ferone D, de Herder WW, Kros JM, De Caro ML, Arvigo M, et al. Dopamine receptor expression and function in corticotroph pituitary tumors. J Clin Endocrinol Metab. 2004;89(5):2452–62.

30. Bertagna X, Bertagna C, Laudat MH, Husson JM, Girard F, Luton JP. Pituitary-adrenal response to the antiglucocorticoid action of RU 486 in Cushing's syndrome. J Clin Endocrinol Metab. 1986;63(3): 639–43.

31. Nieman LK, Chrousos GP, Kellner C, Spitz IM, Nisula BC, Cutler GB, et al. Successful treatment of Cushing's syndrome with the glucocorticoid antagonist RU 486. J Clin Endocrinol Metab. 1985;61(3): 536–40.

32. Castinetti F, Fassnacht M, Johanssen S, Terzolo M, Bouchard P, Chanson P, et al. Merits and pitfalls of mifepristone in Cushing's syndrome. Eur J Endocrinol. 2009;160(6):1003–10.

33. Fleseriu M, Biller BM, Findling JW, Molitch ME, Schteingart DE, Gross C, SEISMIC Study Investigators. Mifepristone, a glucocorticoid receptor antagonist, produces clinical and metabolic benefits in

patients with Cushing's syndrome. J Clin Endocrinol Metab. 2012;97(6):2039–49.

34. Batista DL, Zhang X, Gejman R, Ansell PJ, Zhou Y, Johnson SA, et al. The effects of SOM230 on cell proliferation and adrenocorticotropin secretion in human corticotroph pituitary adenomas. J Clin Endocrinol Metab. 2006;91(11):4482–8.

35. Boscaro M, Ludlam WH, Atkinson B, Glusman JE, Petersenn S, Reincke M, et al. Treatment of pituitary-dependent Cushing's disease with the multireceptor ligand somatostatin analog pasireotide (SOM230): a multicenter, phase II trial. J Clin Endocrinol Metab. 2009;94(1):115–22.

36. Colao A, Petersenn S, Newell-Price J, Findling JW, Gu F, Maldonado M, et al. A 12-month phase 3 study of pasireotide in Cushing's disease. N Engl J Med. 2012;366(10):914–24.

Prolactinoma Presenting with Galactorrhoea and Secondary Amenorrhoea: Diagnosis and Management

Case 7

Jubbin J. Jacob, Alex J. Graveling, and John S. Bevan

Abstract

A 35-year-old woman was referred with secondary amenorrhoea and galactorrhoea. She had been trying to conceive since stopping the combined oral contraceptive 18 months earlier. Serum prolactin was found to be grossly elevated with low oestradiol. MRI demonstrated a pituitary macroadenoma in contact with the optic structures. Dopamine agonist therapy was commenced and a pregnancy was achieved after an appropriate length of treatment and interval barrier contraception. This chapter explores the differential diagnosis of secondary amenorrhoea and galactorrhoea, together with discussion of the investigation and management of prolactinomas; with special focus on pre-pregnancy planning and management during pregnancy.

Keywords

Galactorrhoea • Secondary amenorrhoea • Prolactin • Macroprolactinoma • Infertility • Dopamine agonists • Cabergoline • Pregnancy

J.J. Jacob, MD, DNB
Department of Endocrinology, J.J.R. Macleod
Centre for Diabetes, Endocrinology and Metabolism
(Mac-DEM), Aberdeen Royal Infirmary, Aberdeen, UK

Endocrine and Diabetes Unit, Department
of Medicine, Christian Medical College and Hospital,
Ludhiana, Punjab, India

A.J. Graveling, MBChB, MRCP (UK)
Department of Endocrinology, J.J.R. Macleod Centre
for Diabetes, Endocrinology and Metabolism
(Mac-DEM), Aberdeen Royal Infirmary, Aberdeen,
Aberdeenshire, UK

J.S. Bevan, BSc, MBChB, MD, FRCP (✉)
Department of Endocrinology, J.J.R. Macleod
Centre for Diabetes, Endocrinology and Metabolism
(Mac-DEM), Aberdeen Royal Infirmary, Aberdeen, UK

Aberdeen University, Aberdeen, Grampian, UK
e-mail: johnbevan@nhs.net

Case

Case Study: Part 1

A 35-year-old woman was referred to the Endocrine Clinic by her general practitioner with secondary amenorrhoea and episodes of galactorrhoea. The case study attained menarche at 15 years and this was followed by regular menses. For 18 years she had regular withdrawal bleeds during treatment with a combined oral contraceptive (OCP). Eighteen months prior to referral she had stopped oral contraception; she was in a stable relationship and wished to get pregnant. However she had had no periods since stopping the OCP and a recent pregnancy test was negative. For 12 months she had noticed occasional spontaneous milky discharge from both breasts staining her undergarments.

What are the important points to elicit from the history?

Does she have secondary amenorrhoea?

Amenorrhoea is the absence of menstrual bleeding in a woman. Secondary amenorrhoea is defined as cessation of the menstrual cycle after a woman has attained menarche. Oligomenorrhoea is defined as menstrual cycles that occur at intervals longer than 35 days. There is no consensus as to the period of time that should pass before oligomenorrhoea is labelled as amenorrhoea. However, cessation of periods for over 90 days should prompt concern and absence of menstrual flow for over 6 months can be labelled as amenorrhoea. The history of spontaneous menarche and cessation of periods for over 18 months in our case study confirmed secondary amenorrhoea.

How is galactorrhoea defined?

Galactorrhoea is defined as inappropriate lactation (i.e., beyond 6 months post-partum in a non-breastfeeding woman) [1]. It is always pathological in a man but may be physiological in a woman. The colour and consistency should be documented. A bloody or purulent discharge should not be regarded as galactorrhoea and care needs to be taken to exclude local breast pathology. A history of repeated nipple stimulation from breast self-examination or during physical intimacy should be sought. Chest wall irritation can lead to an increase in prolactin and may be caused by tight clothing. Skin conditions over the chest wall including herpes zoster, burns-related scarring and atopic dermatitis can lead to prolactin hypersecretion and galactorrhoea. Milky

discharge may also follow breast operations, including breast augmentation surgery.

Any additional information from the case study's history?

It is important to exclude pregnancy in any patient presenting with secondary amenorrhoea and galactorrhoea; already excluded by a negative pregnancy test in our case study. In the absence of pregnancy, hyperprolactinaemia should be suspected.

Symptoms of oestrogen deficiency including a decrease in libido, vaginal dryness, dyspareunia and recurrent urinary infection should be noted. **A careful drug history is mandatory**. Enquiry should be made regarding prescription drugs, contraceptives, "over the counter" medications (especially anti-sickness medications and anti-migraine tablets containing anti-emetics), dietary supplements (including herbs) and illicit drug use (Table 7.1).

What additional features in the history would increase the likelihood of a pituitary tumour as the cause of her symptoms?

Symptoms of an intracranial mass lesion including headache and visual disturbances would be suggestive. Clinical features of acromegaly may rarely be associated with pituitary adenomas that co-secrete growth hormone and prolactin. Large tumours producing prolactin may compress the normal pituitary gland leading to pituitary hormone deficiencies and their associated clinical features.

Prolactinomas are usually sporadic tumours but can occasionally occur as part of multiple endocrine neoplasia type 1; a family history of pituitary adenoma, parathyroid dysfunction or other 'endocrine tumours' should be sought [2].

What are the physical signs to look for?

Table 7.1 Drugs and herbs causing hyperprolactinaemia [2, 3]

Herbs and natural agents	Illicit drugs	Prescription medications		
		Anti-depressants and anti-psychotics	Hormonal agents	Others
Anise	Cannabis	Selective Serotonin	Conjugated Oestrogen and	Anti-emetics and motility
Blessed thistle	Cocaine	Reuptake inhibitors	Medroxyprogesterone	agents
Fennel	Amphetamines	(SSRI)	combinations	Domperidone (+++)
Fenugreek	Benzodiazepines	Citalopram (±)	Medroxyprogesterone	Metoclopromide (+++)
seeds		Fluoxetine (CR)	contraceptive depot	Chlorpromazine (+++)
Marshmallow	Opiates	Paroxetine (±)	injections (Depo-Provera)	Prochlorperazine (+++)
Nettle		Monoamine Oxidase	Danazol	Cisapride (+)
Red Clover		inhibitors (+++)		H₂ receptor blockers
Red Raspberry		Tricyclic		Methyldopa (+)
		anti-depressants (+++)		Sumatriptan (+)
		Alprazolam (±)		Sodium Valproate
		Buspirone (+++)		Opiates
		Anti-psychotics		Reserpine
		Resperidone (+++)		Verapamil
		Haloperidol (+++)		Isoniazid
		Clozapine (0)		
		Olanzapine (+)		

(+++) abnormal in over 50 % of patients, (+) abnormal in a small percentage, (*CR*) case reports only, (+) minimal effect, (0) no effects

Physical examination would include general examination, breast examination, examination of the thyroid and visual assessment. Breast examination should include inspection of chest wall to look for any skin lesions and scarring. Asking the patient to perform gentle, segmental, massage of the breast towards the nipple (in the presence of a chaperone) will often produce milk. When in doubt about the nature of discharge from the nipple, the expressed secretions can be examined under low power with a microscope. True milky secretions will contain easily seen fat globules and scanty cellular material. If microscopy proves inconclusive or contains abundant cellular material then the secretions can be sent for cytological examination. Goitre and signs of hypothyroidism should be looked for. Assessment of vision should include visual acuities, visual fields by confrontation and fundoscopy.

Case Study: Part 2

Further questioning did not reveal any positive drug history. There was no history to suggest nipple stimulation, chest wall irritation, symptoms of an intracranial mass or features of

hormonal deficiency. There was no family history of pituitary or other endocrine problems. Apart from expressible galactorrhoea; examination was normal with intact visual fields and no goitre. Differential diagnosis at this stage would include many of the causes of hyperprolactinaemia listed in Tables 7.1 and 7.2.

> What biochemical tests and radiological investigations are needed to reach a diagnosis?

Biochemical Tests

The first step would be ruling out pregnancy with urine or serum estimation of human chorionic gonadotropins. Complete blood count, renal function, liver function test and urinalysis help exclude systemic disease. Endocrine evaluation should include thyroid function tests, prolactin, gonadotrophins and oestradiol. Prolactin estimation should not be performed immediately following breast examination. Borderline prolactin values should be reconfirmed by repeat testing because of the significant variability of prolactin levels across the day and its response to stressful stimuli. All patients with unexplained hyperprolactinaemia

Table 7.2 Differential diagnosis of hyperprolactinaemia [2, 3]

Physiological	Pharmacological	Pathological		Systemic disorders
		Pituitary	Hypothalamic pituitary stalk compression/damage	Systemic disorders
Coitus	**See** Table 7.1.	**Prolactinoma**	Granulomas	**Primary hypothyroidism**
Exercise		**Non-functioning pituitary macroadenoma**	Infiltrations	Neurogenic chest wall trauma
Lactation		Acromegaly	Irradiation	Thoracic surgery
Pregnancy		Lymphocytic hypophysitis	Rathke's cyst	Herpes zoster (thoracic)
Sleep		Trauma	Trauma	Chronic renal failure
Stress			Tumours (e.g., craniopharyngioma, germinoma, hypothalamic metastasis or meningioma)	Cirrhosis
				Cranial irradiation
				Epileptic seizure
				Polycystic ovarian syndrome

Common or important causes are listed in **bold**

require MRI (magnetic resonance imaging). Serum prolactin above 2,000 mU/l is almost always associated with pituitary or sellar tumours and a prolactin >5,000 mU/l is virtually diagnostic of a macroprolactinoma.

When evaluating prolactin results the clinician needs to be aware of assay "interferences" due to the presence of macroprolactin and the "prolactin hook effect." Macroprolactin is a complex of prolactin with IgG antibody found in about 1 % of normal individuals resulting in artificially elevated measurements of serum prolactin. Macroprolactin is a physiologically inactive complex and therefore **not** associated with clinical symptoms of hyperprolactinaemia. Re-assay of serum after polyethylene glycol treatment usually confirms the presence of macroprolactin. Large tumours producing exceedingly high concentrations of prolactin and this may saturate both the capture and signal antibodies in immunoassays. This is known as the "hook effect" and results from blockage of the capture antibody-prolactin-signal antibody "sandwich" formation, leading to misleadingly low prolactin values, very rarely within the normal range, in automated immunometric assays. Re-assay of diluted serum will resolve the problem leading to accurate determination of the prolactin level. Patients with galactorrhoea and apparently normal serum prolactin should have prolactin levels verified after sample dilution.

Dynamic Testing with Metoclopramide

Whilst not in routine use, this can provide useful information in patients with mild to moderate elevations in serum prolactin that may be medication related or due to a microprolactinoma too small to be seen on MRI. The intravenous administration of a dopamine antagonist in normal subjects produces a marked rise in prolactin and only a mild increase in thyrotropin stimulating hormone (TSH). Patients with a microprolactinoma exhibit a blunted prolactin response and an exaggerated TSH response.

Imaging

Pituitary imaging provides information about the size of the tumour and its relationship to the optic pathways; it is also useful in the follow up of patients with larger tumours. Imaging is best performed using MRI of the pituitary and hypothalamus with gadolinium contrast enhancement. For patients unable to tolerate or too large to fit in the MRI tunnel, computed tomography scanning of the pituitary can be useful but provides inferior resolution of the pituitary.

Indications for MRI pituitary would include:
- Sustained hyperprolactinaemia (at any level) after other causes have been excluded.
- Headache and visual field defects.

Visual Assessment

Formal visual field testing using Goldmann perimetry should be performed if the adenoma is touching or in close proximity to optic structures.

Case Study: Part 3

Initial investigations revealed normal blood count and renal/liver functions. Baseline hormone levels showed normal thyroid profile, low oestradiol, undetectable luteinising hormone (LH), unremarkable follicle-stimulating hormone (FSH) and grossly elevated prolactin 30,800 mU/L (Table 7.3). Short *Synacthen* test was sub-optimal with baseline cortisol 163 nmol/L and post *Synacthen* value of 450. MRI showed a pituitary macroadenoma measuring 23 mm vertically, 22 mm transversely and 14 mm in antero-posterior diameter. The suprasellar component was causing displacement of the optic chiasm. There were multiple foci of low signal intensity within the gland consistent with areas of cystic change or necrosis (Fig. 7.1a, b). Visual fields assessed by perimetry were normal (Fig. 7.2).

The imaging results and biochemistry in our case study were consistent with a prolactin producing macroadenoma resulting in secondary amenorrhoea, galactorrhoea and infertility. There was no evidence of visual field defects despite the proximity of the tumour to the optic chiasm. Anterior pituitary functions were essentially intact apart from suppression of the hypothalamo-pituitary-gonadal axis secondary to hyperprolactinaemia.

Table 7.3 Endocrine investigations at diagnosis

Hormone	Value	Reference range with units
Prolactin	30,890	50–520 mU/L
Oestradiol	70	Varies during menstrual cycle but usually >200 pmol/L
LH	<1.0	4–10 U/L
FSH	5.0	4–10 U/L
Free T4	11[a]	10–25 nmol/L
Free T3	4.2	3–7 pmol/L
TSH	1.9	0.3–4.5 mU/L
Cortisol (baseline)	163	nmol/L
Cortisol (30 mins post *Synacthen*)	450	Normal peak >550
Insulin-like growth factor 1 (IGF-1)	10[b]	9–42 nmol/L

[a]Thyroid profile improved after 2-months cabergoline: free T4 15, free T3 4.3 and TSH 1.8
[b]Likely growth hormone deficiency but dynamic testing of growth hormone reserve not undertaken

How would you manage this patient?

Medical therapy with dopamine agonists (DA) is the first-line treatment for all patients with macroprolactinomas, including those with visual compromise. In the majority of patients, DAs induce reduction in tumour size and prolactin levels, and relieve pressure symptoms, soon after starting therapy.

Case Study: Part 4

Dopamine agonist therapy was initiated with cabergoline 0.25 mg twice a week, increased to 0.5 mg twice a week after 2 weeks. The drug was recommended to be taken at bedtime with a snack to minimise any symptomatic postural hypotension or nausea. She was warned to report any clear nasal discharge which might indicate the rare development of a cerebrospinal fluid (CSF) leak following shrinkage of her adenoma. She was advised to use barrier contraception for at least the first 6 months of therapy to avoid the risk of early pregnancy leading to leading to prolactinoma expansion. No steroid replacement was recommended and it was planned to repeat the short *Synacthen* test after an interval.

Four weeks after starting cabergoline she was tolerating treatment well and repeat prolactin was 11,880 mU/L — one-third of her pre-treatment levels. Two months later prolactin had fallen into the normal range (290 mU/L). Five months after commencing treatment, serum prolactin remained normal and menstruation resumed. Repeat MR imaging (4 months after starting treatment) revealed marked shrinkage of the enhancing and non-enhancing components of the sellar mass and the remnant measured 7×9×3 mm (Fig. 7.1c, d). Cabergoline was continued at the same dose. The case study conceived after withdrawing contraception following 6 months of cabergoline treatment. This occurred before her hypothalamic-pituitary-adrenal axis was reassessed so paired early morning samples for cortisol and adrenocorticotropic hormone (ACTH) were used as an alternative to

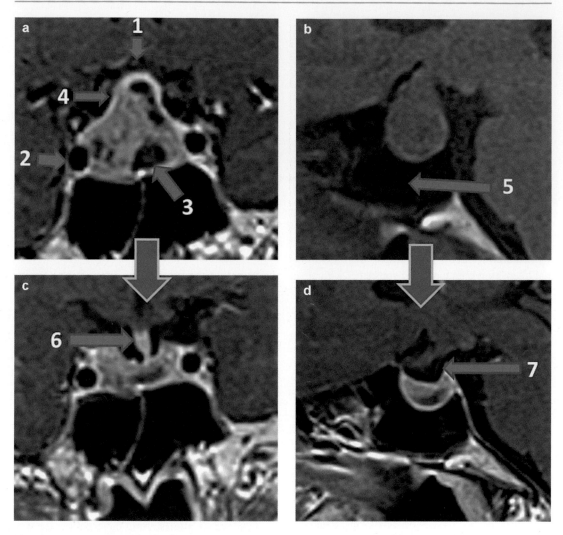

Fig. 7.1 MR imaging showing dramatic shrinkage of macroprolactinoma. (**a, b**) Pre-treatment. (**c, d**) After 4-months cabergoline therapy. *Blue arrows*: (*1*) optic chiasm; (*2*) internal carotid artery; (*3*) cystic area within prolactinoma; (*4*) suprasellar extension; (*5*) sphenoid sinus; (*6*) pituitary stalk; (*7*) concave upper tumour margin after cabergoline treatment

Synacthen testing during pregnancy. Cabergoline has been continued throughout the pregnancy which is presently without complication. Visual field perimetry will be performed each trimester. The case study has been asked to urgently report any visual disturbance or unusual headache, which might suggest prolactinoma expansion. MR imaging will not be performed unless there is visual compromise during pregnancy. The case study has been informed that continuous cabergoline treatment makes it less likely she will have the option of breastfeeding her child.

Issues Considered in the Management of This Case Study

Choosing the Best Dopamine Agonist

The three currently available DAs are bromocriptine, cabergoline and quinagolide. Bromocriptine is the longest established but is used much less frequently nowadays due to a higher incidence of side effects, particularly gastrointestinal. However, it does have the largest and longest pregnancy safety record. Bromocriptine has to be administered two to three times daily, at least at the start of treatment. When used to treat

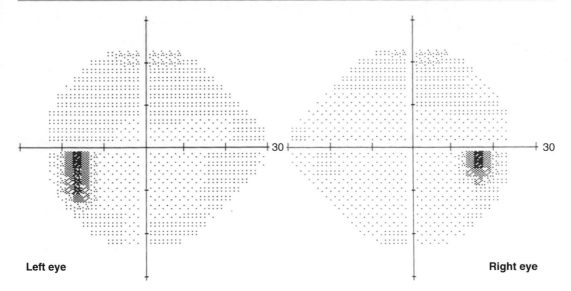

Left eye

Right eye

Fig. 7.2 Visual fields at baseline

large prolactinomas (>4 cm in size), Bromocriptine achieved normal prolactin levels in 33 % of patients [4].

Cabergoline is now the first choice DA for medical management of prolactinomas. A large trial demonstrated that cabergoline is superior to bromocriptine in terms of tolerance (12 % stopped taking bromocriptine compared with 3 % taking cabergoline), patient convenience and efficacy [5]. Cabergoline achieved normalisation of prolactin in around 60 % of patients with large prolactinomas. Cabergoline's safety record during pregnancy is now reasonably substantial, although the data sheet still recommends drug withdrawal 1 month before intended conception (which is impractical for most patients). Pregnancy safety data for quinagolide are limited and less reassuring; the manufacture recommends drug withdrawal in those who become pregnant. Cabergoline was therefore a straightforward choice for our case study.

Minimising Adverse Effects from Dopamine Agonists

Adverse effects of dopamine agonists can be minimised by starting with a low dose and gradually up-titrating, as in the case study. The most common adverse effects are gastrointestinal (especially nausea - vomiting is less common) and postural hypotension leading to dizziness

and occasional syncopal episodes. These problems can be minimized by asking the patient to take the DA at bedtime with a light snack. Other potential side effects to warn patients about are dry mouth, constipation, Raynaud's phenomenon and somnolence. Most minor side effects tend to occur at the beginning of treatment and often resolve with time.

Shrinkage of an inferiorly invasive prolactinoma can rarely result in a CSF leak. Patients with macroprolactinomas should be instructed to report promptly any clear fluid leaking from the nostril. Rarely, tumour shrinkage may cause distortion of optic structures leading to visual disturbance (traction ophthalmopathy) so patients should be asked to report *any* changes in vision during treatment. Pituitary apoplexy has also been reported in patients with macroprolactinoma during DA treatment.

Long-term use of DA therapy has occasionally been associated with psychiatric symptoms, an unusual increase in gambling and similar obsessive behaviours, dyskinesias, nightmares and paraesthesiae. The use of high-dose DA therapy in patients with Parkinson's disease has been associated with clinically significant cardiac valve fibrosis; this finding has not been found in patients on low-dose DA therapy for prolactinoma [6]. Current MHRA guidelines still suggest that patients on cabergoline therapy should have an echocardiogram done within the first 6 months of starting therapy and thereafter at least once a year. However, in the light of recent reassuring studies, many clinicians do not undertake surveillance echocardiograms on patients taking less than 2 mg cabergoline per week.

Assessing Tumour Responses to Dopamine Agonist Treatment

Serum prolactin levels fall quickly, often within hours of taking the first tablet of DA. It is therefore reasonable to re-measure serum prolactin at 2, 4 and 12 weeks after the start of therapy in a typical case to assess response. Repeat MR imaging to assess tumour shrinkage is best done after 3–4 months, by which time most tumour shrinkage has already occurred. Imaging can then be repeated after a year. Some tumours show much slower progressive shrinkage but they are in the minority.

If vision is impaired at outset, recheck visual fields by perimetry after a week and repeat again at the end of the second week. They can then be done less frequently if improvements in the fields have been documented. It is prudent to recheck rest of pituitary function at intervals to see if deficiencies (often subtle) improve as the normal pituitary is de-compressed secondary to tumour shrinkage.

> How do you manage patients on medical treatment for macroprolactinoma who become pregnant?

Effect of Dopamine Agonists on Foetal Development

Foetal exposure to any medication, including DAs, should be minimised. Whilst all patients with microprolactinomas can have DAs stopped on confirmation of pregnancy, this may not be possible in patients with large macroprolactinomas where the drug may have to be continued through the entire gestation. This is particularly true for patients with large residual tumour remnants after tumour shrinkage or for those in whom DA therapy has been commenced relatively recently (<1 year, as in our case study) and for whom the risk of tumour re-expansion is significant.

Data available for over 6,000 pregnancies exposed to bromocriptine and over 700 pregnancies exposed to cabergoline in the first trimester showed no increase in adverse pregnancy or foetal outcomes compared to population based controls (Table 7.4). Experience of patients exposed to DAs throughout the pregnancy is more limited but is increasing [8]. Quinagolide use is not recommended for patients desiring pregnancy. Long-term follow-up of cognitive performance for children born to mothers treated with bromocriptine during pregnancy is reassuring [9].

Effect of Pregnancy on Prolactinoma Size

The oestrogenic milieu of normal pregnancy stimulates pituitary lactotrophs to gradually increase prolactin production as pregnancy progresses. This physiological increase in prolactin prepares the breasts for lactation. Pituitary imaging demonstrates lactotroph hyperplasia with a gradual increase in pituitary volume through the course of pregnancy (more than doubles) which peaks in the first week post-partum. Data summarising symptomatic increase in sizes of macroprolactinomas in pregnancy showed that in patients with no prior definitive treatment (surgery or radiotherapy) there was a 23 % chance of an

Table 7.4 Pregnancy outcomes in women exposed to bromocriptine and cabergoline in early pregnancy compared to normal American population data [7]

	Bromocriptine (%) (n=6,239)	Cabergoline (%) (n=789)	Normal (%)
Spontaneous abortions	9.9	7.6	10–15
Terminations	1.2	7.5	20
Ectopic pregnancy	0.5	0.4	1–1.5
Hydatiform moles	0.2	0.1	0.1–0.15
Preterm birth (<37 weeks)	12.5	11.6	12.7
Multiple pregnancies	1.7	1.7	3.2
Foetal malformations	1.8	3.2	3.0

increase in size during pregnancy and in those who received prior definitive treatment there was a 5 % chance of a symptomatic increase in size [7]. Taking into account the fact that our case study had received primary medical therapy with cabergoline for just over 6 months before falling pregnant (with excellent tumour shrinkage) we estimated her risk of tumour enlargement during pregnancy, off cabergoline, to be at least 10 %.

Current Recommendations for Managing Macroprolactinomas in Pregnancy

- Pre-pregnancy planning is an essential part of management for patients with macroprolactinomas who desire pregnancy. A small subset of patients cannot tolerate DA or do not achieve significant tumour size reduction. Hence, non-hormonal, barrier contraception should be used during the first few months of DA therapy when drug tolerance and tumour response can be assessed. In our case study, good tolerance and an excellent response was established following 4 months of cabergoline therapy. Unresponsive or intolerant patients may need considered for transsphenoidal surgical debulking prior to pregnancy.
- In patients who have had previous pituitary surgery or radiotherapy, medical therapy can usually be safely stopped on confirmation of pregnancy (nowadays, these will comprise a small number since most will have received primary DA therapy)
- In patients without previous surgery or radiotherapy (as for our case study) there are two options. First, to continue cabergoline therapy throughout pregnancy or, second, to stop DA therapy and monitor carefully for features of tumour expansion. The risk of tumour growth during pregnancy in these patients depends on the duration and type of DA therapy, and residual tumour size at the start of the pregnancy. Regardless of which option is chosen, patients need careful follow-up for symptoms of tumour growth with visual field assessments every trimester, as a minimum.

- Most patients with symptomatic tumour growth can be treated successfully with reinstitution of DA therapy or increasing the drug dose.
- Patients who are diagnosed with symptomatic macroprolactinoma for the first time during pregnancy can usually be treated successfully with DAs rather than surgery.
- In the rare patient with extreme dopamine intolerance or resistance, together with symptomatic growth of a macroprolactinoma, surgery may be needed during pregnancy. Any major surgery is associated with a 1.5-fold increase in foetal losses in the first trimester and a five-fold increase in foetal losses in the second trimester [7].

References

1. Leung AK, Pacaud D. Diagnosis and management of galactorrhea. Am Fam Physician. 2004;70(3): 543–50.
2. Bevan JS. Prolactinomas and hyperprolactinaemia (including macroprolactinaemia). In: Wass JAH, editor. Oxford textbook of endocrinology and diabetes. 2nd ed. Oxford: Oxford University Press; 2011. p. 187–97.
3. Melmed S, Casanueva FF, Hoffman AR, Kleinberg DL, Montori VM, Schlechte JA, Wass JA; Endocrine Society. Diagnosis and treatment of hyperprolactinemia: an Endocrine Society clinical practice guideline. J Clin Endocrinol Metab. 2011;96(2):273–88.
4. Moraes AB, Silva CM, Vieira Neto L, Gadelha MR. Giant prolactinomas: the therapeutic approach. Clin Endocrinol (Oxf). 2013;79(4):447–56.
5. Webster J, Piscitelli G, Polli A, Ferrari CI, Ismail I, Scanlon MF. A Comparison of cabergoline and bromocriptine in the treatment of hyperprolactinemic amenorrhea. Cabergoline Comparative Study Group. N Engl J Med. 1994;331(14):904–9.
6. Drake WM, Stiles CE, Howlett TA, Toogood AA, Bevan JS, Steeds RP, UK Dopamine Agonist Valvulopathy Group. A cross-sectional study of the prevalence of cardiac valvular abnormalities in hyperprolactinemic patients treated with ergot-derived dopamine agonists. J Clin Endocrinol Metab. 2014;99(1):90–6.
7. Molitch ME. Prolactinoma in pregnancy. Best Pract Res Clin Endocrinol Metab. 2011;25(6):885–96.
8. Lebbe M, Hubinont C, Bernard P, Maiter D. Outcome of 100 pregnancies initiated under treatment with cabergoline in hyperprolactinaemic women. Clin Endocrinol (Oxf). 2010;73(2):236–42.
9. Raymond JP, Goldstein E, Konopka P, Leleu MF, Merceron RE, Loria Y. Follow-up of children born of bromocriptine-treated mothers. Horm Res. 1985;22(3): 239–46.

A 25-Year-Old Woman with Headache and Joint Pain

Case 8

Nigel G.L. Glynn and Márta Korbonits

Abstract

A 25-year-old woman is referred by her primary care provider with headache, arthralgia and sweating. Systematic history and clinical examination suggest growth hormone excess – acromegaly. The diagnosis is confirmed on biochemical testing. This chapter discusses the appropriate investigation and management of patients with acromegaly, with particular emphasis on recent advances in clinical care and insights provided by contemporary research.

Keywords

Acromegaly • Growth hormone • Insulin-like growth factor-1 • Pituitary tumour

Case

Tamara is 25-year-old hairdresser with a 2-year history of gradually worsening headache. This has been accompanied by 6 months of widespread arthralgia.

> What questions would you ask and what diagnoses would you consider at this stage?

N.G.L. Glynn, MB, BCh, BAO
Department of Endocrinology, Barts and The London School of Medicine, Queen Mary University of London, London, UK

M. Korbonits, MD, PhD (✉)
Department of Endocrinology, William Harvey Research Institute, Barts and the London School of Medicine, Queen Mary University of London, Charterhouse Square, London EC1M 6BQ, UK
e-mail: m.korbonits@qmul.ac.uk

Chronic headache in a young person is usually due to tension headache or migraine. Benign intracranial hypertension should be considered in obese young women. Space-occupying lesions are less common. However, the concurrent history of joint pains suggests that a systemic disease may be the cause of her symptoms.

A detailed medical history is taken to enquire about other systemic symptoms:

Her only medical history is of a kidney stone 2 years ago that was treated with extracorporeal shock wave lithotripsy.

On review of systems she reports a number of other longstanding complaints:

- She has a tendency to sweat profusely. This has been problematic for over 5 years. She attended her GP on a number of occasions, but no cause or remedy could be found. She does not report any weight loss or palpitations.

- She has been attending her dentist for the last year due to difficulty with her bite and pain in her lower jaw.
- Her menstrual cycle has been irregular for 2 years and she complained of oily skin and mild acne.

The history of headache, arthralgia and sweating raises the possibility of growth hormone excess or acromegaly. This is almost always due to a growth hormone (GH) secreting tumour of the pituitary gland (95 % of cases). In addition, the dental difficulties may be due malocclusion of the teeth which can occur in acromegaly. Similarly, oligomenorrhoea can occur in the presence of a pituitary tumour due to either prolactin release from the tumour, hyperprolactinaemia due to stalk disruption or direct damage to gonadotroph cells. GH excess can also induce a PCOS-like phenotype possibly due to increased circulating insulin levels.

What examination findings would support a diagnosis of GH excess?
- Enlargement of the hands and feet
  - The patient may have had to remove rings or change shoe size
- Positive Tinel's or Phalen's sign consistent with carpal tunnel syndrome
- Skin thickening
- Hypertension
- Axillary skin tags suggestive of insulin resistance
- Dental spacing
- Prognathism
- Bitemporal hemianopia
  - A suprasellar tumour may compress the optic chiasm and typically compromises the temporal field of vision initially. Failure of visual acuity and optic atrophy may also occur.
- Frontal bossing
- Deep, cavernous voice due to enlargement of frontal sinuses and soft tissue of the larynx

- Macroglossia – often indicated by tooth marks on the side of the tongue
- Organomegaly – in particular goitre or hepatosplenomegaly
- Galactorrhoea
- Signs of heart failure including raised venous pressure, basal lung crackles, lower limb oedema

Review of a series of old photographs reveals that the patient has been developing coarser facial features for approximately 7 years.

The diagnosis of acromegaly is often delayed by up to a decade. The symptoms and signs develop so slowly that the patient and his/her family don't notice them until complications arise or they develop pain.

What blood tests would you request to confirm a diagnosis of acromegaly?

Growth hormone: GH is normally released in short pulses between prolonged periods of relatively low levels of secretion. Random GH levels can be variable but undetectable GH would make acromegaly unlikely. A glucose load will suppress GH to almost undetectable levels in normal individuals. Therefore, a 75-g oral glucose tolerance test (OGTT) is considered the gold standard test for diagnosis of acromegaly. Traditionally, suppression below 1 µg/L was considered normal when using a radioimmunoassay to measure GH. However, modern immunochemiluminescent GH assays are more sensitive. Failure to suppress serum GH below 0.4 µg/L after OGTT is diagnostic of acromegaly, if the patient has clinical symptoms and signs of the disease. Premenopausal women are relatively GH resistant and a higher cut-off of 0.7 µg/L may be appropriate. GH assay standardisation is still suboptimal internationally and locally appropriate cut-offs may differ slightly. This should be discussed with the endocrine laboratory in your institution.

The OGTT will also give information about the patient's glucose tolerance which is often (up to 40 %) impaired in acromegaly.

Insulin-like growth factor 1 (IGF-1): IGF-1 production from the liver is stimulated by GH and this peptide mediates most of the effects of GH peripherally. Its concentration in the plasma is much more stable than GH and therefore IGF-1 levels are almost invariably elevated in active acromegaly. Age-specific normal ranges should be provided by the laboratory.

Prolactin: Hyperprolactinaemia is observed in 30 % of patients with acromegaly. Some GH producing tumours co-secrete prolactin. However, prolactin may be elevated due to compression of the pituitary stalk. An enlarging tumour can disrupt inhibitory dopamine supply to the anterior pituitary which has a permissive effect on prolactin secretion.

Assessment of the remainder of the pituitary function: Thyroid function tests, gonadotrophins (and menstrual history) and early morning cortisol. Dynamic assessment of ACTH reserve may be appropriate if the cortisol level is equivocal.

Her basal GH level is 35.6 µg/L and does not suppress with an OGTT. IGF-1 level is elevated 890 µg/L (age-related reference range 149–332). She has impaired glucose tolerance.

Her prolactin level is mildly elevated at 720 mU/L (range 0–496).

Thyroid function test are normal and early morning cortisol is healthy at 825 nmol/L.

What test would you order next?

MRI pituitary with intravenous contrast enhancement (Fig. 8.1).

MRI shows a homogenous pituitary macroadenoma measuring 2 cm in craniocaudal diameter. It extends into the suprasellar cistern but does not compress the optic chiasm. The tumour invades the left cavernous sinus.

What is the diagnosis?

Acromegaly due to a GH secreting pituitary tumour (somatotroph adenoma). The raised prolactin level may be due to pituitary stalk distortion or co-secretion of prolactin from the tumour (somatomammotroph adenoma).

What treatment would you recommend?

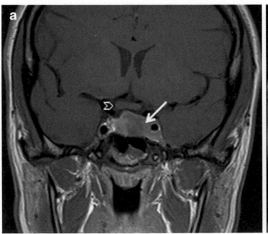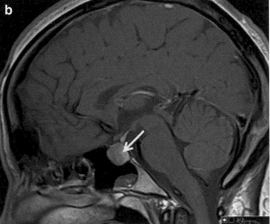

Fig. 8.1 Pre-operative MRI pituitary. Pre-contrast T1 weighted images in the coronal (**a**) and sagittal (**b**) plain show a homogenous mass arising from the pituitary fossa and invading the left cavernous sinus (*arrow*). The tumour extends into the suprasellar cistern. It encroaches upon but does not compress the optic chiasm (*arrowhead*)

Surgical resection: This is the primary treatment for most patients. Rates of postoperative remission are dependent on the tumour size and the experience of the surgeon. Tumours which invade the cavernous sinus are difficult to completely resected due to the risk of bleeding from the highly vascular sinus.

Pre-operative somatostatin analogue (SSA) treatment (see below) may be beneficial in reducing soft tissue swelling and reduce the risk of anaesthetic complications in patients with severe macroglossia and enlarged laryngeal tissues. In the case of very large tumours, pre-operative SSA may also improve the surgical outcome and increase the likelihood of post-operative remission. However, this is controversial and the results of prospective clinical trials evaluating this approach are awaited.

The patient undergoes transsphenoidal surgery to debulk the pituitary tumour. Histological analysis confirms a pituitary adenoma with a low ki-67 index (proliferative index) of less than 1 %. Immunohistochemical staining is weakly positive for GH and negative for all other anterior pituitary hormone. This suggest a sparsely granulated somatotroph adenoma which could be confirmed with electron microscopy.

Post-operative testing shows that her GH and IGF-1 levels have declined but remain elevated. The remainder of her pituitary function is preserved.

Medical

SSA are the most commonly used medical therapy for acromegaly. They have both anti-tumour and anti-secretory effects on somatotroph adenomas. Long-acting formulations are usually administered monthly by intramuscular injection. This treatment will normalise IGF-1 in approximately 60 % of patients. Tumour shrinkage is less predictable but up to 80 % of patients are reported to display at least 20 % tumour volume reduction. Sparsely granulated tumours may be more resistant to SSA therapy.

Pegvisomant prevents GH binding to its receptor and producing IGF-1. This drug can normalise IGF-1 in the majority of patients with acromegaly, if used in sufficient doses. Serum GH levels rise during therapy and the drug cross reacts with many GH assays. Therefore, serum GH levels should not be measured while taking pegvisomant, but IGF-1 concentration should be used to titrate the appropriate dose. It is administered daily (or on alternate days) by deep subcutaneous injection.

Dopamine agonists can also lower GH levels and may cause modest tumour shrinkage. They are administered orally. A higher weekly dose, than used in prolactinoma, is often required for clinical effectiveness.

Radiotherapy

External beam radiotherapy is a long-established and effective treatment of acromegaly. Treatment results in stabilisation of tumour size more commonly than shrinkage. GH levels decline slowly and it may take 10 years for the maximal biochemical effect to be seen. Radiotherapy may damage the normal pituitary gland resulting in hypopituitarism in 50 % of treated subjects after 10 years. This may have significant implications for young patients who wish to preserve fertility.

The patient is planning to start a family; therefore, it is decided to use medical therapy to control acromegaly for now.

> What side effects may be encountered with medical therapy for acromegaly?

SSA can cause nausea and diarrhoea. Gallstones commonly develop when using long term SSA. However, these are typically asymptomatic unless the drug is stopped suddenly.

Dopamine agonists can cause nausea, postural hypotension, constipation and rarely psychological symptoms such as depression or impulse control disorders. Also, they occasionally induce

Raynaud's phenomenon. Long-term use of high-dose dopamine agonist in Parkinson's disease has been associated with valvular heart disease. However, it is controversial whether this risk applies to patients with patients with pituitary tumours.

Pegvisomant can cause derangement of liver biochemistry in 2–3 % of patients. This should be monitored regularly, particularly with concurrent use of SSA. It normally improves with dose reduction or discontinuation. Initial concerns about enlargement of the tumour remnant while taking pegvisomant have not been borne out with clinical experience.

The patient is commenced on a long-acting somatostatin analogue. Her GH and IGF-1 decline further but she continues to have active acromegaly.

Can combinations of medical treatment be used?

There is increasing experience with the use of combination medical therapy in acromegaly. SSA and pegvisomant or SSA and cabergoline are the most commonly used combinations. This appears safe and effective but derangement of liver biochemistry is more common with the former combination. This may necessitate dose reduction or cessation of some medications.

What GH and IGF-1 levels should be targeted?

International consensus guidelines recommend that treatment of acromegaly should aim to reduce GH levels to less than 2.5 µg/L. A 5-point day curve is very useful for estimating average daily GH exposure. However, random, basal GH levels, particularly if measured on more than one occasion, may suffice. Standardised mortality in patients with acromegaly equates to the normal population at GH levels below this target. Treatment should also aim to lower IGF-1 levels into the age-related reference range.

What should be done when there is discordance between GH and IGF-1 levels?

Up to one-third of patients have discordant GH and IGF-1 levels during follow-up of acromegaly. The most common pattern encountered is a safe GH level (<2.5 µg/L) in the presence of a persistently elevated IGF-1 concentration. This is often observed in patients who have had pituitary radiotherapy. While there is no consensus on the best approach in this situation, the patient's clinical status is often a good guide to whether acromegaly is still active. Persistent sweating and joint pain is consistent with active disease.

On combination SSA and low-dose pegvisomant the patient's IGF-1 level are within the age related reference range. Her headache, sweating and arthralgia resolve. Her menstrual cycle is now regular.

Does the patient require any further pituitary imaging?

An MRI scan should be repeated 6–12 weeks after surgery to define the size and location of any tumour remnant. A further MRI is indicated 3–6 months after commencing medical therapy to assess the anti-tumour response. The frequency of further interval scans will depend on the clinical course and any other treatments which have been given eg. radiotherapy.

What clinical issues will be important during long-term follow-up?

In addition to monitoring GH/IGF-1 levels and tumour size, it is important to monitor the end organ effects of long-term GH excess.

Glucose metabolism: Overt diabetes occurs in 15 % of patients with acromegaly while 40 % have impaired glucose tolerance. In general, glucose levels decline and are easier to control once

GH/IGF-1 levels are lowered. However, use of SSA may cause deterioration in glycaemic control as they antagonise insulin and incretin hormones.

Heart: Hypertension is also common in acromegaly with the consequent risk of stroke and hypertensive cardiomyopathy. Curiously, patients with acromegaly do not commonly develop coronary artery disease. GH & IGF-1 have direct effects on the heart which are toxic in excess. Left ventricular hypertrophy and diastolic dysfunction develop prior to systolic failure. Careful blood pressure management is essential. Echocardiogram should be performed at diagnosis.

Gastrointestinal: Colonic polyps appear to be more common in acromegaly. It is controversial whether the rate of malignant transformation is truly increased. However, the prognosis from colorectal cancer has traditionally been poor in acromegaly. Colonoscopy should be considered at diagnosis.

Bones and joints: Patients with acromegaly often suffer from joint deformities. Progressive arthropathy of the axial skeleton can lead to spinal deformity, a major cause of morbidity in acromegaly. GH excess has been associated with bone overgrowth (diffuse idiopathic skeletal hyperostosis). The risk of fracture may also be increased.

> Is the patient's history of urolithiasis of any clinical relevance?

Previous diagnosis of a kidney stone raises the possibility of hypercalcaemia and hyperparathyroidism. The combination of primary hyperparathyroidism and a pituitary tumour should, in turn, raise the clinical suspicion of multiple endocrine neoplasia (MEN) type 1 syndrome. This syndrome is due to a mutation in the gene encoding the menin protein on chromosome 11. It is characterised by a triad of hyperparathyroidism (typically due to parathyroid hyperplasia), pituitary adenomas and pancreatic neuroendocrine tumours. Adrenocortical adenomas and cutaneous lipomas are also common in this condition.

Her serum calcium is normal, ruling out hyperparathyroidism. Nonetheless, kidney stones are more common in sporadic acromegaly. GH excess causes hyperphosphataemia and hypercalciuria. This is mainly due to enhanced intestinal calcium absorption secondary to increased renal 1,25 dihydroxy vitamin D synthesis.

> Other than MEN 1, should any other genetic cause of pituitary adenomas be considered in young patients with acromegaly?

Diagnosis of acromegaly in a child or young adult should prompt a thorough family history. Recently, it has been recognised that some young patients diagnosed with pituitary tumours have a family history of isolated pituitary adenomas, a syndrome now known as Familial Isolated Pituitary Adenoma (FIPA). This is an autosomal dominant condition but the penetrance is incomplete. Approximately 20 % of families with FIPA have a heterozygous germline mutation in the aryl hydrocarbon receptor-interacting protein (AIP) gene. Patients with acromegaly who have this mutation typically have large invasive tumours which are partially resistant to medical therapy.

Germline AIP mutations can be identified in patients with pituitary adenomas who have no known family history of the disease – approximately 20 % of childhood onset cases and 11 % of young onset (<30 years) pituitary macroadenomas.

Our patient had no known family history of pituitary adenoma and sequencing of the AIP gene does not reveal any pathogenic mutation.

Case Review

Tamara is young lady with headache, joint pain, sweating and dental malocclusion. The clinical suspicion of acromegaly is reinforced by review of the patient's photo album which displays gradual development of acral features over several years. The diagnosis is confirmed by failure to suppress serum GH to normal levels following an oral glucose load. This is supported by an elevated IGF-1 level. MRI scan shows a pituitary macroadenoma. Primary surgical debulking does not result in disease remission. Combination medical therapy with somatostatin analogue and GH receptor antagonist, pegvisomant, is used to normalise IGF-1 level. Radiotherapy has been reserved for now and will be reconsidered when she has completed her family. Screening for genetic causes of pituitary tumours was negative.

Key Points

- Growth hormone excess can present with a constellation of symptoms, which have typically developed over many years. Comparison of serial photographs of the patient's face is often helpful when the symptoms or signs are subtle.
- The diagnosis of acromegaly should be confirmed biochemically before proceeding to pituitary imaging.
- Surgical debulking is recommended for most patients with acromegaly, as it may result in disease remission.
- Patients with persistently active disease following surgery should be offered medical therapy to reduce GH to safe levels and IGF-1 concentration into the age-related normal range.
- Radiotherapy is an effective second or third line treatment but it may take 10 years for its maximal effect to be observed.

- Patients should be monitored for long-term complications of growth hormone excess including hypertension and glucose intolerance.
- Genetic causes of acromegaly should be considered in young patients and those with a family history of pituitary tumours.

Suggested Reading

Besser GM. Comprehensive clinical endocrinology. London: Mosby; 2002.

Feenstra J, de Herder WW, ten Have SM, van den Beld AW, Feelders RA, Janssen JA, et al. Combined therapy with somatostatin analogues and weekly pegvisomant in active acromegaly. Lancet. 2005;365(9471): 1644–6.

Giustina A, Chanson P, Bronstein MD, Klibanski A, Lamberts S, Casanueva FF, et al. A consensus on criteria for cure of acromegaly. J Clin Endocrinol Metab. 2010;95(7):3141–8.

Kamenicky P, Blanchard A, Gauci C, Salenave S, Letierce A, Lombès M, et al. Pathophysiology of renal calcium handling in acromegaly: what lies behind hypercalciuria? J Clin Endocrinol Metab. 2012;97(6):2124–33.

Korbonits M, Storr H, Kumar AV. Familial pituitary adenomas – who should be tested for AIP mutations? Clin Endocrinol (Oxf). 2012;77(3):351–6.

Melmed S, Colao A, Barkan A, Molitch M, Grossman AB, Kleinberg D, et al. Guidelines for acromegaly management: an update. J Clin Endocrinol Metab. 2009;94(5):1509–17.

Trainer PJ, Drake WM, Katznelson L, Freda PU, Herman-Bonert V, van der Lely AJ, et al. Treatment of acromegaly with growth hormone-receptor antagonist pegvisomant. N Engl J Med. 2000;342(16):1171–7.

Recent-Onset Visual Field Loss and Raised Prolactin Level (Non-functioning Pituitary Tumour)

Case 9

Nick Phillips and Stephen M. Orme

Abstract

Non-functioning pituitary adenomas can exert their effects in a number of ways. They can lead to pressure on the optic chiasm, and this can produce visual field defects. More rarely the tumour extends laterally into the cavernous sinus and leads to cranial nerve palsies. Pituitary tumours may expand and therefore stretch the overlying dura and cause pressure effects around the pituitary fossa, leading to the development of headaches.

Because of the tumour mass and other factors, hypopituitarism can occur, which usually follows a classic pattern. Growth hormone secretion is more readily affected, followed by gonadotrophin (LH and FSH) and ACTH secretion, with TSH secretion being most likely to be preserved.

Lactotrophs (anterior pituitary cells which produce prolactin), are the most abundant cells in the anterior pituitary. They tonically secrete high levels of prolactin, and this is inhibited by the hypothalamic release of dopamine, which passes down the portal hypophysial tract, within the pituitary stalk, so that physiological prolactin secretion maintained. When there is a physical disruption of the delivery of dopamine to the lactotrophs of the anterior pituitary, then hyperprolactinaemia ensues, this is termed the 'stalk disconnection effect'.

Keywords

Non-functioning pituitary adenoma • Visual field defects • Hypopituitarism • Prolactin • Stalk disconnection effect

Presenting History

A 36-year-old woman presents with a 9-month history of supra-orbital headaches which she has put down to work stress. She also had suffered from chronic, nonspecific headaches for a number of years, for which she occasionally took paracetamol. She has previously been on the oral

N. Phillips, MBChB, FRCS, FRCS (SN) PhD (✉)
Department of Neurosurgery, Leeds General Infirmary, Leeds, West Yorkshire LS21 2NU, UK
e-mail: nickphill@gmail.com

S.M. Orme, MBChB, MD, FRCP
Department of Endocrinology, St. James's Hospital, Leeds, West Yorkshire, UK

R. Ajjan, S.M. Orme (eds.), *Endocrinology and Diabetes: Case Studies, Questions and Commentaries*,
DOI 10.1007/978-1-4471-2789-5_9, © Springer-Verlag London 2015

contraceptive pill and had normal menstrual periods, but had a Mirena coil fitted 3 years ago and had no menstrual periods over this time. She has not been aware of any deterioration in visual acuity or visual fields. Her prolactin level is raised at 1,345 miu/L.

> What additional questions would you ask?

When evaluating a patient with pituitary disease, one must determine whether the pituitary adenoma has led to a reduction in visual fields or any evidence of hypopituitarism. One has to determine whether potentially rather vague symptoms have come on over a prolonged period of time (remember pituitary adenomas tend to be very slow growing), or whether there has been a sudden change in symptoms, perhaps due to a pituitary apoplexy (a very rare event).

Presentation of Patients with Non-functioning Pituitary Adenomas

Pituitary adenomas are relatively common and have a prevalence of 78–94 cases per 1,000,000 population. They cause their effects by pressure on the visual apparatus, cranial nerves, and adjacent pituitary gland. This pressure may cause disorders of the cranial nerves, hormonal problems and headache.

Pituitary tumours that extend above the diaphragma sella will cause some element of visual deficit. Some patients will seek ophthalmological examination and be referred from that route, but many patients will not have noticed visual symptoms, and will have tumours found incidentally.

The cranial nerves in and around the cavernous sinus are exposed to pressure from a large pituitary tumour and may cause a more rapid sequence of referral through the ophthalmological services or neurology after the investigation of ophthalmoplegia.

Pressure on the normal pituitary gland, its stalk or the hypothalamus may impair the normal secretory function of these structures and cause hormonal insufficiency. The first hormone affected is growth hormone, and in children this will cause growth failure. In adults the symptoms may well be somewhat vague and contribute to non-specific effects on well-being and energy. The gonadotrophins are next affected. In premenopausal women disorders of the menstrual cycle and infertility will result. In men impotence and infertility are common with a reduction in male secondary sexual characteristics such as beard growth, being a relatively late event. ACTH deficiency, can present with tiredness, weight loss and dizziness on standing. In older patients, particularly it may present with somewhat vague symptoms and hyponatraemia is a not uncommon finding. Deficiencies in TSH are rare even with large tumours.

Not all patients with pituitary tumours have symptoms of headache even when the tumour is large. Those patients who do have headache tend to have a relatively vague and non-specific headache, though it occasionally may be retro-orbital.

> What will you ask in the history regarding vision?

Visual field problems in relation to pituitary tumours take the form of visual field defects and disorders of ocular motility.

Many pituitary tumours can cause visual field deficits that are asymptomatic, especially if the progression has been slow. The patient may not report any symptoms related to vision; these patients usually are referred after optometric examination. It is worth asking when the last normal eye test was and if they had visual fields performed.

Conversely, symptomatic patients may report bumping into objects. This may be unilateral or bilateral and usually implies temporal field loss. The duration of such a symptom is important, as long-standing visual loss has reduced prognosis for recovery after the relief of compression by surgery.

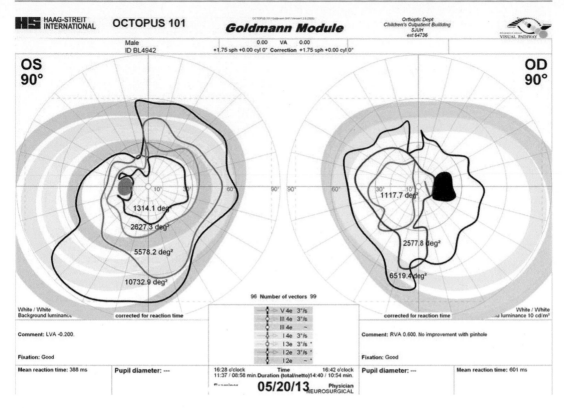

Fig. 9.1 Goldman visual fields showing severe bitemporal hemianopia from chiasmal compression, worse on the *right*

Sudden or rapid onset of visual field defects associated with headache and ophthalmoplegia suggests pituitary apoplexy, which of course is an emergency.

> What sorts of patterns of visual field loss can occur in pituitary tumours?

Bitemporal hemianopia is the classic picture of visual field loss, – this will rarely be symmetrical or complete (Fig. 9.1). The superior temporal fields are more frequently affected then the inferior temporal fields. Pressure on the optic chiasm is dependent on the anatomical location of the chiasm in relation to the pituitary gland and tumour. In about 70 % of cases the optic chiasm is above the pituitary gland in the normal position. In the remainder the chiasm may be more anteriorly placed near the tuberculum sella (prefixed), or more posteriorly placed (post fixed). In patients with a postfixed chiasm, the intracranial length of optic nerve is longer and affected by the tumour, causing field defects related to optic nerve compression such as junctional scotoma and monocular blindness. Junctional scotoma is due to compression at the junction of the optic nerve and chiasm and is a superior temporal field.

Visual field deficits relating to a prefixed chiasm are rare and would result in a homonymous field defect which is seen in about 4.2 % of patients with pituitary adenomas.

> What questions will you ask regarding ocular motility?

Disorders of ocular motility in pituitary tumours are relatively rare and are reported at between 1 and 6 %. The third (oculomotor) nerve is usually affected, causing diplopia and drooping of the eyelid.

Which other tumours and pathologies could cause visual defects in this region?
• Meningioma, craniopharyngioma, hypothalamic tumour (glioma, astrocytoma)
• Optic nerve glioma, chordoma, germinoma, dermoid, metastasis
• Inflammatory pathology such as Langerhan's cell histiocytosis, sarcoid, and lymphocytic hypophysitis

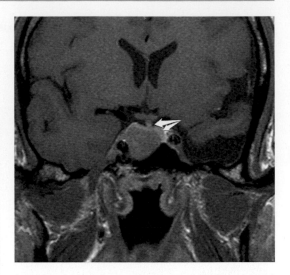

Fig. 9.2 A T1 MRI scan showing a pituitary adenoma distorting the distal pituitary stalk and gland (*white arrows*)

Which blood tests, radiological tests, and other tests should now be performed after an initial assessment?

Pituitary region tumours sufficiently large to cause a visual deficit usually require some consideration of surgery, with the notable exception of those tumours secreting prolactin. It is important to establish the serum prolactin level early in the assessment as a prolactinoma is eminently treatable medically without the risks of surgery. The prolactin level should be interpreted with the size of the tumour.

What is the stalk effect?

Secretion of prolactin by the pituitary gland is inhibited tonically by dopamine which is transferred to the anterior pituitary down the pituitary stalk from the hypothalamus in the hypophyseal portal system.

The stalk effect is seen when the serum prolactin level is elevated beyond normal to a level of not more than 4,000 mU/L. It is thought to be

due to the tumour causing pressure on or distorting the pituitary stalk and inhibiting the secretion or transport of the inhibitory factor dopamine to the pituitary (Fig. 9.2).

What other hormone assessments are necessary before considering surgery?

It is important to establish if the patient has hypothyroidism before anaesthesia and a free T4 level should be measured. Patients about to have surgery should have empirical glucocorticoid replacements, and the adrenal axis should be assessed post-operatively. The gonadal hormones and growth hormone can be assessed post-operatively. Patients with pituitary adenomas are very unlikely to have diabetes insipidus preoperatively. Were this to occur, one should entertain an alternative diagnosis, such as a craniopharyngioma or a dysgerminoma.

What scans should be arranged?

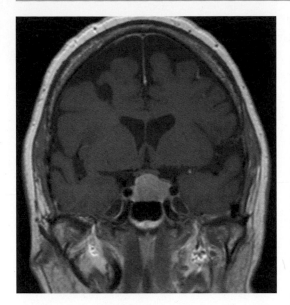

Fig. 9.3 T1 weighted, post gadolinium contrast enhanced scan in the coronal plane showing a pituitary adenoma touching the optic chiasm

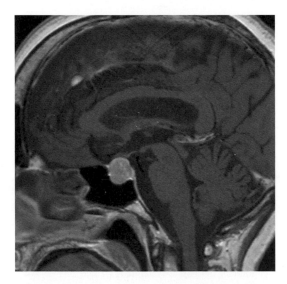

Fig. 9.4 T1 weighted post gadolinium contrast enhanced scan in the sagittal plane of the same tumour seen in Fig. 9.3

A targeted MRI with T1 sequences pre and post contrast, in the coronal, sagittal and axial planes should be requested (Figs. 9.3 and 9.4). If the patient has a pacemaker. a CT scan with contrast should be requested.

> What tests of vision should be arranged?

Formal examination of the visual fields is important for many reasons and can be done either using automated Humphrey perimetry or Goldman perimetry. Humphrey automated perimetry produces dark areas graphically to represent visual loss in each eye. Statistics such as mean standard deviation and pattern standard deviation from the normal age-matched controls are calculated. In Goldman perimetry, which is the reference standard, Isopters are produced graphically that follow a normal pattern unless there is significant visual field defects in which case they will diverge from that pattern.

> Having established the diagnosis of a non-functioning pituitary adenoma what would your management plan be?

If blood tests do not show that the adenoma is a prolactinoma then consideration of surgery is important. The timescale of referral to a specialist multidisciplinary pituitary surgery meeting should be days rather than weeks or months if there is a documented visual field defect. The primary treatment is likely to be trans-nasal surgery to remove as much tumour as possible. Eighty percent of patients have very early improvement in their vision after surgery. Surgery rarely results in complete resection of the tumour because of its location in close proximity to vital structures. Debulking the tumour is usually sufficient to relieve pressure on the optic chiasm and therefore potentially result in an improvement in visual fields. After a radiological evaluation of the extent of resection patients may need either further surgery or adjuvant therapy in the form of radiotherapy which can be fractionated or given by stereotactic radiosurgery in a single session.

What is the role of the endocrinologist in the post-operative management of patients with pituitary adenoma?

The degree of tumour resection will be assessed radiologically by an MRI scan at 3 months. During this time the patient should have a full endocrine assessment. Preoperative endocrine deficiencies can sometimes be reversed by surgery. In general, surgical extirpation does not result in deterioration in anterior pituitary function. But, this can happen on occasion. Diabetes insipidus can occur post-operatively, but is not found in pituitary adenomas pre-operatively.

A formal evaluation of the visual fields should also be arranged using the same modality of assessment as was done preoperatively.

Summary

The initial history and examination should establish if there are any features of pituitary apoplexy (sudden onset of symptoms, rapid loss of vision, headache, cranial nerve palsies). Thereafter an assessment of the time scale and progression of the visual loss in the history will give an idea of the likely recovery of vision with treatment. Examination findings should reveal if there are any clinical signs such as a third nerve palsy which would indicate a larger tumour. Examination of the visual fields by confrontation should be performed before more formal testing to give an idea of the degree of visual loss, and this will contribute to the urgency of the case.

Pituitary adenoma is the commonest tumour to cause mass effect in this region. Evaluation of pituitary hormone status is desirable, before surgery, but a concern about a patient's vision is of

prime importance. Patients should have an assessment as to whether they have a hormone secreting tumour (such as a prolactinoma) and should be treated empirically with steroid hormone replacement over the peri-operative period. It must be remembered that a tumour may cause an elevation of serum prolactin by the stalk effect.

Visual field testing will show the extent of any visual field deficit, most commonly hemianopia. This can be correlated with the MRI appearances of a pituitary adenoma which is largely hyperintense on T1 scanning, relatively homogeneous and if sufficiently large to cause a visual field defect will extend above the boundaries of the sella.

Formal pituitary function testing can be performed in the post-operative period, when evaluation of posterior pituitary function can be undertaken (if needs be), particularly if there is evidence of polyuria and possibly hypernatraemia peri-operatively.

Suggested Reading

Dersu I, Wiggins MN, Luther A, Harper R, Chacko J. Understanding visual fields, part I; Goldmann perimetry. J Ophthalmol Med Technol. 2006;2:1–10.

Fernandez-Balsells MM, Murad MH, Barwise A, Gallegos-Orozco JF, Paul A, Lane MA, et al. Natural history of nonfunctioning pituitary adenomas and incidentalomas: a systemic review and metaanalysis. J Clin Endocrinol Metab. 2011;96(4): 905–12.

Fraser CL, Biousse V, Newman NJ. Visual outcomes after treatment of pituitary adenomas. Neurosurg Clin N Am. 2012;23(4):607–19. doi:10.1016/j.nec.2012.06.004.

Kreitschmann-Andermahr I, Siegelt S, Carneiro RW, Maubach JM, Harbeck B, Brabant G. Headache and pituitary disease: a systemic review. Clin Endocrinol (Oxf). 2013;79:760–9.

Powell M, Lightman SL, Laws ER. Management of pituitary tumors: the clinician's practical guide. 2nd ed. Totowa: Humana Press; 2003.

Case 10

Deepak Chandrajay and Julian H. Barth

Abstract

The delicate balance of water homeostasis and osmolality of body fluids in man is regulated by antidiuretic hormone (ADH) secreted from the posterior pituitary. Inadequate secretion or inappropriate peripheral action of ADH leads to diabetes insipidus (DI). Patients present with polyuria and polydipsia. Biochemically they have hyperosmolar plasma and hypoosmolar urine. The water deprivation test is an established test to differentiate between cranial and renal DI. Psychological conditions such as primary polydipsia have to be considered while evaluating patients with polyuria and polydipsia. Metabolic conditions such as diabetes mellitus and electrolyte abnormalities such as hypokalaemia and hypercalcaemia can cause similar symptoms. Synthetic ADH still remains the treatment of choice for cranial DI. Drugs are the most common cause of renal DI. In renal DI, the primary aim should be to treat the underlying abnormality such as correction of electrolyte abnormalities or withdrawal of offending drugs.

Keywords

Polyuria • Polydipsia • Diabetes insipidus • Antidiuretic hormone • Water deprivation test • Desmopressin

D. Chandrajay, MBBS, MRCP, FRCPath (✉)
Metabolic Medicine and Chemical Pathology,
Leeds Teaching Hospitals NHS Trust,
Great George Street, Leeds,
West Yorkshire LS1 3EX, UK
e-mail: drdeepakcj@doctors.org.uk

J.H. Barth, FRCP, FRCPath, MD
Chemical Pathology/Metabolic Medicine,
Department of Blood Sciences,
Leeds Teaching Hospitals NHS Trust,
Leeds, West Yorkshire, UK

Case

Thirty year old man underwent trans-sphenoidal surgery for cystic pituitary adenoma. Three weeks post operation he developed increasing thirst and was drinking 4–5 l of fluid in 24 h. He was waking up four to five times at night to pass urine. He had no history of visual disturbances, headache, loss of libido or weight loss. His medications included hydrocortisone and levetiracetam.

R. Ajjan, S.M. Orme (eds.), *Endocrinology and Diabetes: Case Studies, Questions and Commentaries*,
DOI 10.1007/978-1-4471-2789-5_10, © Springer-Verlag London 2015

Table 10.1 Biochemical results for the patient

	Serum/ plasma	Spot urine	24-h urine
Osmolality (mOsmol/kg)	298	86	–
Sodium (mmol/L)	147	16	114
Potassium (mmol/L)	4.1	3	21
Urea (mmol/L)	2.5	30	215
Creatinine (µmol/L)	58	1.9	13.6
Adjusted calcium (mmol/L)	2.34	–	–
ALT (iu/L)	35	–	–
TSH (miu/L)	1.5	–	–
Glucose (mmol/L)	5.1	–	–
Urine volume (L)	–	–	7.2

Table 10.2 Water deprivation test results

Time	Urine volume (mL)	Urine osmolality (mOsm/kg)	Plasma osmolality (mOsm/kg)
0800 am	0	94	295
0900 am	430	103	299
1000 am	460	84	300
1100 am	380	113	298
1200 pm	375	117	302
1230 pm	Desmopressin ®administered 1 µg intramuscularly		
1300 pm	110	246	299
1400 pm	60	758	296

There is no family history of diabetes mellitus, hypertension or malignancy.

On examination BP 134/82 mmHg, arterial pulse rate 88/min, systemic examination was unremarkable.

What are the initial investigations for polyuria in this patient?

The presence of low urine osmolality with high plasma osmolality and hypernatraemia is suggestive of DI (Table 10.1). In primary polydipsia, patients usually have low/normal sodium with low urine osmolality. Other abnormalities such as hyperglycaemia, hypercalcaemia and hypokalaemia can lead to DI.

How would you exclude adrenal insufficiency in this patient?

Glucagon stimulation test. A 9 am cortisol of 402 nmol/L which peaked to 650 nmol/L at 150 min during an intra-muscular glucagon stimulation test, confirms adequate cortisol reserve. Subsequently, oral hydrocortisone was stopped. Cortisol deficiency reduces glomerular filtration and may lead to reduced water excretion hence, DI may be masked. A short Synacthen® test should not be used within 2 weeks of pituitary

surgery as it may give a false positive result because the adrenal glands have not had a chance to atrophy.

How would you make the diagnosis of DI?

Water deprivation test. Water restriction in the normal individual results in secretion of ADH by the posterior pituitary in order to reclaim water from the distal renal tubules. Failure of this mechanism results in a rise in plasma osmolality due to water loss, and the production of a dilute urine with low osmolality. Response to administration of synthetic ADH, Desmopressin®, helps differentiate cranial DI from nephrogenic DI.

During water deprivation the patient did not conserve water and passed dilute urine. After administration of Desmopressin®, the urine osmolality increased to 758 mOsm/kg, confirming a diagnosis of cranial DI. A normal person will reduce their urine volume to less than 50 mL after 4 h of fluid restriction (unpublished data) and the urine osmolality approaches 750–1,000 mOsm/Kg. See Table 10.2.

How do you treat the patient?

Patients with intact thirst mechanism are able to compensate for the fluid loss. However, inadequate thirst mechanism can lead to severe dehydration and hypernatremia. Hence, monitoring of fluid balance is essential. Desmopressin® 100 µg tablets once a day (perhaps given at night in the first instance) and titrated depending on the response. Intranasal and parenteral preparations are also available. The duration of action after oral administration ranges from 6 to 12 h. The response is seen as a decrease in urine output within 1–2 h.

Review of Diabetes Insipidus

Water constitutes approximately 50–60 % of total body weight in human adults. It is distributed between the extracellular and intracellular compartments.

There is a two part system regulating water and salt homeostasis. Antidiuretic hormone (ADH) is mainly involved in the regulation of water homeostasis and osmolality of body fluids. ADH is primarily under osmoregulation but is also stimulated by hypovolaemia or hypotension. The renin-angiotensin-aldosterone system (RAAS) is a more sensitive mechanism to restore changes in blood pressure and total body volume [1]. Other natriuretic peptides such as atrial natriuretic peptide and brain natriuretic peptide have been identified in water overload.

ADH also known as vasopressin, arginine vasopressin (AVP) is synthesised in the hypothalamus and stored in the posterior pituitary as a prohormone. It is released as an active hormone in response to changes sensed by central and peripheral osmoreceptors [2, 3]. The osmolality of extracellular fluid is maintained between 285 and 295 mOsm/kg of water in normal subjects through close interaction between the osmoreceptors and the hypothalamus. In the kidneys, ADH acts on the collecting duct and increases the permeability of water through aquaporin channels [4] in the apical plasma membrane of the principal cells. This results in increased water retention but since no ions are reabsorbed, the reduced urine volume has an increased osmolality. In response to high plasma osmolality the hypothalamus also stimulates the thirst mechanism to induce water consumption.

In diabetes insipidus (DI) patients are unable to secrete ADH and thereby conserve water and consequently produce large volume of dilute, tasteless (*insipid*) urine. Patients will experience extreme thirst and drink copious amount of water to maintain their water homeostasis. In diabetes mellitus, which is one of the most common causes of polyuria and polydipsia, the urine is sweet and hypertonic. DI is caused by two different mechanisms:

1. Cranial DI – Inadequate synthesis of ADH in the hypothalamus or release from pituitary
2. Renal DI – Inadequate renal response to ADH.

In cranial DI there is lack of ADH in the plasma, whereas in renal DI the ADH concentration in both plasma and urine is high.

Central DI

Central DI is caused by inadequate synthesis, storage or release of ADH. Disease affecting hypothalamus and/or pituitary can result in this condition. An intact thirst mechanism keeps the patient hydrated and their serum sodium concentration within the reference interval. During a water deprivation test there is no improvement in urine osmolality on dehydration, however, after the administration of Desmopressin® there is a marked increase in urine osmolality. Imaging of the brain is important to look for a lesion of the pituitary or the hypothalamus. The common pathological diseases in the brain causing central DI are listed in Table 10.3. More than half of the patients undergoing pituitary surgery develop transient DI within 24 h post-surgery and resolve spontaneously [5].

Treatment- Desmopressin®, a synthetic analogue, remains the treatment of choice [6, 7]. It is available as tablets (60,100 and 200 μg) or nasal spray (10 μg per meter spray). The duration of action is 6–12 h and a decrease in urine output can be noted within 1–2 h of administration of the drug. There is marked variation in the pharmacokinetics of desmopressin, hence, it is recommended to establish a customised regimen for each individual [8, 9].

Other agents such as thiazides and chlorpropamide are useful when there is some residual ADH secretion. The action of chlorpropamide

Table 10.3 Causes of DI

Cranial DI	Nephrogenic DI
Idiopathic	Drug induced
Tumour	Lithium
Craniophayringioma	Carbamazepine
Meningioma	Foscarent
Germinoma	Clozapine
Metastatic disease	Orlistat
Breast	Loop diuretics
Lung	Electrolyte disorders
Colon	Hypokalaemia
Kidney	Hypercalcaemia
Melanoma	Renal disorders
Lymphoma and Leukaemia	Polycystic kidney
Trauma	Renal infarct
Head injury	CKD
Post pituitary surgery	RTA
Infection	Post obstructive
Encephalitis	uropathy
Meningitis	Genetic
Tuberculosis	V2 ADH receptor
Infiltrative disease	mutation
Histiocytosis	Aquaporin 2
Sarcoidosis	receptor gene
Lymphocytic hypophysitis	mutation
Pregnancy	**Other causes**
Transient DI due to placental	Diabetes mellitus
vasopressinase	Diuretic abuse
Genetic	Psychogenic
DIDMOAD syndrome	polydipsia
Mutation of arginine	Hypothyroidism
vasopressin-neurophysin	Hypoadrenalism
II gene	

[10] is through increasing the sensitivity of the epithelial cells of collecting ducts to smaller concentrations of ADH. Thiazide diuretics inhibit the NaCl co-transporter in the renal distal convoluted tubule and sodium loss leading to contraction of extracellular volume and low glomerular filtration and subsequent increased proximal tubular sodium and water reabsorption [11, 12]. Hence, less water and solutes are delivered to the distal tubule and collecting duct.

Nephrogenic DI

Impaired response of the renal tubules to the effect of ADH leads to production of large volume of dilute urine. There is stimulation of posterior pituitary by plasma hyperosmolality causing continued release of ADH. The loop of Henley in the renal nephron creates a hyperosmolar state in the renal medulla. ADH acts on the principal cells of the collecting duct and increases permeability of water establishing equilibrium between urine and hyperosmolar medullary interstitium. This process reduces water content in urine and increases urinary osmolality.

Electrolyte imbalances such as hypercalcaemia or hypokalaemia cause down regulation of aquaporins [7, 13]. Structural diseases of the kidney such as polycystic kidneys, renal infarcts, or renal calcification distort the medullary architecture, thus interfering in establishing permeability of water. Medications like lithium causes reduction in the aquaporin levels [12, 14].

Treatment- Maintenance of adequate water intake, correction of electrolyte imbalance and preventing further exposure to medications and toxins causing nephrogenic DI is considered as a priority. Thiazides have shown to partially recover the aquaporin channel lost by lithium therapy [15]. Amiloride inhibits lithium reabsorption by blocking sodium channel in the collecting ducts [12]. Prostaglandin inhibitor, Indomethacin also improves the hydro-osmotic effect of ADH [16] and hence co-administration with a thiazide improves the effect.

> What are the main differential diagnoses of polydipsia?

Hypercalcaemia and diabetes mellitus are relatively easy to diagnose. Psychogenic (or primary) polydipsia can represent a diagnostic challenge in some cases.

Psychogenic or primary polydipsia is more commonly seen in patients with psychiatric disorders. Anxiety, stress, compulsive behaviour, dry mouth due to the use of anti-cholinergic agents [17] and cigarette smoking [18] may be contributory factors. Patients present with water intoxication and hyponatraemia. Any structural lesion to hypothalamus may induce polydipsia and hence it is essential to differentiate it from DI.

The biochemistry shows low plasma osmolality with low urine osmolality. Treatment includes water restriction, behavioural therapy and pharmacotherapy. Propranolol [19] and angiotensin converting enzyme inhibition [20] have been used

Table 10.4 Biochemical changes in DI

High or high normal plasma sodium concentration

Inability to concentrate urine in water deprivation test

Administration of synthetic vasopressin analogue improves urine concentrating ability by the kidney in cranial DI

In nephrogenic DI, there is no increase in urine osmolality after vasopressin administration.

Increase in plasma ADH with an increase in plasma osmolality excludes cranial DI.

Increase in urine osmolality with increasing concentration of plasma ADH excludes nephrogenic DI.

AVP is unstable in plasma [21] and can give rise to falsely low or high result depending on sample handling [22, 23].

if there were suggestions of activation of renin angiotensin system.

If there is acute-onset hyponatraemia with clinic symptoms, saline infusion with regular monitoring is required.

> What is solute diuresis?

In certain pathological conditions, presence of osmotically active substance in the renal tubules, filtered through the glomeruli, lead to incomplete reabsorption of fluid leading to excessive urine volume. Glycosuria in uncontrolled diabetes mellitus is a common cause. Excessive urea excretion in catabolic state or on high protein nutrition supplementation may also lead to solute diuresis. Treatment with intravenous mannitol or sodium chloride may also cause diuresis. The urine osmolality is usually more than 300 mOsm/kg in solute diuresis.

> What are the main laboratory tests for polyuria and polydipsia?

Urine Osmolality

DI is present if urine osmolality is low (below 200 mOsm/kg of water) in a patient with symptoms of polyuria and polydipsia. It is recommended to proceed to water deprivation test to differentiate between cranial and renal DI. See Table 10.4.

Water Deprivation Test

Indication

For the diagnosis of suspected cranial or nephrogenic diabetes insipidus and primary polydipsia.

Contraindications

Diabetes mellitus, hypoadrenalism, hypercalcaemia, hypokalaemia, hypothyroidism, urinary infections, chronic renal failure and therapy with carbamazepine, chlorpropamide or lithium therapy. If there is evidence for the ability to concentrate urine, e.g., spot urine osmolality >750 mOsm/kg.

Caution

Patients with true DI may become severely water depleted during water deprivation and should be carefully monitored throughout the procedure.

Preparation

Patients should not fast and can have access to food and drink till the beginning of the test.

Procedure

At 0800 am weigh the patient and begin fluid restriction. Ask the patient to empty bladder and measure the urine output and specific gravity. Take blood sample for sodium, potassium, calcium, glucose, urea and plasma osmolality.

At 0900 am, weigh the patient and measure urine output and urine osmolality.

At 1000 am, weigh the patient and measure urine output and urine osmolality.

At 1100 am, weigh the patient and measure urine output and urine osmolality. Blood test for plasma osmolality and sodium.

At 1200 pm, weigh the patient and measure urine output and urine osmolality.

At 1300 pm, weigh the patient and measure urine output and urine osmolality.

At 1400 pm, weigh the patient and measure urine output and urine osmolality. Blood test for plasma osmolality and sodium

At 1500 pm, weigh the patient and measure urine output and urine osmolality.

At 1600 pm, weigh the patient and measure urine output and urine osmolality. Blood test for plasma osmolality and sodium.

Table 10.5 Guide to interpretation of water deprivation test

Post-dehydration osmolality (mOsm/kg)		Post DDAVP osmolality (mOsm/kg)	
Plasma	Urine	Urine	Diagnosis
283–293	>750	>750	Normal
>293	<300	<300	Nephrogenic diabetes insipidus
>293	<300	>750	Cranial diabetes insipidus
<293	300–750	<750	Chronic polydipsia
<293	300–750	<750	Partial nephrogenic DI or primary polydipsia
>293	300–750	>750	Partial cranial DI

Fluid restriction should be stopped if plasma osmolality >300 mOsm/kg or there is a fall in weight >5 %.

Proceed to Desmopressin® administration if urine osmolality rises <30 mOsm/kg (in toto) over three successive urine samples. The test should be terminated if urine osmolality rises >750 mOsm/kg.

Table 10.5 presents a guide to interpretation of the water deprivation test.

References

1. Thrasher T. Baroreceptor regulation of vasopressin and renin secretion: low-pressure versus high-pressure receptors. Front Neuroendocrinol. 1994;15(2):157–96.
2. Bourque CW. Central mechanisms of osmosensation and systemic osmoregulation. Nat Rev Neurosci. 2008;9:519–31. doi:10.1038/nrn2400.
3. Lechner SG, Markworth S, Poole K, Smith ES, Lapatsina L, Frahm S, et al. The molecular and cellular identity of peripheral osmoreceptors. Neuron. 2011;69:332–44. doi:10.1016/j.neuron.2010.12.028.
4. Brown D. The ins and outs of aquaporin-2 trafficking. Am J Physiol Renal Physiol. 2003;284(5):893–901.
5. Verbalis J, Robinson A, Moses M. Postoperative and post traumatic diabetes insipidus. In: Czernichow P, Robinson A, editors. Diabetes insipidus in man. Basel: Karger; 1985. p. 247–67.
6. Robertson G. Diabetes insipidus. Endocrinol Metab Clin North Am. 1995;24(3):549–72.
7. Robinson A, Verbalis J. Diabetes insipidus. Curr Ther Endocrinol Metab. 1997;6:1–7.
8. Richardson D, Robinson A. Desmopressin. Ann Intern Med. 1985;103(2):228–39.
9. Lam K, Wat M, Choi K, Pang RWC, Ip TP, Kumana CR. Pharmacokinetics, pharmacodynamics, long-term efficacy and safety of oral 1-deamino-8-d-arginine vasopressin in adult patients with central diabetes insipidus. Br J Clin Pharmacol. 1996;42(3):379–85.
10. Pokracki F, Robinson A, Seif S. Chlorpropamide effect: measurement of neurophysin and vasopressin in humans and rats. Metabolism. 1981;30(1):72–8.
11. Knoers NV, Deen PM. Molecular and cellular defects in nephrogenic diabetes insipidus. Pediatr Nephrol. 2001;16:1146–52.
12. Nguyen MK, Nielsen S, Kurtz I. Molecular pathogenesis of nephrogenic diabetes insipidus. Clin Exp Nephrol. 2003;7(1):9–17.
13. Nielson S, Frokiaer J, Marples D, Kwon TH, Agre P, Knepper MA. Aquaporins in the kidney: from molecules to medicine. Physiol Rev. 2002;82(1): 205–44.
14. Marples D, Frokiaer J, Knepper M, Nielsen S. Disordered water channel expression and distribution in acquired nephrogenic diabetes insipidus. Proc Assoc Am Physicians. 1998;110(5):401–6.
15. Kim G-H, Lee JW, Oh YK, Chang HR, Joo KW, Na KY, et al. Antidiuretic effect of hydrochlorothiazide in lithium-induced nephrogenic diabetes insipidus is associated with up regulation of aquaporin-2, Na-Cl cotransporter and epithelial sodium channel. J Am Soc Nephrol. 2004;15:2836–43.
16. Hochberg Z, Even L, Danon A. Amelioration of polyuria in nephrogenic diabetes insipidus due to aquaporin-2 deficiency. Clin Endocrinol (Oxf). 1998;49(1):39–44.
17. Kruse D, Pantelis C, Rudd R, Quek J, Herbert P, McKinley M. Treatment of psychogenic polydipsia: comparison of risperidone and olanzapine, and the effects of an adjunctive angiotensin-II receptor blocking drug (irbesartan). Aust N Z J Psychiatry. 2001;35(1):65–8.
18. Sklar AH, Schrier RW. Central nervous system mediators of vasopressin release. Physiol Rev. 1983;63(4):1243–80.
19. Kishy T, Kurosawa H, Endo S. Is propranolol effective in primary polydipsia? Int J Psychiatry Med. 1998;28:315–25.
20. Sebastian CS, Bernardin AS. Comparison of enalapril and captopril in the management of self-induced water intoxication. Biol Psychiatry. 1990;27(7):787–90.
21. Robertson GL, Mahr EA, Athar S, Sinha T. Development and clinical application of a new method for the radioimmunoassay of arginine vasopressin in human plasma. J Clin Invest. 1973;52:2340–52.
22. Preibisz JJ, Sealey JE, Laragh JH, Cody RJ, Weksler BB. Plasma and platelet vasopressin in essential hypertension and congestive heart failure. Hypertension. 1983;5(2 Part 2):I129–38.
23. Kluge M, Riedl S, Erhart-Hofmann B, Hartmann J, Waldhauser F. Improved extraction procedure and RIA for determination of arginine8-vasopressin in plasma: role of premeasurement sample treatment and reference values in children. Clin Chem. 1999;45: 98–103.

Hypertension in the Young Adult

Case 11

Klaus K. Witte and Haqeel A. Jamil

Abstract

Hypertension is the most common cardiovascular condition to be seen in primary care. It also represents the strongest single modifiable risk factor with regards to future morbidity and mortality. The incidence of hypertension is predicted to continue to increase, being contributed to by an ageing population.

The major consequence of this largely asymptomatic condition is the development of cardiovascular sequelae. The aim of early diagnosis is to provide an opportunity to intervene in order to prevent or delay the onset of overt vascular disease. The positive effects of treatment have been proven in numerous randomised placebo-controlled trials. However since hypertension is usually asymptomatic and treatment is aimed at prevention of complications, targeting patients at highest risk while avoiding 'medicalisation' and causing side effects in people at low risk is challenging. This is especially the case in young people for whom a diagnosis of hypertension entails life-long treatment, based upon studies performed in older people. Using a clinical example we will review some of those challenges and how to deal with them in this chapter.

Keywords

Hypertension • Young adult • Blood pressure • Essential hypertension • Primary hypertension • Secondary hypertension

Case: The Tense Technician

A Caucasian patient in his early-30s attended his primary care physician for the fourth time in 6 months. John had initially presented with coryzal symptoms, which had since resolved but had left him feeling tired, with a non-specific headache that was affecting his concentration at work. He was anxious that this could represent something

K.K. Witte, MD, FRCP (✉)
H.A. Jamil, MBChB, MRCP
Division of Cardiovascular and Diabetes Research,
University of Leeds, LIGHT laboratories,
Clarendon Way, Leeds LS16 5AR, UK
e-mail: k.k.witte@leeds.ac.uk

R. Ajjan, S.M. Orme (eds.), *Endocrinology and Diabetes: Case Studies, Questions and Commentaries*,
DOI 10.1007/978-1-4471-2789-5_11, © Springer-Verlag London 2015

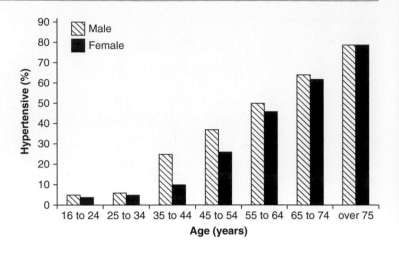

Fig. 11.1 NHS National Statistics (2010) data showing the increasing incidence of hypertension with age (Reproduced with permission from National Statistics [3]. Copyright © 2011, Re-used with the permission of the Health and Social Care Information Centre. All rights reserved)

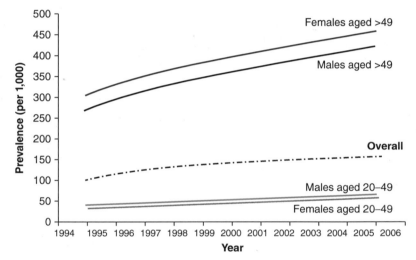

Fig. 11.2 Prevalence of hypertension by gender and age (Data adapted from the Canadian Hypertension Education Program 10-year population study [4])

serious, but the only worrying feature so far was a slightly raised blood pressure.

Why is hypertension important?

Hypertension is the leading contributor to global mortality [1, 2]. The increase in worldwide childhood and adult obesity, along with an ageing and increasingly sedentary population means that the incidence and prevalence is likely to continue to grow (Figs. 11.1 and 11.2) [3–5].

It is also the most significant reversible cause for cardiovascular disease with numerous studies proving that the control of hypertension can lower the risk of cardiovascular events and mortality [6]. Screening and effective control of raised blood pressure has public health benefits and is cost-effective [7], and is therefore endorsed by the British National Institute for Health and Clinical Excellence (NICE) [8]. Both the guidelines and the data are limited to patients within certain age groups and it is unclear whether the benefits of treatment extend to the young [9], in whom prevalence is estimated to be between 5 and 20 % for those aged between 24 and 32 [10]. However, it is generally assumed that earlier treatment is associated with greater benefits in terms of longevity and life free from disease [2, 11].

Hypertension is often classed as "primary" or "secondary," with the latter being due to some specific identifiable additional condition (see below). On the other hand the pathogenesis of primary hypertension is often multifactorial,

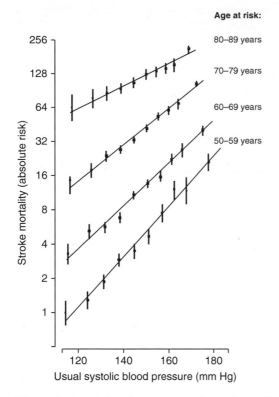
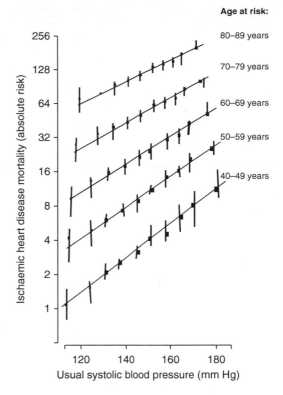

Fig. 11.3 Association between mortality and systolic blood pressure separated by age (Data adapted with permission from a meta-analysis of individual data for one million adults. Adapted from Lewington et al. [17], Copyright 2002, with permission from Elsevier)

although the diagnosis and complications are known to be associated with several risk factors such as race, family history, diabetes mellitus, obesity, inactive lifestyle, high sodium intake and excessive alcohol consumption [8, 12, 13]. Psychosocial factors and depressive illnesses may increase the risk of chronically raised blood pressure [14, 15]. Recent evidence also links severe vitamin D deficiency with the subsequent development of hypertension [16].

Although it is usually asymptomatic in its early stages, untreated chronic hypertension contributes to the early development of cardiovascular disease, renal impairment and disability, regardless of the aetiology. There is a 7 % incremental risk of mortality from ischaemic heart disease (and 10 % from stroke) for every 2 mmHg step in systolic blood pressure [17].

Epidemiological studies suggest that a 10 mmHg lower systolic blood pressure (or 5 mmHg lower diastolic blood pressure) is associated with a 50 % reduction in the risk of death from coronary artery disease or stroke (Fig. 11.3) [17]. Hypertension therefore is an important condition to recognise and address even in young adults and both lifestyle modification and antihypertensive therapies to achieve blood pressure reduction are a priority to reduce risk. However, treatment goals should be individualised to take patient characteristics and co-morbidities into account. Recently, there has been limited evidence to suggest that excessive lowering of the diastolic blood pressure to below 70 mmHg in the high-risk elderly population with co-existing severe coronary artery disease or diabetes, may be associated with an increase in cardiovascular complications [6, 18–20].

John's general practitioner (GP) arranged for him to have a series of blood tests (full blood count, urea/electrolytes, glucose, thyroid function

Fig. 11.4 Blood pressure definitions. National Institute for Health and Clinical Excellence (2011) (Adapted from NICE guidance [8]. Available from http://guidance.nice. org.uk/CG127 Reproduced with permission)

	Clinic blood pressure		ABPM / home blood pressure
Normotensive	Less than 140/90	or	Less than 135/85
Hypertension stage 1	≥140/90	and	≥135/85
Hypertension stage 2	≥160/90	and	≥150/95
Severe hypertension	≥180/110	–	–

tests and estimated glomerular filtration rate), urinalysis and electrocardiogram. She also arranged for 24-h blood pressure monitoring in order to confirm the diagnosis.

How should a clinician proceed?

The use of ambulatory blood pressure monitoring (ABPM) is currently recommended by the NICE guidelines in order to confirm the diagnosis, when there are persistently elevated clinic blood pressure (BP) readings (between 140/90 and 180/110 mmHg) and an absence of end-organ damage (Fig. 11.4) [8]. Where ABPM is not available, home BP monitoring should be used since this shows a stronger correlation to daytime ABPM measurements than clinic BP readings [21, 22]. If clinic BP is the only available test, then this should be measured on at least three to six visits spanning a period of 3 months [23].

The following ABPM cut-offs have been recommended by both the seventh Joint National Committee and the European Societies of Hypertension and Cardiology guidelines to diagnose hypertension [24, 25]:
• 24-h average above 135/85 mmHg
• Daytime average above 140/90 mmHg
• Night-time average above 125/75 mmHg
ABPM can also be used to monitor treatment response, and to clarify the diagnosis of [26]:
• "White-coat" syndrome
• Episodic hypertension (if suspecting a phaeochromocytoma)
• Hypotensive symptoms with anti-hypertensive medications
• Resistant hypertension
Systolic blood pressure readings over 180 or diastolic blood pressure readings over 110 mmHg

suggest severe hypertension. In the presence of hypertensive ophthalmic changes such as retinal haemorrhage, papilloedema or exudates, or symptoms indicative of phaeochromocytoma, such as headaches, palpitations, sweating and labile blood pressure [27], this is termed "malignant" or accelerated hypertension and requires urgent treatment (within 24 h). On the other hand, in asymptomatic patients with no evidence of acute end-organ damage, the short-term risk of severe hypertension is low and there is no proven benefit of rapid in-patient blood pressure reduction [28, 29].

Based on the ABPM results (overall average blood pressure 138/87; daytime average 142/94), John was given a diagnosis of hypertension. Initial examination, blood tests and urinalysis were normal, suggesting no end-organ damage had yet occurred, but given John's young age, his GP performed a more focussed cardiovascular examination and requested some further blood tests to identify whether this could be secondary hypertension (serum calcium, parathyroid hormone, serum lipid profile, aldosterone:renin ratio).

Determining the Cause: What to Look for and What Tests to Do

The main focus of examination is to assess for end-organ damage although a full examination also helps identify potential causes for the hypertension [30]. In most asymptomatic adults, essential hypertension remains the predominant cause for chronic high blood pressure even in the young, with secondary causes only found in less than 10 % of young adults (Fig. 11.5) [31–33]. Extensive testing in those with no risk factors or

Fig. 11.5 Prevalence of essential (primary) hypertension (*hashed columns*) and relative frequency of secondary hypertension within hypertensive cohort stratified by age (*solid columns*), using data from [28–30]

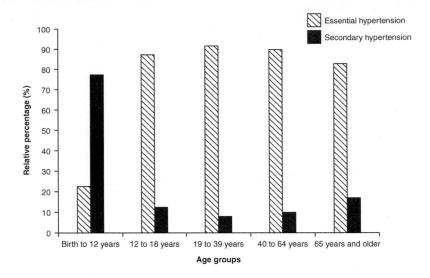

additional features is therefore not indicated or cost effective.

Essential Tests

In the majority of patients without symptoms suggestive of secondary causes, only a limited evaluation is routinely required:

- Confirm near-equal blood pressure in left and right arms (difference of >20 mmHg in systolic blood pressure is significant)
- Fundoscopy to assess for any hypertensive retinal changes
- Blood tests: full blood counts, urea/electrolytes, glucose, thyroid function tests, parathyroid hormone, serum calcium level, serum lipid profile, estimated glomerular filtration rate
- Urinalysis
- Electrocardiogram (Fig. 11.6)

The presence of any of the following general features would justify a work-up for secondary causes of hypertension (Table 11.1 and Fig. 11.7):

- Rapid onset of severe or malignant hypertension (diastolic BP >120 mmHg +/− acute end organ damage)
- Persistently raised blood pressures (diastolic >90 mmHg) despite treatment with three or more antihypertensive agents (inclusive of diuretic use)
- Age of onset before puberty

- Confirmed hypertension at an age less than 30 years with no risk factors (i.e., non-black, no family history, normal BMI, normal plasma cholesterol levels) [34]

No abnormalities were discovered with further testing and a diagnosis of essential hypertension was made. John's GP explained this diagnosis and the potential consequences to John. She then proceeded to discuss risk factors, along with reassurance that dietary and life-style modifications can be sufficient to treat mild hypertension. They also discussed the influence his stressful job may be having on his blood pressure, although the doctor reassured him that work is often indirectly related via lifestyle issues. This led on to a discussion about the adverse effects of smoking, obesity and a sedentary routine. John had recently read a newspaper article about a cure for hypertension called renal denervation and wondered if he might be eligible for this.

> What are the principles with regards to treatment?

The initial treatment approach in mild to moderate uncomplicated essential hypertension is lifestyle modification [8, 35]. The key features of this are increasing daily physical activity levels, with the aim of achieving and maintaining a BMI

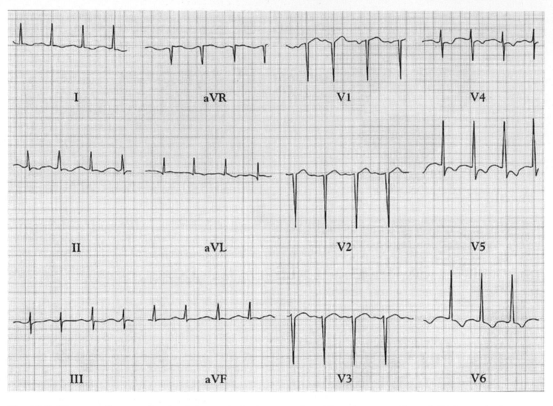

Fig. 11.6 Electrocardiogram showing left ventricular hypertrophy with strain pattern (lateral ST depression)

Table 11.1 Clinical features and diagnostic tests for common secondary causes for hypertension

Secondary causes	Clinical clues	Tests
Primary hyperaldosteronism [52, 53]	Most common (5–10 % of all hypertensive patients)	Classically, unexplained hypokalaemia with urinary potassium wasting (but most have normal potassium levels)
	Headaches, muscle weakness, cramps	
	Causes: Idiopathic or Conn's adenoma	Raised plasma aldosterone to renin ratio (anti-hypertensive therapy does not need to be discontinued prior to testing)
Fibromuscular dysplasia (causing renal artery stenosis) [54]	Most common in young females	Acute serum creatinine increase (>30 % of baseline) with angiotensin-converting enzyme inhibitor or angiotensin II receptor blocker)
	Unknown aetiology	
	Holosystolic renal artery bruit (see below)	Presence of unilateral small kidney or unexplained renal size asymmetry (more than 1.5 cm)
Renovascular disease (causing renal artery stenosis [55, 56]	Occurs in 1 % of all hypertensive patients	
	Moderate to severe hypertension onset in patients over the age of 55	Computed tomography angiography
	Known history of diffuse atherosclerosis	Magnetic resonance imaging with gadolinium contrast media
	Recurrent episodes of flash pulmonary oedema	Doppler ultrasonography of renal arteries (if CT and MRI contraindicated)
	Abdominal bruit (can occur in systole and diastole – low sensitivity)	Renal artery angiography (not first line, but considered the gold standard)
Primary renal disease	Raised pre-treatment serum creatinine	Urinalysis abnormalities
		Renal ultrasonography

Table 11.1 (continued)

Secondary causes	Clinical clues	Tests
Coarctation of the aorta [57]	Delayed or diminished femoral pulses	Upper limb hypertension with reduced lower limb blood pressures (systolic difference >20 mmHg)
	Unequal left and right brachial pulses	Unequal left and right blood pressures
	Usually a systolic murmur in the left infraclavicular area and under the left scapula (can be non-specific)	Magnetic resonance imagining
Thyroid disorders [58]	Signs and symptoms of hypo/hyper-thyroidism	Serum thyroid-stimulating hormone
Primary hyperparathyroidism [59]	Signs and symptoms of hypercalcaemia	Parathyroid hormone and serum calcium levels
Phaeochromocytoma [27, 60]	Rare (0.1–0.6 % of hypertensive patients)	ABPM Plasma free metanephrines (99 % sensitivity)
	Paroxysmal hypertensive episodes with headaches, sweating and palpitations	24-h urinary fractionated metanephrines
Oral contraceptives	Temporary hypertension related to usage	Trial off contraceptive medication
Sleep apnoea syndrome [61]	Mainly affects obese males with a history of snoring, day time somnolence and fatigue	Epworth Sleep Apnoea score and overnight pulse oximetry Polysomnography
Cushing's syndrome [62, 63]	Cushingoid appearance with proximal muscle weakness and central obesity	24-h urinary cortisol
	Can be iatrogenic	Overnight or low-dose dexamethasone suppression

<25. Weight loss lowers systolic blood pressure by 5–20 mmHg per 10 kg lost [36]. Dietary changes with particular attention given to increasing proportionate consumption of fruits, vegetable and low-fat dairy products, and reducing dietary sodium intake to less than 100 mmol/day, can also lead to a 10 mmHg reduction in the systolic blood pressure [37, 38]. Limiting daily alcohol consumption is also an important intervention to ensure good blood pressure control [13]. Vitamin D supplementation could be considered in those with severely reduced 25-hydroxyvitamin D levels, especially patients of South Asian origin who are especially susceptible to vitamin D deficiency [16]. This has been shown to reverse the renin-angiotensin activation that is associated with low vitamin D levels, and can thus improve blood pressure control [39].

At this early point, counselling is essential to ensure long term compliance with lifestyle and medical therapy. It is important to explain that lifestyle modifications are important even if the BP remains elevated. Equally, patients are often reassured to find that if medical therapy is required, a combination of two treatments is not a marker of "difficult hypertension" or "failed" treatments but rather a way to achieve optimal results with fewer side effects.

Lifestyle changes alone can be adequate to treat mild hypertension and lower overall cardiovascular risk but persistently raised blood pressures or evidence of any end-organ damage warrants pharmacological therapy (Fig. 11.8). The reduction in cardiovascular risk is directly related to the magnitude of blood pressure reduction regardless of the agent used, with the goal being to reduce the daytime blood pressure to below 140/90 mmHg (with lower targets in those with concurrent diabetes) (Fig. 11.9) [8, 40].

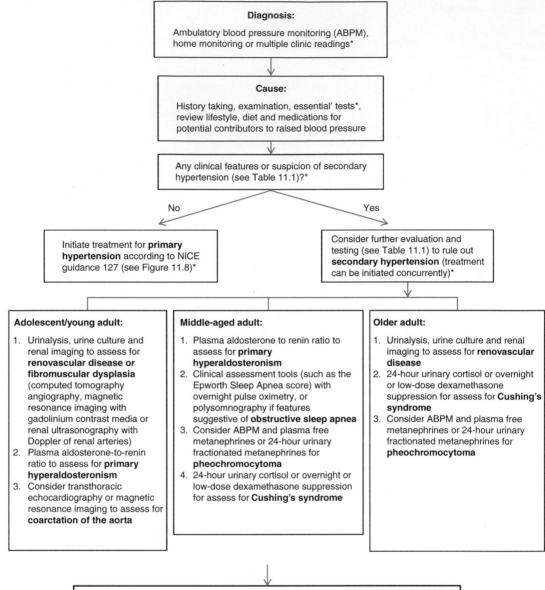

Fig. 11.7 Diagnostic algorithm for the evaluation of primary and secondary hypertension. National Institute for Health and Clinical Excellence (2011) (Adapted from 'CG 127 [8]. Available from http://guidance.nice.org.uk/CG127 Reproduced with permission)

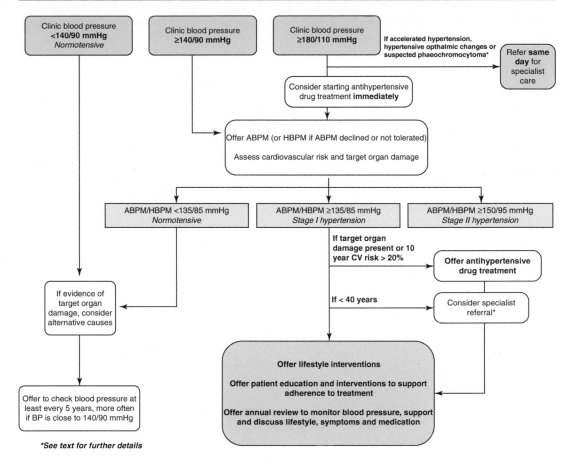

Fig. 11.8 Updated algorithm for the diagnosis of primary hypertension. ABPM, ambulatory blood pressure monitoring; HBPM, home blood pressure monitoring. National Institute for Health and Clinical Excellence (2011) (Adapted from NICE guidelines [8]. Available from http://guidance.nice.org.uk/CG127 Reproduced with permission)

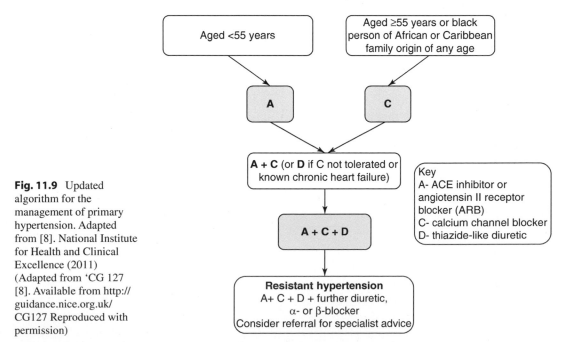

Fig. 11.9 Updated algorithm for the management of primary hypertension. Adapted from [8]. National Institute for Health and Clinical Excellence (2011) (Adapted from 'CG 127 [8]. Available from http://guidance.nice.org.uk/CG127 Reproduced with permission)

Three months later, John attended for a review with Dr Byrom. He had successfully stopped smoking, had lost several kilograms of weight and was now exercising regularly. She re-examined him for any signs of end-organ damage (fundoscopy and urinalysis) and also repeated the ABPM. The results of this showed that John had been successful in controlling his blood pressure, and his 24-h average blood pressure was 130/82. John now attends every year for a blood pressure review with the practice nurse, and is delighted to have avoided long-term pharmacological therapy.

Specialist Insight

What is the strategy for resistant cases?

Failure of the blood pressure to respond to treatment despite the use of three or more anti-hypertensive agents (inclusive of a diuretic) is known as resistant hypertension (as defined by the American Heart Association 2008 guidelines) [41]. Resistant hypertension is commonly due to:
- Suboptimal therapy
- Extracellular volume expansion (due to chronic kidney disease or a high-sodium diet) [42]
- Poor compliance with medical or dietary therapy
- Secondary hypertension (see Table 11.1 and Fig. 11.7)
- "White coat" hypertension [43]
- Ingestion of substances that can elevate the blood pressure (see below)

Patients with resistant hypertension are more likely to have an underlying cause for their hypertension, and are also at a much higher risk of developing cardiovascular complications and end-organ damage [44]. The strategy with such patients should include the following:
- Re-evaluation for potential secondary causes of hypertension
- Assessing for and treating end-organ damage: premature cardiovascular disease, hypertensive

retinopathy, left ventricular hypertrophy, heart failure (either with normal or reduced ejection fraction), chronic kidney disease, transient ischaemic attack or stroke [45, 46].
- Consider stopping any medications or agents that are known to increase the blood pressure such as: non-steroidal anti-inflammatory agents, selective COX-2 inhibitors, decongestants, oral contraceptives (especially oestrogen), herbal remedies (such as ginseng, ephedra), amphetamines, prednisolone, sympathomimetic diet pills, psychiatric medications (including antidepressants), liquorice, cocaine, alcohol [49].
- ABPM (see above) to rule out co-existent 'white coat' hypertension.
- Referral to a hypertension specialist service if the blood pressure remains elevated for over 6 months despite the above measures and three or more anti-hypertensive agents.

What is renal denervation?

Renal denervation is a novel therapy that may be an option for resistant hypertension. It is a percutaneous procedure that involves trans-luminal radiofrequency sympathetic denervation of the renal artery. Early case series and a randomised controlled trial demonstrated safe and significant blood pressure reductions of around 25/11 mmHg [47, 48]. However, the recent and only randomised, *blinded* placebo controlled study of renal denervation for hypertension (Symplicity HTN-3) failed to show any significant additional blood pressure lowering at 6 months [49]. This trial has fortunately tempered the previously unfettered enthusiasm for this intervention.

Blood pressure control is merely a surrogate for morbidity or mortality. New treatments, for hypertension, especially irreversible device-based therapies, must not just demonstrate better blood pressure control but also improved efficacy in lowering stroke or heart attack rates over current treatments before being accepted as routine. At present renal denervation is not routinely commissioned by the National Health Service (NHS) in England, ands trials with hard endpoints are currently ongoing [50, 51].

References

1. Ezzati M, Lopez AD, Rodgers A, Vander Hoorn S, Murray CJ, Comparative Risk Assessment Collaborating Group. Selected major risk factors and global and regional burden of death. Lancet. 2002;360(9343):1347–60.
2. Taylor BC, Wilt TJ, Welch HG. Impact of diastolic and systolic blood pressure on mortality: implications for the definition of "normal". J Gen Intern Med. 2011;26:685.
3. National Statistics. Health Service for England 2010—trend tables. NHS Information Centre. 2011. Available at http://www.ic.nhs.uk/statistics-and-data-collections/health-and-lifestyles-related-surveys/health-survey-for-england/health-survey-for-england–2010-trend-tables. Accessed 1 Dec 2013.
4. Tu K, Chen Z, Lipscombe LL, for the Canadian Hypertension Education Program Outcomes Research Taskforce. Prevalence and incidence of hypertension from 1995 to 2005: a population-based study. CMAJ. 2008;178(11):1429–35.
5. Kotchen TA. Obesity-related hypertension: epidemiology, pathophysiology, and clinical management. Am J Hypertens. 2010;23(11):1170–8.
6. Williams B. Hypertension and "J-curve". J Am Coll Cardiol. 2009;54:1835–6.
7. Krause T, Lovibond K, Caulfield M, McCormack T, Williams B. Management of hypertension: summary of NICE guidance. BMJ. 2011;343:d4891.
8. National Clinical Guideline Centre (NCGC). Hypertension: the clinical management of primary hypertension in adults., Clinical guideline 127. Methods, evidence and recommendations. Commissioned by the National Institute for Health and Clinical Excellence. London: NCGC; 2011.
9. Tirosh A, Afek A, Rudich A, Percik R, Gordon B, Ayalon N, et al. Progression of normotensive adolescents to hypertensive adults: a study of 26,980 teenagers. Hypertension. 2010;56:203–9.
10. Nguyen QC, Tabor JW, Entzel PP, Lau Y, Suchindran C, Hussey J, et al. Discordance in national estimates of hypertension among young adults. Epidemiology. 2011;22(4):532–41.
11. Gaziano TA, Bitton A, Anand S, Weinstein MC, International Society of Hypertension. The global cost of nonoptimal blood pressure. J Hypertens. 2009;27:1472–7.
12. Greenland P, Knoll MD, Stamler J, Naeton JD, Dyer AR, Garsdie DB, et al. Major risk factors as antecedents of fatal and nonfatal coronary heart disease events. JAMA. 2003;290:891.
13. Xin X, He J, Frontini MG, Ogden LG, Motsamai OI, Whelton PK. Effects of alcohol reduction on blood pressure: a meta-analysis of randomized controlled trials. Hypertension. 2001;38:1112.
14. Meng L, Chen D, Yang Y, Zheng Y, Hui R. Depression increases the risk of hypertension incidence: a meta-analysis of prospective cohort studies. J Hypertens. 2012;30:842.
15. Yan LL, Liu K, Matthews KA, Daviglus ML, Freeman T, Kiefe C. Psychosocial factors and risk of hypertension: the Coronary Artery Risk Development in Young Adults (CARDIA) study. JAMA. 2003;290:2138.
16. Burgaz A, Orsini N, Larsson SC, Wolk A. Blood 25-hydroxyvitamin D concentration and hypertension: a meta-analysis. J Hypertens. 2011;29:636.
17. Lewington S, Clarke R, Qizilbash N, Peto R, Collins R, Prospective Studies Collaboration. Age-specific relevance of usual blood pressure to vascular mortality: a meta-analysis of individual data for one million adults in 61 prospective studies. Lancet. 2002;360 (1903):1913. Erratum in Lancet 2003 Mar 22;361 (9362):1060.
18. Chrysant SG. Current status of aggressive blood pressure control. World J Cardiol. 2011;3(3):65–71.
19. Cushman WC, Evans GW, Byington RP, Goff Jr DC, Grimm Jr RH, Cutler JA, et al. Effects of intensive blood-pressure control in type 2 diabetes mellitus. N Engl J Med. 2010;362:1575–85.
20. Moreno G, Mangione CM. Management of cardiovascular disease risk factors in older adults with type 2 diabetes mellitus: 2002–2012 literature review. J Am Geriatr Soc. 2013;61(11):2027–37.
21. Uhlig K, Patel K, Ip S, Kitsios GD, Balk EM. Self-measured blood pressure monitoring in the management of hypertension: a systematic review and meta-analysis. Ann Intern Med. 2013;159:185.
22. Parati G, Stergiou GS, Asmar R, Bilo G, de Leeuw P, Imai Y, et al. European Society of Hypertension practice guidelines for home blood pressure monitoring. J Hum Hypertens. 2010;24:779.
23. O'Brien E, Asmar R, Beilin L, Imai Y, Mancia G, Mengden T, et al. Practice guidelines of the European Society of Hypertension for clinic, ambulatory and self blood pressure measurement. J Hypertens. 2005;23:697.
24. Chobanian AV, Bakris GL, Black HR, Cushman WC, Green LA, Izzo Jr JL, et al. The Seventh Report of the Joint National Committee on Prevention, Detection, Evaluation, and Treatment of High Blood Pressure: the JNC 7 report. JAMA. 2003;289:2560.
25. Mancia G, Fagard R, Narkiewicz K, Redón J, Zanchetti A, Böhm M, et al. ESH/ESC Guidelines for the management of arterial hypertension: the Task Force for the management of arterial hypertension of the European Society of Hypertension (ESH) and of the European Society of Cardiology (ESC). J Hypertens. 2013;31(7):1281–357.
26. de la Sierra A, Segura J, Banegas JR, Gorostidi M, de la Cruz JJ, Armario P, et al. Clinical features of 8295 patients with resistant hypertension classified on the basis of ambulatory blood pressure monitoring. Hypertension. 2011;57:898.
27. Zuber SM, Kantorovich V, Pacak K. Hypertension in pheochromocytoma: characteristics and treatment. Endocrinol Metab Clin North Am. 2011;40(2):295–311.
28. Ahmed ME, Walker JM, Beevers DG, Beevers M. Lack of difference between malignant and accelerated hypertension. Br Med J (Clin Res Ed). 1986; 292:235.

29. Shantsila A, Shantsila E, Lip GY. Malignant hypertension: a rare problem or is it underdiagnosed? Curr Vasc Pharmacol. 2010;8(6):775–9.
30. Severe symptomless hypertension. Lancet. 1989;9(2):1369–70.
31. Yoon EY, Cohn L, Freed G, Rocchini A, Kershaw D, Ascione F, et al. Use of antihypertensive medications and diagnostic tests among privately insured adolescents and young adults with primary versus secondary hypertension. J Adolesc Health. 2014; pii:S1054-139X(13)00800-8.
32. Rimoldi SF, Scherrer U, Messerli FH. Secondary arterial hypertension: when, who, and how to screen? Eur Heart J. 2013. doi:10.1093/eurheartj/eht534.
33. Omura M, Saito J, Yamaguchi K, Kakuta Y, Nishikawa T. Prospective study on the prevalence of secondary hypertension among hypertensive patients visiting a general outpatient clinic in Japan. Hypertens Res. 2004;27(3):193–202.
34. Lurbe E, Torro I, Alvarez V, Nawrot T, Paya R, Redon J, et al. Prevalence, persistence, and clinical significance of masked hypertension in youth. Hypertension. 2005;45:493.
35. Rossi GP, Bernini G, Caliumi C, Desideri G, Fabris B, Ferri C, et al. A prospective study of the prevalence of primary aldosteronism in 1,125 hypertensive patients. J Am Coll Cardiol. 2006;48:2293–300.
36. Mosso L, Carvajal C, Gonzalez A, Barraza A, Avila F, Montero J, et al. Primary aldosteronism and hypertensive disease. Hypertension. 2003;42(2):161–5.
37. Novick AC, Zaki S, Goldfarb D, Hodge EE. Epidemiologic and clinical comparison of renal artery stenosis in black patients and white patients. J Vasc Surg. 1994;20:1.
38. Garovic VD, Textor SC. Renovascular hypertension and ischemic nephropathy. Circulation. 2005;112:1362–74.
39. Textor SC, Lerman L. Renovascular hypertension and ischemic nephropathy. Am J Hypertens. 2010;23:1159.
40. Betensky BP, Jaeger JR, Woo EY. Unequal blood pressures: a manifestation of subclavian steal. Am J Med. 2011;124:e1.
41. Streeten DH, Anderson Jr GH, Howland T, Chiang R, Smulyan H. Effects of thyroid function on blood pressure. Recognition of hypothyroid hypertension. Hypertension. 1988;11:78.
42. Kanbay M, Isik B, Akcay A, Ozkara A, Karakurt F, Turgut F, et al. Relation between serum calcium, phosphate, parathyroid hormone and 'nondipper' circadian blood pressure variability profile in patients with normal renal function. Am J Nephrol. 2007;27:516.
43. Eisenhofer G, Lenders JW, Goldstein DS, Mannelli M, Csako G, Walther MM, et al. Pheochromocytoma catecholamine phenotypes and prediction of tumor size and location by use of plasma free metanephrines. Clin Chem. 2005;51:735–44.
44. Somers VK, White DP, Amin R, Abraham WT, Costa F, Culebras A, et al. Sleep apnea and cardiovascular disease: an American Heart Association/American College of Cardiology Foundation Scientific Statement from the American Heart Association Council for High Blood Pressure Research Professional Education Committee, Council on Clinical Cardiology, Stroke Council, and Council on Cardiovascular Nursing. J Am Coll Cardiol. 2008;52:686.
45. Saruta T, Suzuki H, Handa M, Igarashi Y, Kondo K, Senba S. Multiple factors contribute to the pathogenesis of hypertension in Cushing's syndrome. J Clin Endocrinol Metab. 1986;62:275.
46. Mancini T, Kola B, Mantero F, Boscaro M, Arnaldi G. High cardiovascular risk in patients with Cushing's syndrome according to 1999 WHO/ISH guidelines. Clin Endocrinol (Oxf). 2004;61:768.
47. Elmer PJ, Obarzanek E, Vollmer WM, Simons-Morton D, Stevens VJ, Young DR, et al. Effects of comprehensive lifestyle modification on diet, weight, physical fitness, and blood pressure control: 18-month results of a randomized trial. Ann Intern Med. 2006;144:485.
48. Carnethon MR, Evans NS, Church TS, Lewis CE, Schreiner PJ, Jacobs Jr DR. Joint associations of physical activity and aerobic fitness on the development of incident hypertension: coronary artery risk development in young adults. Hypertension. 2010;56:49.
49. Sacks FM, Svetkey LP, Vollmer WM, Appel LJ, Bray GA, Harsha D, et al.; DASH-Sodium Collaborative Research Group. Effects on blood pressure of reduced dietary sodium and the Dietary Approaches to Stop Hypertension (DASH) diet. DASH-Sodium Collaborative Research Group. N Engl J Med. 2001;344(1):3–10.
50. Forman JP, Stampfer MJ, Curhan GC. Diet and lifestyle risk factors associated with incident hypertension in women. JAMA. 2009;302:401.
51. Schroten NF, Ruifrok WP, Kleijn L, Dokter MM, Silljé HH, Lambers Heerspink HJ, et al. Short-term vitamin D3 supplementation lowers plasma renin activity in patients with stable chronic heart failure: an open-label, blinded end point, randomized prospective trial (VitD-CHF trial). Am Heart J. 2013;166(2):357–64.
52. Blood Pressure Lowering Treatment Trialists' Collaboration, Turnbull F, Neal B, Ninomiya T, Algert C, Arima H, et al. Effects of different regimens to lower blood pressure on major cardiovascular events in older and younger adults: meta-analysis of randomised trials. BMJ. 2008;336:112.
53. Calhoun DA, Jones D, Textor S, Goff DC, Murphy TP, Toto RD, et al. Resistant hypertension: diagnosis, evaluation, and treatment: a scientific statement from the American Heart Association Professional

Education Committee of the Council for High Blood Pressure Research. Circulation. 2008;117:e510.

54. Pimenta E, Gaddam KK, Oparil S, Aban I, Husain S, Dell'Italia LJ, et al. Effects of dietary sodium restriction on blood pressure in subjects with resistant hypertension: results from a randomized trial. Hypertension. 2009;54:444–6.

55. Verdecchia P, Reboldi GP, Angeli F, Schillaci G, Schwartz JE, Pickering TG, et al. Short- and long-term incidence of stroke in white-coat hypertension. Hypertension. 2005;45:203.

56. Faselis C, Doumas M, Papademetriou V. Common secondary causes of resistant hypertension and rational for treatment. Int J Hypertens. 2011;2011:236239.

57. Sipahi I, Tuzcu EM, Schoenhagen P, Wolski KE, Nicholls SJ, Balog C, et al. Effects of normal, prehypertensive, and hypertensive blood pressure levels on progression of coronary atherosclerosis. J Am Coll Cardiol. 2006;48:833.

58. Asayama K, Ohkubo T, Kikuya M, Metoki H, Hoshi H, Hashimoto J, et al. Prediction of stroke by self-measurement of blood pressure at home versus casual screening blood pressure measurement in relation to the Joint National Committee 7 classification: the Ohasama study. Stroke. 2004;35:2356.

59. Symplicity HTN-1 Investigators. Catheter-based renal sympathetic denervation for resistant hypertension: durability of blood pressure reduction out to 24 months. Hypertension. 2011;57(5):911–7.

60. Symplicity HTN-2 Investigators. Renal sympathetic denervation in patients with treatment-resistant hypertension (The Symplicity HTN-2 Trial): a randomised controlled trial. Lancet. 2010;376:1903–9.

61. Medtronic announces US renal denervation pivotal trial fails to meet primary efficacy endpoint while meeting primary safety end point [press release]. 9 Jan 2014.

62. Sapoval M; Assistance Publique – Hôpitaux de Paris. Renal Denervation in Hypertension (DENER-HTN). In: ClinicalTrials.gov[Internet]. Bethesda: National Library of Medicine (US). 2000-[cited 22 Feb 2014]. Available from: http://clinicaltrials.gov/show/NCT01570777; NLM Identifier NCT01570777.

63. Schlaich M, Baker IDI Heart and Diabetes Institute. Renal Denervation for Resistant Hypertension (RDNP-2012-01). In: ClinicalTrials.gov[Internet]. Bethesda: National Library of Medicine (US). 2000-[cited 10 Mar 2014]. Available from: http://clinicaltrials.gov/show/NCT01865240; NLM Identifier NCT01865240

Weight Loss and Dizziness: Adrenal Failure

Case 12

Wycliffe Mbagaya and Stephen M. Orme

Abstract

The adrenal glands produce corticosteroids, mineralocorticoids and adrenal androgens. Adrenal insufficiency may be caused by primary adrenal failure or by impairment of hypothalamic-pituitary-adrenal axis. Adrenal insufficiency is life threatening when diagnosis is missed. The main symptoms include weight loss, fatigue, anorexia and dizziness. A stepwise diagnostic work up is required to identify the underlying cause of adrenal insufficiency. The treatment of adrenal insufficiency requires glucocorticoid and mineralocorticoid replacement therapy, which requires careful monitoring. The long-term management of patients with adrenal insufficiency requires experienced specialist care. All doctors should know how to diagnose and manage acute adrenal failure.

Keywords

Weight loss • Dizziness • Adrenal insufficiency • Addison's disease • Cortisol • Short corticotropin test • Adrenal crisis

Case

A 38-year-old woman with hypothyroidism presented to her doctor with severe weakness and dizziness. This has been progressive over the last 4 months, and she has been unable to take part in her weekly badminton matches. She also noticed that she had lost 6 kg in the preceding 3 months despite having a good appetite. She noticed that she had general lack of energy and struggled to complete tasks at work. She had nausea but no diarrhoea or vomiting. She had no history of fever or joint pains. She did not have any history suggestive of anorexia or malabsorption.

She has a past medical history of hypothyroidism that was well controlled with levothyroxine 75 μg daily.

Her sister has type 1 diabetes and hypothyroidism while her mother was also hypothyroid.

W. Mbagaya, MBChB, MRCP (UK), FRCPath (✉)
Laboratory Medicine, Leeds Teachings Hospitals NHS Trust, Beckett Street, Leeds, West Yorkshire LS9 7TF, UK
e-mail: mbagaya@doctors.net.uk

S.M. Orme, MBChB, MD, FRCP
Department of Endocrinology, St. James's Hospital, Leeds, West Yorkshire, UK

R. Ajjan, S.M. Orme (eds.), *Endocrinology and Diabetes: Case Studies, Questions and Commentaries*,
DOI 10.1007/978-1-4471-2789-5_12, © Springer-Verlag London 2015

Her blood pressure was 110/75 mmHg lying and 86/55 mmHg standing with a regular resting pulse of 120 per minute. She weighed 51 kg with a body mass index of 18.1 kg/m^2.

> **What other information would you want to know about this patient?**

In this case, it is important to rule out other causes of weight loss such anorexia and malabsorption due to any bowel disease. Other causes of dizziness such as cardiac disease should also be excluded. Even though this patient has been on thyroxine replacement, it is important to establish her current thyroid status.

> **What signs should you look for?**

On examination, she was thin with dry skin; she had increased pigmentation that was pronounced over her palmar creases, knuckles, previous scars and oral mucosa. Examination of her body hair distribution revealed sparse pubic and axillary hair.

Table 12.1 presents the clinical features and Table 12.2, the causes of adrenal sufficiency.

> **What other tests would you consider in this patient?**

In view of the presence of generalised malaise, weight loss, postural hypotension with hyperpigmentation, adrenal insufficiency should be on part of the differential diagnosis. A short corticotropin test should be carried out to confirm this; 250 micrograms (μg) of ACTH should be given to this patient with base line and 30 min cortisol levels measured. A baseline serum ACTH levels should also be measured at the start of the corticotropin test, this will help exclude secondary adrenal insufficiency. There is considerable variability between cortisol results of different assays, thus cortisol results should be interpreted using locally derived cut-off values.

Table 12.1 Clinical features of adrenal insufficiency

Features due to glucocorticoid insufficiency
Weakness
Malaise
Weight loss
Nausea and vomiting
Hypoglycaemia
Myalgia
Anaemia
Features due to mineralocorticoid insufficiency
Hypotension
Dehydration
Hyponatraemia
Features due to reduced adrenal androgens
Decreased body hair
Decrease libido, especially in females
Dry itchy skin
Features due to increased ACTH (adrenocorticotrophic hormone) secretion
Increased pigmentation over sun exposed areas, knuckles, palmar creases
Increased pigmentation of mucous membranes such as oral mucosa.

Table 12.2 Causes of adrenal sufficiency

Autoimmune destruction of the adrenal glands
Polyglandular deficiency type I
Polyglandular deficiency type II
Sporadic autoimmune destruction of the adrenals
Infective adrenalitis
Tuberculosis
HIV
Intra-adrenal haemorrhage
Metastatic cancer to the adrenals
Infiltrative disease
Haemochromatosis
Amyloidosis
Sarcoidosis

Antibodies to 21-hydroxylase enzyme may be present in patients with Addison's disease.

Plasma renin activity and aldosterone should be measured. In patients with Addison's disease, plasma renin activity will be high while the plasma aldosterone will be low.

Imaging of the adrenal glands using CT scan or MRI scan may be helpful in determining the cause of adrenal insufficiency. This may identify any infiltration, calcification and haemorrhage.

Table 12.3 Biochemical results for the patient

	Serum/plasma	Spot urine
Sodium (mmol/L)	128	46
Potassium (mmol/L)	4.8	11
Urea (mmol/L)	7.2	
Creatinine (μmol/L)	126	
TSH (miu/L)	1.1	
T4 (pmol/L)	17.6	
Osmolality (mOsmol/kg)	278	390
Glucose (mmol/L)	4.3	
Adjusted Calcium (mmol/L)	2.55	
9 am Cortisol (nmol/L)	136	
FSH iu/L	13.1	
LH iu/L	9	
Haemoglobin (g/L)	100	
MCV (fl)	84	
Platelet count ($\times 10^{12}$)	327	
RBC count ($\times 10^{9}$)	6.8	

The low baseline cortisol, suboptimal 30-min cortisol value, high ACTH, high urine sodium and hyponatraemia confirm the diagnosis as Addison's disease.

Biochemical results for the patient are presented in Table 12.3.

> How would you treat this patient?

Acute adrenal insufficiency is a life threatening condition and patients should be treatment immediately without any delays in getting a definitive diagnosis. Intravenous hydrocortisone 100 mg every 6 h should be given. Blood samples for electrolytes, cortisol and ACTH should be taken before administering hydrocortisone. Intramuscular hydrocortisone may be used if intravenous access is not available. Shocked patients will need fluid and electrolyte replacement while those with hypoglycaemia will also need dextrose. Stable patients may be given oral hydrocortisone.

Patients with primary adrenal failure will also require mineralocorticoid replacement given as fludrocortisone 0.05–0.1 mg/day. Patients with adrenal insufficiency should be aware that their corticosteroid and mineralocorticoid replacement will continue for life.

Adrenal crises occur due to glucocorticoid dose reduction or lack of dose adjustment in times of stress. In order to avoid an adrenal crisis, patients with adrenal failure should be advised to increase their steroid requirements during stress, intercurrent illness and pregnancy.

Background

The adrenal glands are important endocrine organs that produce glucorcorticoids, mineralocorticoids and androgens. The adrenal gland is composed of an outer cortex and an inner medulla. The outer cortex is divided in three parts: the outer zona glomerulosa, the mid zona fasciculata and an inner zona reticularis [1]. Mineralocorticoids which are produced by the outer zona glomerulosa are predominantly involved in sodium and potassium balance. Glucocorticoids, which are produced by the fasciculate, are predominantly involved in carbohydrate metabolism but also have some effect in salt and electrolyte balance. The zona reticularis produces adrenal androgens which are metabolised peripherally to testosterone and dihydrotestosterone [2]. The adrenal gland is under hypothalamic-pituitary control to produce glucocorticoids and the renin angiotensin system to produce mineralocorticoids.

Addison's disease is a disorder of the adrenal glands that causes decreased production of adrenal hormones. This was named after Thomas Addison who was the first physician to make a connection between adrenal disease and the clinical signs and symptoms of adrenal failure. This may be as a result of a destructive process such as autoimmune disease, infiltrative disease such as tuberculosis, haemochromatosis, sarcoidosis or amyloidosis [3, 4]. Adrenal insufficiency occurs when more than 90 % of the adrenal cortex is destroyed resulting in minimal adrenal hormone production. Patients with pituitary or hypothalamic disease with decreased ACTH production develop secondary adrenal insufficiency.

Addison's disease has a prevalence of about 140 per million in developed countries with a female preponderance [5]. Autoimmune disease is the most common cause of Addison's in the developed world while tuberculosis the most common cause in developing countries. Other causes of Addison's disease include drugs such as ketoconazole and metyrapone, adrenal infarction secondary to haemorrhage and conditions that interfere with adrenal hormone synthesis [6].

Patients with Addison's disease may present with weight loss, fatigue, dizziness, exhaustion and anorexia. These symptoms are as a result of reduced corticosteroid and mineralocorticoid production. The clinical signs and symptoms of Addison's disease usually develop gradually. The non-specific nature of these symptoms means that they are likely to be ignored, missed or attributed to other conditions. Mineralocorticoid deficiency may result in urinary sodium loss, hyponatraemia with mild hyperkalaemia and intravascular volume depletion that causes postural hypotension. Addison's disease patients have increased pigmentation over sun-exposed areas, friction areas, creases and the mucous membranes [7]. The increased pigmentation is postulated to be a consequence of the increased ACTH, which has melanocyte stimulating hormone like sequences that cause hyperpigmentation. A small proportion of patients will develop salt craving. Female patients may have loss of libido as well as loss of pubic and axillary hair. This is attributed to the loss of production of adrenal androgens. Some patients may have other autoimmune diseases such as coeliac disease, hypothyroidism or vitiligo [7].

Some patients with adrenal insufficiency may have an initial presentation with an adrenal crisis. These patients will present with persistent vomiting, profound muscle weakness, shock, acute abdominal pain, extreme sleepiness and hypoglycaemia or even coma. This may be precipitated by stressful conditions such as surgery, intercurrent illness, hyperthyroidism and treatment with enzyme inducing agents (such as rifampicin) or commencement of thyroid hormone replacement; both of which increase cortisol metabolism.

Laboratory Investigations

The aim of diagnosis in adrenal insufficiency include demonstration of low cortisol secretion, to differentiate primary and secondary adrenal insufficiency as well establish the cause of the insufficiency [6, 7].

Patients with Addison's disease may present with hyponatraemia with slight increase in serum potassium levels. Some patients may have raised calcium as well. Urine sodium will reveal excessive renal sodium loss. These electrolyte changes demonstrate reduced mineralocorticoid activity.

Cortisol and ACTH concentrations, which have a diurnal variation, change throughout the day due to their coupled pulsatile release. This makes random cortisol and ACTH samples to be of limited value in the diagnosis of adrenal disease. However, early morning cortisol of <80 nmol/L may strongly suggests adrenal insufficiency while values greater than 415 nmol/L predict a normal response to the corticotropin or insulin induced hypoglycaemia [8–10]. The short corticotropin test is a safe and reliable test with high predictive value in the diagnosis of adrenal insufficiency. There is considerable variability in the cortisol values measured by different cortisol assays, thus locally derived cut-off values should be used. Most healthy individuals will have a cortisol level of greater than 500 nmol/L 30 min after 250 µg of ACTH [11]. The short corticotropin test can be performed at any time of the day due to its reproducibility at different times [12]. The standard short corticotropin test should not be undertaken 4–6 weeks after pituitary or hypothalamic insult as the adrenal gland may still respond to ACTH leading to a false normal result [11, 13]. Similarly, patients with early adrenal disease may have an adequate cortisol response to ACTH. Cortisol results may be affected by certain conditions such as oral contraceptive use that increase cortisol binding globulin and liver cirrhosis, which reduces cortisol binding globulin. These conditions should be considered when interpreting cortisol results in these patient groups.

Measurement of serum ACTH can help distinguish between primary adrenal insufficiency and secondary adrenal insufficiency [9]. Serum ACTH levels of < 22 pmol/L at baseline of the short corticotropin test excludes Addison's disease [14, 15]. Patients with Addison's disease will have increased ACTH production while secondary adrenal insufficiency patients will have an inappropriately low ACTH for the low cortisol.

When secondary adrenal insufficiency is suspected, the insulin tolerance test, which tests the entire hypothalamic-pituitary-adrenal axis, is the gold standard [16]. Insulin produces hypoglycaemia that results in the release of anterior pituitary hormones including ACTH and growth hormone. This test is associated with many side effects and should be avoided in patients with ischaemic heart disease and epilepsy.

In patients with inappropriately low ACTH in the presence of cortisol deficiency, a complete endocrine pituitary profile as well as pituitary MRI should be arranged. This may identify pituitary adenomas, cranipharyngiomas and granulomatous pituitary disease.

Patients with autoimmune adrenal failure may have autoantibodies to the adrenal cortex or 21-hydroxylase enzyme. Patients with suspected autoimmune adrenal failure should also be screened for premature ovarian failure and thyroid disease.

Plasma renin activity and aldosterone levels should be measured in patients with adrenal insufficiency. This may show increased plasma renin activity with reduced plasma aldosterone.

Adrenal CT scan or MRI may identify infiltrating adrenal disease such as haemochromatosis, amyloidosis, TB adrenalitis, adrenal metastasis and adrenal lymphoma.

Male patients with adrenal failure without other autoimmune diseases should have measurement of plasma very long fatty acids to exclude adrenoleukodystrosphy.

Table 12.4 is a summary of the investigations in adrenal insufficiency.

Table 12.4 Summary of investigations in adrenal insufficiency

	Primary adrenal insufficiency	Secondary adrenal insufficiency
↓↓Cortisol	↓↓	↓
30 min cortisol after corticotropin	↓↓	↓
ACTH	↓↓	↑ or →
Plasma renin	↓↓	→
Aldosterone	↓↓	→
DHEA	↓↓	↓

Treatment

Addison's disease is potentially life-threatening and treatment should commence immediately the diagnosis is confirmed. In patients with suspected adrenal crisis, immediate treatment should be started even without a definitive laboratory diagnosis. In these patients, rapid intravenous fluid and electrolyte replacement as well as intravenous hydrocortisone 100 mg every 6 h should be administered. One litre of normal saline should be given rapidly followed by 2–4 l over 24 h. The patient's blood pressure, fluid status and electrolytes should be monitored closely. Patients without intravenous access should be given intramuscular injection and central intravenous access sought. Oral hydrocortisone may be administered once the patient is able to take orally [17, 18]. It is important to treat any associated condition that may have precipitated the adrenal crisis.

In patients with chronic adrenal insufficiency, lifelong corticosteroid treatment is given, with short acting steroids such as hydrocortisone as treatment of choice. Hydrocortisone 15–20 mg in divided doses should be administered daily. Cortisol levels peak after an oral dose, followed by a rapid decline to less than 100 nmol/L in 5–7 h. The current oral corticosteroid administration is unable to mimic the pattern of normal cortisol secretion. Diurnal variability in glucocorticoid sensitivity has been found in the past. Similarly, unfavourable metabolic response to evening hydrocortisone administration has been demonstrated while high glucocorticoid levels disrupt sleep. Late-evening hydrocortisone administration should therefore be avoided. The patient's current medication should be considered when deciding the hydrocortisone dose. Patients taking drugs known to induce CYP3A4 hence cortisol inactivation, such as phenobarbital, rifampicin, phenytoin will require increased glucocorticoid dose. Conversely, patients taking drugs that inhibit CYP3A4 such as antiretrovirals would require a reduction in their dose.

There is no reliable biomarker to monitor glucocorticoid replacement, thus monitoring is dependent on clinical grounds. These include monitoring weight, checking for signs of overreplacement and underreplacemnt. Glucocorticoid overreplacement may lead to osteoporosis, impaired glucose tolerance and obesity while underreplacemnt increases risk of adrenal crisis. Some experts however recommend use of hormone cortisol day profiles as a measure of adequacy of treatment.

Glucocorticoid dose should be increased during periods of stress such as intercurrent illness, major surgery, trauma and pregnancy [17, 18]. Addison's disease patients with hyperthyroidism should receive higher hydrocortisone doses as hyperthyroidism increases cortisol clearance. Patients with hypothyroidism should start thyroxine replacement after hypoadrenalism has been excluded or adequately treated. Patients with primary adrenal insufficiency will also require mineralocorticoid replacement, normally as fludrocortisone 100 µg as a single dose daily. There is a good interindividual variability in the mineralocorticoid requirements of Addison's patients. Patients with Addison's disease will require a 50 % increase in fludrocortisone dose in summer and tropical climate due to increased salt loss through perspiration. The adequacy of the fludrocortisone dose can be assessed by blood pressure monitoring; presence of peripheral oedema, presence of hypernatraemia and plasma renin activity.

Addison's disease patients should be informed of the risk of adrenal crisis and how to avoid this. Many crises are due to glucocorticoid dose reduction and lack of glucocorticoid dose adjustment in stress. All patients should have knowledge of the sick day rules; this should also be extended to family members and partners. All patients should have a bracelet or steroid emergency card and instructions on dose adjustments during stress. It is advisable that the glucocorticoid dose is doubled during respiratory infections until recovery or parenteral hydrocortisone for gastrointestinal infections. Patients with limited access to acute medical services should receive a hydrocortisone self-injection kit.

References

1. Miller WL, Auchus RJ. The molecular biology, biochemistry, and physiology of human steroidogenesis and its disorders. Endocr Rev. 2011;32:81–151.
2. Charmandari E, Tsigos C, Chrousos G. Endocrinology of the stress response. Annu Rev Physiol. 2005;67:259–84.
3. Erichsen MM, Løvås K, Skinningsrud B, Wolff AB, Undlien DE, Svartberg J, et al. Clinical, immunological, and genetic features of autoimmune primary adrenal insufficiency: observations from a Norwegian registry. J Clin Endocrinol Metab. 2009;94:4882–90.
4. Mason AS, Meade TW, Lee JA, Morris JN. Epidemiological and clinical picture of Addison's disease. Lancet. 1968;2:744–7.
5. Lovas K, Husebye ES. High prevalence and increasing incidence of Addison's disease in western Norway. Clin Endocrinol (Oxf). 2002;56:787–91.
6. Bornstein SR. Predisposing factors for adrenal insufficiency. N Engl J Med. 2009;360:2328–39.
7. Neary N, Nieman L. Adrenal insufficiency: etiology, diagnosis and treatment. Curr Opin Endocrinol Diabetes Obes. 2010;17:217–23.
8. Hägg E, Asplund K, Lithner F. Value of basal plasma cortisol assays in the assessment of pituitary-adrenal insufficiency. Clin Endocrinol (Oxf). 1987;26:221–6.
9. Le Roux CW, Meeran K, Alaghband-Zadeh J. Is a 0900-h serum cortisol useful prior to a short synacthen test in outpatient assessment? Ann Clin Biochem. 2002;39:148–50.
10. Schmidt IL, Lahner H, Mann K, Petersenn S. Diagnosis of adrenal insufficiency: evaluation of the corticotropin-releasing hormone test and Basal serum cortisol in comparison to the insulin tolerance test in patients with hypothalamic-pituitary-adrenal disease. J Clin Endocrinol Metab. 2003;88:4193–8.
11. Arlt W. The approach to the adult with newly diagnosed adrenal insufficiency. J Clin Endocrinol Metab. 2009;94:1059–67.
12. Azziz R, Bradley Jr E, Huth J, Boots LR, Parker Jr CR, Zacur HA. Acute adrenocorticotrophin (1-24) (ACTH)adrenal stimulation in eumenorrheic women: reproducibility and effect of ACTH dose, subject

weight, and sampling time. J Clin Endocrinol Metab. 1990;70:1273–9.

13. Grossman AB. Clinical Review: The diagnosis and management of central hypoadrenalism. J Clin Endocrinol Metab. 2010;95:4855–63.

14. Charmandari E, Nicolaides NC, Chrousos GP. Adrenal insufficiency. Lancet. 2014;383:2152–67.

15. Grinspoon SK, Biller BM. Clinical review 62: laboratory assessment of adrenal insufficiency. J Clin Endocrinol Metab. 1994;79:923–31.

16. Wallace I, Cunningham S, Lindsay J. The diagnosis and investigation of adrenal insufficiency in adults. Ann Clin Biochem. 2009;46:351–67.

17. Hahner S, Allolio B. Therapeutic management of adrenal insufficiency. Best Pract Res Clin Endocrinol Metab. 2009;23:167–79.

18. Quinkler M, Hahner S. What is the best long-term management strategy for patients with primary adrenal insufficiency? Clin Endocrinol (Oxf). 2012;76: 21–5.

Diagnosis and Management of Polycystic Ovary Syndrome (PCOS)

Case 13

Ioannis Kyrou, Martin O. Weickert, and Harpal Singh Randeva

Abstract

Polycystic ovary syndrome (PCOS) is the most common endocrine disorder in reproductive-age women (5–15 %). All PCOS definitions include hyperandrogenism and oligo/anovulation in the proposed diagnostic criteria. Polycystic ovary morphology on ultrasound was not part of the initial definition and is not considered necessary for diagnosis if the patient meets the other two criteria. PCOS remains a diagnosis of exclusion and other disorders which are associated with symptoms/signs of androgen excess in women must be excluded. The clinical expression of PCOS is variable with hirsutism representing the most common clinical manifestation (65–75 %). Moreover, there is a strong link between PCOS and metabolic syndrome manifestations, including obesity, insulin resistance, type 2 diabetes mellitus (T2DM), dyslipidaemia, hypertension and non-alcoholic fatty liver disease (NAFLD). PCOS women exhibit increased incidence of obesity (30–75 %) and central adiposity even within the normal BMI range (50–70 %). In the spectrum of PCOS phenotypes, presence of hyperandrogenism is associated with a more adverse cardiometabolic profile, whereas menstrual irregularity and polycystic ovary morphology are more closely linked to infertility problems. Oral contraceptives are recommended as first-line treatment for hirsutism/acne in PCOS. Lifestyle modifications for weight loss are also essential in overweight/obese PCOS women. Metformin therapy may improve metabolic and reproductive outcomes in selected PCOS women and is recommended in PCOS patients

I. Kyrou, MD, PhD • M.O. Weickert, MD, FRCP
Endocrinology and Metabolism (WISDEM),
Warwickshire Institute for the Study of Diabetes,
University Hospitals Coventry and Warwickshire
NHS Trust, Coventry, UK

Division of Metabolic and Vascular Health,
Warwick Medical School,
University of Warwick, UHCW, Coventry, UK

H.S. Randeva, MBChB, PhD, FRCP (✉)
Endocrinology and Metabolism (WISDEM),
Warwickshire Institute for the Study of Diabetes,
University Hospitals Coventry and Warwickshire
NHS Trust, Coventry, UK
e-mail: Harpal.Randeva@warwick.ac.uk

R. Ajjan, S.M. Orme (eds.), *Endocrinology and Diabetes: Case Studies, Questions and Commentaries*,
DOI 10.1007/978-1-4471-2789-5_13, © Springer-Verlag London 2015

with T2DM or impaired glucose tolerance who are failing lifestyle modification. Clomiphene citrate is mainly used for ovulation induction in anovulatory PCOS women without other infertility factors. The long-term management plan for the care of PCOS women must include regular screening and follow-up in order to prevent, diagnose and treat T2DM, cardiovascular risk factors, NAFLD, obstructive sleep apnea, eating disorders, depression/anxiety, endometrial hyperplasia/cancer and pregnancy complications.

Keywords

Polycystic ovary syndrome (PCOS) • Hyperandrogenism • Hirsutism • Anovulation • Oligomenorrhea • Amenorrhea • Infertility • Central obesity • Insulin resistance

Case: Female Patient with Hirsutism and Oligomenorrhea

A 21-year-old white Caucasian woman presents to clinic after a referral from her primary care physician due to hirsutism and oligomenorrhea. Her main complaint is excessive growth of coarse dark hair on her face and to a lesser degree on her chest, midline abdomen and thighs.

How would you proceed?

A detailed history is needed, initially establishing the severity/progression of her hirsutism and obtaining a thorough menstrual history.

She mentions that her hirsutism has been gradually worsening over the last year and that she has tried waxing and shaving, but without lasting results. Moreover, she noted facial acne recently for the first time since her teenage years. She also finds very distressing that her frontal hairline appears to be thinning in the temporal areas.

In addition, she mentions that her menstrual periods have been irregular since stopping her oral contraceptive pill more than a year ago. Since then she has been menstruating once every 2–3 months. Her last period was 2 months ago without significant premenstrual symptoms. She reports that this did not alarm her because she had irregular menses during most of her teenage years (menarche at age 13; followed by irregular

menses for the next 3 years which became regular when she was prescribed an oral contraceptive pill). A home pregnancy test which she recently did was negative. She has not noticed any nipple discharge. She got married about a year ago and at that time she stopped her oral contraceptive pill, but she admits that she is not planning to become pregnant in the near future.

What other questions would you ask?

Given that polycystic ovary syndrome (PCOS) is a common cause of menstrual irregularities, the patient should be also asked about changes in her weight and other features that can be associated with this condition.

She reports that her weight has increased by 12 kg over the past 3 years which she attributes to poor dietary habits and a sedentary lifestyle. Overall, she describes that it has been a stressful period with finishing her studies and applying for jobs. She also notes that she often tends to get tired easily and feel sleepy during the day. Furthermore, her husband has mentioned to her that she has been snoring on several occasions over the past few months.

Her past medical history is unremarkable, she has never smoked or used recreational drugs and her alcohol intake is less than 10 units/week.

Family history includes type 2 diabetes mellitus (T2DM) in both her parents and a myocardial infarction in her father aged 50 years. She further mentions that, her mother did not have menstrual problems but had a history of miscarriages and was diagnosed with gestational diabetes mellitus (GDM) when she was pregnant with her. She has no siblings.

> **What would you do next?**

The patient requires a full physical examination.

She is 169 cm tall, weighs 92 kg (body mass index [BMI]: 32.2 kg/m^2) and her waist circumference is 98 cm. Her resting blood pressure was 120/80 mmHg with regular pulse. She has dark hair and a light skin tone. Excessive growth of terminal dark hair was noted on her face, chest, midline abdomen, lower back and upper thighs, with a Ferriman-Gallwcy hirsutism score of >7 (total score calculated by assessing nine androgen-sensitive body areas [i.e., upper lip, chin, chest, arms, upper abdomen, lower abdomen, upper back, lower back and thighs] each with a score ranging from 0 [no terminal hair] to 4 [frankly virile]); however, it was not possible to obtain an accurate total score due to previous hair removal from some of these areas with cosmetic measures. Mild degree of acne vulgaris was also present on the face and upper back. There was no diffuse hair loss, but slight thinning of the hairline was noted in the temporal areas of the scalp. Breast exam was remarkable only for periareolar hair growth bilaterally without expressible galactorrhoea. Mild acanthosis nigricans was evident in her axillae bilaterally. Her thyroid was not palpable. On abdominal exam, central adiposity was noted with a few silver/white coloured, narrow (<1 cm wide) striae scattered at her lower abdomen and hips, while there were no palpable masses or hepatomegaly. The rest of the physical examination was unremarkable.

Summarise the Pertinent Symptoms/Signs

This young woman presents with clinical hyperandrogenism, oligomenorrhea and central obesity. Clinical hyperandrogenism is established in this patient by the presence of hirsutism, acne and androgenic alopecia. Insulin resistance signs are also present manifesting as acanthosis nigricans.

- Hirsutism. Hirsutism is defined as excessive growth of terminal dark hair characterised by a male distribution pattern in women (e.g., facial hair above the upper lip, on the chin, cheeks and sideburns; midline chest/abdomen/lower back hair; hair on the inner thighs [male escutcheon]). Clinicians should distinguish hirsutism from hypertrichosis in women. The latter is not caused by excess androgens, although hyperandrogenaemia may aggravate its clinical presentation. Hair growth in hypertrichosis is typically not restricted to androgen-sensitive areas, but is rather diffuse and consists mainly of vellus or lanugo-type hair (short [<0.5 cm], fine, unpigmented hair]. Hypertrichosis can be hereditary/congenital or acquired due to various medical conditions (e.g., anorexia nervosa, cancer) or medications (e.g., phenytoin, diazoxide, minoxidil). The modified Ferriman-Gallwey scoring system is often used to diagnose and quantify hirsutism (hirsutism: score >7; mild hirsutism: score 8–15; severe hirsutism: score >15). However, this scoring system has limitations (e.g., lack of normative data for ethnic populations) and does not assess the impact of hirsutism on the psychological well-being and quality of life. Furthermore, it is often not practical to utilise such scores in clinical practise because patients frequently apply cosmetic hair removal methods before an initial assessment. Regardless of scoring methods, a thorough medical history with details about the onset and progression of excessive growth of terminal hair and about any previous treatments is essential to provide diagnostic clues and guide laboratory testing in hirsute women. Clinicians should further look for other signs of hyperandrogenism (e.g., acne, seborrhoea, male pattern hair loss, virilization) and insulin resistance, such as skin tags and acanthosis nigricans. Accordingly, testing for elevated androgen levels is suggested: (1) in women with moderate or severe hirsutism and (2) in women with hirsutism of any degree when it is characterised by sudden onset and/or rapid progression, or when it is associated with any of the following: menstrual irregularity or infertility; clitoromegaly; central obesity; acanthosis nigricans.

- Oligomenorrhea. Oligomenorrhea is defined as ≤8 menstrual periods per year (or cycle length of >35 days) and typically reflects anovulatory cycles (chronic oligo-ovulation or anovulation). A thorough menstrual history must be obtained with details about menarche, menstrual cyclicity, the last menstrual period date, and previous treatments, pregnancies, abortions, miscarriages and infertility problems. Clinicians should further ask about premenstrual symptoms (e.g., fluid retention, cramps, breast swelling and tenderness) which could indicate ovulation. It is usually normal for a woman to experience menstrual irregularity and anovulatory cycles for up to 2 years after menarche and for several years before menopause. However, predictable and regular cycles should be expected during the rest of the reproductive years (normal cycle range: 25–35 days).

What are the differential diagnoses?

In the context of the above symptoms and signs, there is high clinical suspicion of PCOS in our case patient which is the most frequent cause of androgen excess in women of reproductive age (70–75 %). Common disorders that are also associated with symptoms/signs of androgen excess in reproductive-age women and should be considered in the differential diagnosis of PCOS are listed in Table 13.1. According to the current clinical practise guidelines for PCOS diagnosis by the Endocrine Society, hyperprolactinaemia, thyroid disease (particularly hypothyroidism), and nonclassic congenital adrenal hyperplasia (primarily 21-hydroxylase deficiency) must be ruled out in all women presenting with suspected PCOS.

- Hyperprolactinaemia. Measurement of early morning prolactin levels is essential to exclude hyperprolactinaemia. Clinicians should also look for symptoms/signs indicating a prolactinoma (e.g. galactorrhoea).

- Primary hypothyroidism. Measurement of thyroid-stimulating hormone (TSH) plasma levels is usually sufficient to exclude hypothyroidism.

- Nonclassic congenital adrenal hyperplasia (NC-CAH; 21-hydroxylase deficiency). Early morning plasma levels of 17-hydroxyprogesterone (17-OHP) should be measured to rule out NC-CAH due to 21-hydroxylase deficiency. NC-CAH can be detected in approximately 1.5–6.8 % of women presenting with androgen excess. Its clinical presentation may not differ from that of PCOS and heightened clinical suspicion is required in women with a positive family history or in those of high-risk ethnic group (e.g., Ashkenazi Jewish ancestry). Early morning 17-OHP levels in the range of 200–400 ng/dL are considered abnormal (this applies to the early follicular phase of a normal menstrual cycle, because 17-OHP levels increase with ovulation, and also depends on the assay). However, if the early morning 17-OHP levels are at the lower end of this range, an ACTH stimulation test should be used for diagnosis (stimulated increase to 17-OHP levels of >1,000 ng/dL 60 min after the intravenous injection of ACTH).

- Androgen-secreting tumours. Androgen-secreting tumours are present in about 0.2 % of women with androgen excess (more frequently are ovarian; >50 % are malignant). Markedly increased testosterone levels that exceed two to three times the upper limit of the laboratory reference range suggest an androgen-secreting tumour (testosterone reference ranges vary depending on the lab/method). Significantly raised testosterone levels with acute onset and rapid progression of clinical hyperandrogenism should be evaluated as an androgen-secreting tumour until proven otherwise. Virilization can develop in less than a few months with marked androgen excess, while a longer period might be required in the presence of persistent modest hyperandrogenaemia. Rapid progression of

Table 13.1 Common disorders to consider in the differential diagnosis of the polycystic ovary syndrome (PCOS)

Differential diagnoses	Hirsutism and/or hyperandrogenaemia	Oligomenorrhoea or amenorrhoea	Distinctive characteristics — Clinical features	Laboratory tests
Hyperprolactinaemia; prolactinoma	Mild or absent	Present	Galactorrhoea; macroprolactinomas may cause visual disturbances headache, cranial nerve palsies and hypopituitarism symptoms	Increased plasma levels of prolactin
Primary hypothyroidism	Mild or absent	Potentially present	Slow relaxing tendon reflexes; periorbital oedema; bradycardia; hypothermia; dry-coarse skin; deep voice-hoarseness; potentially thyroid goitre	Increased plasma levels of TSH; decreased T4 levels; potentially increased prolactin levels (in secondary hypothyroidism TSH levels can be low or normal)
Nonclassic (late-onset; adult onset) congenital adrenal hyperplasia (21-hydroxylase deficiency)	Present	Not often present	Common in women of Ashkenazi Jewish, Hispanic, Slavic and central European ancestry; family history of hirsutism and/or infertility	Increased levels of 17-hydroxyprogesterone at 8 am or after stimulation (60 min after intravenous ACTH)
Androgen-secreting adrenal or ovarian tumours	Markedly present	Present	Virilization with severe manifestations (e.g., clitoral enlargement, male pattern alopecia, deepening of voice, decreased breast size, increased muscle mass); usually recent/sudden onset and rapid progression of symptoms	Markedly increased levels of testosterone (>2–3 upper normal range) and androstenedione; markedly increased DHEAS levels suggest an adrenal tumour and should prompt imaging of the adrenals (CT or MRI)
Cushing's syndrome	Present	Present	Facial plethora; cervical, thoracic, and/or central obesity; violaceous/red striae >1 cm wide; easy bruising; progressive proximal muscle weakness; thin skin especially in young patients	24-h urinary free cortisol levels and midnight salivary cortisol levels are increased; failure to suppress morning plasma cortisol by an overnight dexamethasone suppression test
Acromegaly	Mild or absent	Often present	Prognathism; tooth separation; gradual acral enlargement (e.g., increased shoe/glove size); coarsening of facial features (e.g., lower lip and nose); hypertension; potentially compressive effects from a macroadenoma	Increased plasma levels of insulin-like growth factor-1 and failure to suppress GH levels or paradoxical rise in GH levels after an oral glucose tolerance test
Premature ovarian failure	Absent	Present	Estrogen deficiency symptoms (e.g., hot flashes, urogenital atrophy); potential presence of other autoimmune endocrinopathies (e.g., autoimmune thyroiditis, autoimmune adrenal failure)	Increased plasma levels of FSH with normal or decreased estradiol levels
Simple obesity	Often present	Not often present	Diagnosis of exclusion	Absent

(continued)

Table 13.1 (continued)

Differential diagnoses	Hirsutism and/or hyperandrogenaemia	Oligomenorrhea or amenorrhea	Distinctive characteristics	
			Clinical features	Laboratory tests
Idiopathic hirsutism (hirsutism with regular menstrual cycles and without increased circulating androgens)	Present	Absent	Diagnosis of exclusion; usually mild hirsutism (Ferriman-Gallwey hirsutism score: 8–15); more common in women of Mediterranean heritage	Absent
Drug-induced androgen excess (e.g., anabolic or androgenic steroids, danazol, valproic acid)	Often present	Potentially present	Detailed history to rule out exogenous androgen use and drug-induced androgen excess	Absent

Routinely assess: (1) Prolactin early in the morning; (2) Thyroid-stimulating hormone (TSH) (3) 17-hydroxyprogesterone early in the morning (before 8 am; follicular phase; 17-hydroxyprogesterone levels 60 min after stimulation with intravenous ACTH might be additionally required)

Testosterone measurement based on clinical features: Total testosterone early in the morning (in regularly cycling women best assess on day 4–10 of the menstrual cycle) with sex hormone binding globulin (SHBG) levels for calculation of the Free Androgen Index (FAI: 100 × total testosterone/SHBG); or free testosterone depending on the available lab/method

Further laboratory tests based on clinical features: (1) Cortisol in the morning (8 am) after 1 mg dexamethasone at midnight; (2) Androstenedione; (3) Dehydroepiandrosterone sulfate (DHEAS); (4) Follicle stimulating hormone (FSH) and luteinizing hormone (LH) in the morning (8 am)

Human Chorionic Gonadotropin (hCG): Pregnancy should also be excluded first by urine or serum hCG in all women of reproductive age that present with amenorrhea or an irregular uterine bleeding pattern (irregular uterine bleeding is frequently caused by complications of pregnancy such as threatened or incomplete miscarriage and ectopic pregnancy) clinical hyperandrogenism and virilization are rarely seen in PCOS. In PCOS the ovarian secretion of both androstenedione and testosterone is increased, while the adrenal synthesis of dehydroepiandrosterone sulfate (DHEAS) may also be enhanced. DHEAS is secreted almost exclusively from the adrenals and should be measured if there is clinical suspicion of an androgen-secreting tumour. Markedly increased plasma DHEAS levels must prompt imaging studies of the adrenals.

> What laboratory tests would help in confirming the diagnosis?

Clinicians must first exclude (1) pregnancy by a urine or serum test for human chorionic gonadotropin (hCG); and (2) exogenous androgen use and drug-induced androgen excess by asking the patient to list all prescribed and over the counter medications, including any herbal supplements and injections. Our case patient listed only a multivitamin tablet and denied any other medications or supplements. Furthermore, her urine hCG test was negative. Thus, a set of biochemical and hormonal assessments, including a standard 2 h oral glucose tolerance test (OGTT), was requested for this patient and was subsequently done early in the morning (8 am) after overnight fasting.

- Biochemical hyperandrogenism. Testosterone is found in the circulation in three fractions: (1) tightly bound to sex hormone binding globulin (SHBG; 65–68 % of the total testosterone); (2) weakly bound to albumin (30–33 %); and (3) free testosterone (1–2 %). The latter two fractions constitute the bioavailable testosterone (non SHBG-bound) which can be readily diffused into target tissues where it is converted to dihydrotestosterone by the enzyme 5α-reductase. Thus, SHBG is a crucial regulator of the bioavailable testosterone levels. SHBG is synthesised primarily in the liver and high levels of testosterone and insulin suppress its production, whereas thyroxine and estrogen enhance it. Accordingly, circulating SHBG levels are decreased in hyperandrogenaemia and hyperinsulinaemia, leading

to increased free/bioavailable testosterone levels. In PCOS this creates a feed-forward vicious cycle between androgen excess, hyperinsulinaemia and low SHBG levels. Measurement of circulating androgens may not be necessary for PCOS diagnosis in cases of clinical hyperandrogenism without any signs of virilization, since either clinical or biochemical hyperandrogenism satisfy the PCOS diagnostic criteria. Establishing biochemical hyperandrogenism for the diagnosis of PCOS has limitations because there is no diagnostic level of circulating testosterone, while the existing normative data in women are not clearly defined. Furthermore, the different assays for testosterone measurement in women are not standardised across laboratories. Particularly measurement of free testosterone with direct tracer immunoassays can be problematic compared to the gold standard methods (e.g., equilibrium dialysis). If a reliable measurement of free testosterone cannot be obtained, the free androgen index (FAI) can be calculated based on total testosterone and SHBG levels (FAI: 100 × total testosterone/SHBG; levels in nmol/L). FAI has been shown to correlate well with the free testosterone levels measured by equilibrium dialysis.

- Gonadotropins. Luteinizing hormone (LH) and follicle stimulating hormone (FSH) are not necessarily required for the diagnosis of PCOS, since neither their ratio nor their absolute circulating levels are included in PCOS diagnostic criteria. Raised LH levels with low-normal FSH levels and an increased LH/FSH ratio (>2) are more frequently noted in lean PCOS women. These findings are less common in overweight/obese PCOS women, presumably due to effects of hyperinsulinaemia on LH secretion. Thus, a high LH/FSH ratio supports the diagnosis of PCOS but the absence of such findings has no diagnostic value.

- Glucose tolerance. The current PCOS clinical practice guidelines by the Endocrine Society recommend an initial assessment of glucose tolerance by a standard OGTT in PCOS patients. Measurement of fasting glucose levels may not be sufficient to detect impaired

Table 13.2 Definitions and proposed criteria for establishing the diagnosis of the polycystic ovary syndrome (PCOS)

NIH [6]	Rotterdam ESHRE [9]	AE-PCOS society [1]
(A) BOTH of the following:	**(A) At least TWO of the following:**	**(A) BOTH of the following:**
Hyperandrogenism: clinical and/or biochemical (not specified)	**Hyperandrogenism:** clinical (hirsutism) and/or biochemical (free testosterone or FAI)	**Hyperandrogenism:** clinical (hirsutism) and/or biochemical (free testosterone by sensitive assays)
Ovarian dysfunction: Chronic anovulation or oligo-ovulation (≤6 menses per year)	**Ovarian dysfunction:** oligo- or anovulation	**Ovarian dysfunction:** oligo- or anovulation **and/or** polycystic ovary morphology on ultrasound
	Polycystic ovary morphology on ultrasound: at least one ovary with ≥12 follicles of 2–9 mm and/or ovarian volume >10 ml in the absence of a dominant follicle >10 mm	
(B) Plus exclusion of other androgen excess or related disorders (e.g., hyperprolactinaemia, hypothyroidism and nonclassic congenital adrenal hyperplasia must be excluded in all cases)		

Clinical hyperandrogenism: hirsutism (excessive terminal hair with a male distribution pattern); acne; male pattern alopecia

Biochemical hyperandrogenism: typically increased total or free testosterone. FAI: Free androgen index (100 × total testosterone/SHBG)

Anovulation: may manifest with menstrual bleeding at intervals of >35 days or <21 days. For women with menstrual bleeding within the normal interval range (25–35 days) ovulation can be verified by a luteal phase day 7 (midluteal) progesterone level [>5 ng/mL – luteal phase day 7 (midluteal) corresponds to cycle day 21 for 28-day intervals and cycle day 28 for 35-day intervals]

Polycystic ovary morphology on ultrasound: ≥12 follicles of 2–9 mm and/or ovarian volume >10 ml. Only one ovary fitting these criteria is sufficient. These ultrasound criteria do not apply to women on oral contraceptive treatment, because it can affect ovarian morphology. If there is evidence of a dominant follicle (>10 mm) or a corpus luteum the ultrasound scanning should be repeated during the next cycle

Abbreviations: *NIH* National Institutes of Health, *ESHRE* European Society of Human Reproduction and Embryology, *AE-PCOS* Androgen Excess-Polycystic Ovary Syndrome Society

glucose tolerance (IGT) in PCOS women. In patients that are unable or unwilling to complete an OGTT, measurement of haemoglobin A1c (HbA1c) is recommended instead, although it appears less sensitive for detecting IGT.

In our case patient, testosterone levels were 2.5 nmol/L (local laboratory normal reference: <1.8 nmol/L) with normal levels of prolactin, TSH, 17-OHP, DHEAS, androstenedione, LH and FSH. SHBG levels were at the lower limit of the laboratory reference range. Normal complete blood count, liver enzymes, and fasting lipid panel were also noted. Based on the OGTT results, plasma glucose increased from fasting levels of 5 mmol/L (90 mg/dL) to 8.6 mmol/L (155 mg/dL) after 2 h. Finally, pelvic ultrasonography revealed: (1) left ovary of $24 \times 20 \times 22$ mm with 12 follicles of 2–9 mm; and (2) right ovary of $18 \times 16 \times 18$ mm with 4 follicles of 2–9 mm (with absence of a dominant follicle >10 mm;

and without any visible endometrial or adrenal pathology).

> How would you interpret these results and what is the final diagnosis?

To date, there are three definitions that can be used to establish the diagnosis of PCOS (Table 13.2). PCOS remains a diagnosis of exclusion, hence all definitions require the exclusion of other disorders which are associated with symptoms/signs of androgen excess in women (see Tables 13.1 and 13.2). According to current guidelines by the Endocrine Society, early morning plasma levels of prolactin, TSH and 17-OHP should be routinely measured in the diagnostic evaluation of PCOS in order to exclude hyperprolactinaemia, thyroid disease (particularly hypothyroidism), and NC-CAH (primarily 21-hydroxylase deficiency), respectively. Depending on the clinical suspicion and presenting symptoms/signs, further laboratory tests may be required in selected patients to exclude other relevant disorders (see Table 13.1).

In our case patient early morning plasma levels of prolactin, TSH and 17-OHP were normal. Furthermore, the assessment of biochemical hyperandrogenism revealed marginally increased levels of total testosterone and normal levels of androstenedione/DHEAS. Based on this, together with the relatively gradual progression of the presenting symptoms/signs, the absence of significant virilization and the results from pelvic ultrasonography further testing to pursue the diagnosis of an androgen-secreting adrenal or ovarian tumour was not considered necessary. In addition, the clinical presentation of our case patient did not prompt investigations for Cushing's syndrome or acromegaly (see Table 13.1).

Finally, PCO morphology was noted on ultrasound in our case patient that satisfied the ultrasound criteria incorporated in the two most recent PCOS definitions (see Table 13.2). In clinical practice, ultrasound scanning of the ovaries is not necessary for the diagnosis of PCOS if the patient already meets the criteria of hyperandrogenism (clinical and/or biochemical) and oligo- or anovulation. Clinicians should recognise that ovarian morphology is affected by age and that PCO morphology can be detected in approximately 20 % of normal women of reproductive age and in 40–50 % of normal adolescents (multifollicular ovaries are a feature of normal puberty that over time subsides with regular menstrual cycling). Furthermore, transvaginal ultrasounds may raise ethical and practical issues in some patients, while the accuracy of transabdominal ultrasound scanning is limited in severely obese patients.

In the context of the above results, the diagnosis of PCOS can be established in our case patient based on any of the three existing PCOS definitions. In addition, the results of the standard OGTT revealed IGT, but not impaired fasting glucose (IFG), based on the current criteria by the American Diabetes Association (ADA) [IFG: fasting glucose of 100–125 mg/dL (5.6–6.9 mmol/L); IGT: 2-h glucose in the OGTT of 140–199 mg/dL (7.8–11.0 mmol/L)].

> **What are the treatment options in this patient?**

Aims of treatment are to ameliorate symptoms of hyperandrogenism, restore menstrual cyclicity, address anovulation and infertility, and prevent/treat complications. Patients should be advised that long-term management will be required because the treatment will not be curative. Accordingly, the treatment plan in PCOS women of reproductive age can include one or more of the following options:

Oral Contraceptives

Monotherapy with oral contraceptives is recommended as first-line treatment for hirsutism/acne in reproductive-age PCOS women who do not desire pregnancy. The use of oral contraceptives in these patients additionally provides adequate contraception and regulates the menstrual bleeding pattern reducing the risk of endometrial hyperplasia. Combined oral contraceptive pills (COCP) contain a potent, synthetic estrogen (ethinyl estradiol) and a progestin component. COCP decrease hyperandrogenism mainly by (1) stimulating hepatic SHBG synthesis and, thus, decreasing the bioavailable levels of androgens; and (2) suppressing pituitary LH secretion and, thus, decreasing ovarian androgen synthesis. COCP formulations have different progestin components with various degrees of androgenicity. Progestins derived from testosterone have mild androgenic activity, while progestins that are not structurally related to testosterone act as androgen receptor antagonists (e.g., norgestimate and desogestrel belong to third generation progestins and are considered non-androgenic). Cyproterone acetate (CPA) is a synthetic antiandrogen progestin (COCP with a daily dose of 2 mg CPA and 35 μg ethinyl estradiol). Furthermore, the progestin drospirenone is a spironolactone analogue that has antiandrogenic (weak antiandrogen; 3 mg used in COCP are approximately equivalent to 1 mg CPA and

25 mg spironolactone) and anti-mineralocorticoid activity (potassium monitoring is required). The existing clinical evidence is not sufficient to suggest one COCP formulation over another or over other hormonal contraceptives (i.e., patch and vaginal ring) in PCOS. Both the efficacy and safety (metabolic and thromboembolic risk) profile of different formulations should be considered in each patient before prescribing a COCP regimen. Screening for contraindications to hormonal contraceptives is also essential; absolute contraindications to COCP include: smoking ≥15 cigarettes per day in women ≥35 years old, blood pressure ≥160/100 mmHg; diabetes with vascular disease or neuropathy/retinopathy; multiple CVD risk factors including evidence of vascular disease or history of ischemic heart disease; history of or acute venous/arterial thrombosis or pulmonary embolism; known thrombogenic mutation; systemic lupus erythematosus with antiphospholipid antibodies; acute active liver disease; and migraine headaches with aura. Currently there are insufficient data to support a recommendation regarding the optimal duration of oral contraceptive treatment in PCOS women, hence patients can potentially continue on their regimen until pregnancy is desired or a contraindication becomes evident.

Antiandrogens

Antiandrogens (i.e., androgen receptor blockers and 5α-reductase inhibitors) are used in combination with COCP for the treatment of moderate/severe hirsutism in PCOS. Monotherapy with antiandrogens may be also used for hirsutism when hormonal contraceptives are contraindicated, but this is not recommended unless another reliable contraception method (e.g., intrauterine device) is ensured due to the risk of fetal male pseudohermaphroditism [in utero feminisation of a 46,XY (male) fetus]. Spironolactone, CPA and finasteride can be prescribed with relatively similar efficacy in PCOS, while the use of flutamide is not recommended because of its potential severe hepatotoxicity.

Spironolactone acts as an androgen antagonist and significantly inhibits the 5α-reductase activity. Spironolactone doses of 100 mg per day (divided to twice daily) are usually effective for hirsutism treatment, but higher doses (e.g., 200 mg per day) may be required. Spironolactone-related hyperkalaemia is rare in patients with normal renal function, but an initial transient diuretic effect is usually noted and may cause postural hypotension and dizziness. Careful monitoring of electrolytes, renal function and blood pressure is required within the first fortnight of treatment at initiation and at each dose increment.

Cyproterone acetate (CPA; not available in the US) acts as an antiandrogen mainly by inhibiting the androgen receptor via competition with testosterone and dihydrotestosterone for receptor binding. In addition, CPA may less potently inhibit the 5α-reductase activity, while it also suppresses circulating gonadotropin and androgen levels. Due to its slow metabolism and long half-life, CPA is administered in the early phase of the treatment cycle in a reverse sequential regimen. Thus, ethinyl estradiol (doses of 20–50 μg daily) is given for 3 weeks (day 5–25) to ensure normal menstrual cycling, and CPA (doses of 50–100 mg daily) is administered for the first 10 days of the cycle (day 5–15). Once the maximal treatment effect is achieved, lower doses of CPA (e.g. 5 mg daily) can be prescribed for maintenance, while a COCP with a daily dose of 2 mg CPA and 35 μg ethinyl estradiol is also available. CPA is usually well tolerated, but can exhibit dose-dependent metabolic effects similar to those of high-dose COCP.

Finasteride acts as an antiandrogen by inhibiting the type 2 5α-reductase. Because clinical manifestations of hyperandrogenism appear to depend on the combined activity of type 1 and type 2 5α-reductase, finasteride is considered partially effective. Despite its partial inhibitory effect, prolonged treatment with finasteride at doses of 2.5–5 mg daily is shown to have practically equal efficacy to other antiandrogens. Significant improvement of hirsutism is usually noted after 6 months of treatment with a finasteride dose of 5 mg daily which is the most frequently used dose in clinical practise. A potential advantage of finasteride is its benign safety profile with no major side/adverse effects and good tolerance by patients.

Flutamide is a pure antiandrogen that acts by inhibiting the androgen receptor in a dose-response manner. Flutamide doses of 250 top 500 mg daily have similar efficacy to other antiandrogens, but flutamide treatment is not recommended because of its potential severe hepatotoxicity. If flutamide is prescribed the lowest effective dose should be used and the patient must be closely monitored.

Topical antiandrogen creams (e.g., 5 % canrenone [the active metabolite of spironolactone] and 0.25–0.5 % finasteride) appear to have limited efficacy for hirsutism with inconsistent results from clinical trials.

Direct Hair Removal/Reduction Methods

Removal of excessive terminal hair by direct methods can be used for hirsutism in PCOS, usually in combination with pharmacotherapy. While the latter restricts hair regrowth, existing terminal hair should be removed by direct methods once androgen suppression is achieved. Among direct methods, photoepilation therapy with laser or intense pulsed light treatments is currently suggested.

Temporary Methods of Direct Hair Removal

Epilation methods involve the removal of the intact hair with its root (e.g., plucking, tweezing, waxing) and can be used in addition to pharmacotherapy in the first months of hirsutism treatment until the drug effects become clinically apparent. These methods are inexpensive and relatively safe, usually causing only transient discomfort. Depilation methods (e.g., shaving) remove the hair shaft from the skin surface and the effect usually lasts only for a few days. Patients should be assured that shaving does not increase the growth (rate and/or duration of the anagen phase) or thickness (diameter) of hair, which is a common misconception. Chemical depilatory products are also often used to separate the hair from its follicle and dissolve it. Irritant contact dermatitis and folliculitis may occur with such agents.

Permanent Methods of Hair Reduction

Electrolysis and photoepilation therapy with laser or intense pulsed light are used for "permanent"

hair reduction which is defined as >30 % reduction in the number of terminal hairs after a treatment regimen that is stable for a period longer than the complete growth cycle of hair follicles (4–12 months depending on body area).

Electrolysis treats each hair individually since this technique requires the insertion of a fine needle into the hair follicle. Galvanic electrolysis and thermolysis are available, causing destruction of the hair follicle by inducing a chemical reaction or heat, respectively. Electrolysis can be used on any hair/skin colour and is usually applied for localised small areas as a cost-effective option. Electrolysis requires an experienced operator and can be time-consuming and relatively painful. Topical lidocaine/prilocaine anaesthetic creams may be used to reduce pain. Potential local side effects, especially by inexperienced operators, include erythema, post-inflammatory pigment changes and even scarring due to tissue destruction.

Photoepilation (light-assisted hair reduction) methods include laser and intense pulsed light (IPL) therapy which achieve hair removal by selective photothermolysis, using light wavelengths that are absorbed by the melanin of the hair and pulse durations that selectively destroy the hair without damaging the adjacent tissue. Thus, hair follicles are destroyed, but vellus (light-coloured/unpigmented) hair may remain. Of note, the choice of the photoepilation method/device should be made according to the skin and hair colour of the patient. Ideal candidates for laser hair reduction therapy are women with light skin and dark hair. Relatively short wavelength devices (e.g., ruby and alexandrite lasers) are optimal for these women, whereas longer wavelength lasers (e.g., neodymium:yttrium-aluminum-garnet, Nd:YAG, lasers) or IPL appear appropriate for women with dark skin and dark hair. For patients with white/light coloured hair IPL combined with radiofrequency (electromagnetic waves delivered together with the light pulse on the same machine) may be effective. Potential local side effects include dyspigmentation and scarring. Other limitations to photoepilation methods are the need for multiple treatments and the cost of therapy which varies depending mainly on the size of the treated area.

Topical Eflornithine Treatment

A 13.9 % eflornithine hydrochloride cream (Vaniqa) is licensed and is an irreversible inhibitor of the enzyme L-ornithine decarboxylase, which catalyses the conversion of ornithine to putrescine. The latter plays a key role in the regulation of cell growth and differentiation within the hair follicle. Thus, topical eflornithine treatment reduces the hair growth rate locally, but is not a hair removal method. Continuous topical application of eflornithine cream (typically twice daily; at least 8 hours apart) is shown to reversibly slow facial hair growth with clinically significant improvement of facial hirsutism and quality of life. These results are usually noted after 6–8 weeks of treatment, while once the topical administration is discontinued facial hair growth returns to pre-treatment levels after approximately 8 weeks. Topical eflornithine treatment for facial hirsutism in PCOS is usually used in combination with other interventions, such as pharmacotherapy, to achieve a more rapid initial response. Systemic absorption of eflornithine with topical treatment for facial hirsutism is extremely low. Local side effects include itching and dry skin. Patients should be advised that this cream is not licensed for treatment of hirsutism in areas other than the face.

Lifestyle Modification: Weight Loss

Weight loss is recommended in overweight/obese PCOS women. A weight-centric management plan is crucial for these patients in clinical practice to achieve sustained weight loss and prevent T2DM and other manifestations of the metabolic syndrome. Weight management in PCOS should typically follow the clinical guidelines for obesity treatment in the general population, including lifestyle interventions, pharmacotherapy (e.g., Orlistat) and bariatric surgery, based on the BMI and existing comorbidities of each patient.

Metformin

Metformin is increasingly prescribed in PCOS women, even without coexisting T2DM, because it may improve metabolic and reproductive outcomes in selected patients. Metformin therapy for symptomatic treatment of PCOS should be initiated under specialist care. Based on the current clinical practise guidelines by the Endocrine Society metformin is recommended in PCOS women with T2DM or IGT who are failing lifestyle modification, whereas it should not be first-line treatment for hirsutism/acne, weight loss, or prevention of pregnancy complications in PCOS. The optimum use of metformin in PCOS treatment is currently under debate and there are differences among various national guidelines which reflect the need for larger and better designed clinical trials with metformin in different PCOS patient populations (e.g., in ethnic populations and adolescents).

In the treatment of overweight/obese PCOS women, metformin may be used as adjuvant to lifestyle interventions to ameliorate the adverse effects of insulin resistance. Metformin reduces hepatic glucose production, decreases glucose absorption and increases glucose uptake into skeletal muscle. Thus, metformin therapy decreases the overall insulin requirements and may contribute to interrupt the vicious cycle between compensatory hyperinsulinaemia and hyperandrogenism in PCOS. A growing body of evidence indicates that metformin treatment in PCOS may induce significant improvements in glucose and insulin plasma levels, surrogate measures of insulin resistance (e.g., SHBG), lipid profile, blood pressure, as well as slight reduction in BMI and WHR. However, there is inconsistency concerning the reported metabolic outcomes of metformin therapy in PCOS, since other studies, including placebo-controlled randomised clinical trials (RCTs), have failed to reproduce these metabolic effects. A recent systematic review of RCTs reported that metformin has limited effects on weight loss, insulin and lipid profiles in obese PCOS women. This inconsistent and heterogeneous response to metformin therapy may be attributed, at least in part, to the variability in the phenotypic expression of PCOS that is allowed by the different PCOS definitions. Metformin appears to be more effective in PCOS patients at the more severe end of this spectrum. In addition, metformin therapy may have reproductive benefits in

PCOS women by reducing hyperandrogenism and restoring menstrual regularity, ovulation and fertility. Indeed, a significant clinical outcome of metformin therapy in PCOS is improved menstrual cyclicity, although it appears to be less effective than oral contraceptives. Existing data from RCTs also indicate that metformin is associated with improved clinical pregnancy rates in PCOS, but there is no evidence that it improves live birth rates.

Infertility Treatment

PCOS women with chronic oligo/anovulation who desire pregnancy are candidates for medical induction of ovulation. Current guidelines recommend clomiphene citrate (initial dose of 50 mg/day orally; starting on day 3 of the cycle and lasting for 5 days [days 3–7 of the cycle]) as first-line infertility treatment in PCOS women with anovulatory infertility and without other infertility factors. Increasing data also support the role of aromatase inhibitors (e.g., letrozole) as an alternative first-line oral pharmacological treatment for anovulatory infertility in PCOS. If pregnancy is not achieved with these first-line oral treatments, due to either anovulation (resistance to induction of ovulation) or failure to conceive despite induced ovulation, patients should be referred to a specialist infertility clinic for further evaluation and treatment. Failure to conceive despite achieving induced ovulation should prompt a thorough fertility work-up in both partners of the couple, including semen analysis and evaluation of the uterine and tubal anatomy, in order to explore additional infertility factors which might not be related to PCOS. Finally, metformin appears to have an adjuvant role to first-line treatments in induction of ovulation in obese PCOS women and is helpful to prevent the ovarian hyperstimulation syndrome (OHSS) in patients receiving gonadotropin treatment for in vitro fertilisation (IVF).

Do women with PCOS require screening/management of comorbidities long term?

Type 2 Diabetes Mellitus (T2DM) and Cardiovascular Disease (CVD) Risk

PCOS is associated with manifestations of the metabolic syndrome, particularly central obesity, insulin resistance, T2DM, dyslipidaemia and hypertension. PCOS patients typically have higher prediabetes/T2DM prevalence and more CVD risk factors than age- and weight-matched women without PCOS. Thus, PCOS may lead to increased CVD morbidity and mortality later in life, although the documented CVD morbidity and mortality in middle-aged PCOS women is not as increased as would be expected. In clinical practice, it is required to screen all PCOS patients for CVD risk factors by assessing BMI, waist circumference, blood pressure, fasting lipids, glucose tolerance, smoking status and family history of premature CVD (<55 and <65 years of age in male and female relatives, respectively).

Non-alcoholic Fatty Liver Disease (NAFLD) – Non-alcoholic Steatohepatitis (NASH)

NASH corresponds to the most severe histologic form of NAFLD, characterised by steatosis and various degrees of inflammation, hepatocyte injury and fibrosis. NASH may gradually lead to cirrhosis, liver failure and hepatocellular carcinoma. In clinical practice, awareness of the high risk of NAFLD in PCOS women is suggested, particularly if central obesity and insulin resistance is present. However, universal routine screening by serum markers of liver dysfunction (e.g. aminotransferases) and ultrasound scanning of the liver in obese PCOS patients is not currently recommended, because there is no simple screening test for NAFLD with high sensitivity and specificity.

Depression, Anxiety and Eating Disorders

Common psychological disorders are more prevalent in PCOS. Indeed, PCOS women exhibit significantly higher rates of depression (28–64 %) and anxiety (34–57 %) compared to women in the general population (8 and 18 %, respectively). In addition, there are data suggesting an increased risk of psychosexual dysfunction (e.g., loss of feminine identity, reduced sexual satisfaction) and negative body image perception (e.g., feeling less physically attractive or healthy) in PCOS women. Finally, eating disorders (e.g., binge-eating disorder) appear more frequent in PCOS, with reports showing that the prevalence of any eating disorder may reach 21 % in PCOS women. Based on this evidence, the current guidelines by the Endocrine Society and the PCOS Australian Alliance suggest screening of PCOS women for depression, anxiety and eating disorders.

Obstructive Sleep Apnea (OSA)

Overweight/obese PCOS women exhibit increased prevalence of OSA and sleep-disordered breathing, potentially attributed to hyperandrogenism and obesity (particularly central). Clinical studies have shown that PCOS patients, after controlling for BMI, have 30 times the risk of sleep-disordered breathing compared to control women and that OSA is more frequent in obese PCOS women than in weight-matched controls. Thus, it appears that obesity alone is not sufficient to account for the high OSA prevalence in PCOS. OSA may have significant deleterious cardiometabolic effects in PCOS patients, since chronic intermittent hypoxia and disruption of normal sleep patterns increase the sympathetic nervous system activity and oxidative stress and, hence, can progressively induce further weight gain, insulin resistance and hypertension.

Initial screening for OSA is suggested in all overweight/obese PCOS women in order to identify suggestive symptoms (e.g. excessive daytime somnolence, snoring, choking/apnea episodes during sleep). OSA screening can also be performed through validated questionnaires (e.g., Epworth Sleepiness Scale, Berlin Questionnaire) and patients that are positive on this screening should be referred to a specialist in sleep medicine for diagnostic evaluation by polysomnography.

Endometrial Cancer

Current evidence suggests that PCOS women are three times more likely to develop endometrial cancer. Overall, PCOS women with amenorrhea appear to be at a greater risk of endometrial

hyperplasia and cancer which may be higher still in the presence of obesity and/or T2DM. The current guidelines by the Endocrine Society recommend heightened awareness of the increased risk of endometrial cancer in PCOS, particularly in the presence of dysfunctional uterine bleeding, prolonged amenorrhea, obesity or T2DM. However, these guidelines suggest against routine ultrasound screening for endometrial thickness in all PCOS women.

Importantly, in PCOS women with chronic anovulation exposure of the endometrium to unopposed non-fluctuating levels of estradiol in the absence of progesterone increases the risk of endometrial hyperplasia/cancer. In order to decrease this risk, clinicians should offer long-term treatment with a COCP regimen or cyclical progestogen to induce periodic withdrawal bleeding. Regular withdrawal bleeding at least every 3 months is considered to significantly reduce the risk of endometrial hyperplasia and cancer in PCOS.

Pregnancy Complications

PCOS women have higher rates of GDM, pregnancy-induced hypertension, pre-eclampsia and pre-term birth; whilst the infant is also at higher risk of neonatal complications (e.g. small for gestational age infant, increased neonatal ICU admission and mortality rates). Finally, PCOS women have been shown to exhibit higher rates of spontaneous miscarriage after assisted reproduction compared to women without PCOS. This is considered related to the high obesity incidence in PCOS and the type of infertility treatment that PCOS women may receive, because it has been reported that after adjustment for these factors the increase in the risk of spontaneous miscarriage in PCOS women was not significant.

Suggested Reading

1. Azziz R, Carmina E, Dewailly D, Diamanti-Kandarakis E, Escobar-Morreale HF, Futterweit W, et al.; Task Force on the Phenotype of the Polycystic Ovary Syndrome of The Androgen Excess and PCOS Society. The Androgen Excess and PCOS Society criteria for the polycystic ovary syndrome: the complete task force report. Fertil Steril. 2009;91(2):456–88.

2. Diamanti-Kandarakis E, Dunaif A. Insulin resistance and the polycystic ovary syndrome revisited: an update on mechanisms and implications. Endocr Rev. 2012;33(6):981–1030.

3. Escobar-Morreale HF, Carmina E, Dewailly D, Gambineri A, Kelestimur F, Moghetti P, et al. Epidemiology, diagnosis and management of hirsutism: a consensus statement by the Androgen Excess and Polycystic Ovary Syndrome Society. Hum Reprod Update. 2012;18(2):146–70.

4. Fauser BC, Tarlatzis BC, Rebar RW, Legro RS, Balen AH, Lobo R, et al. Consensus on women's health aspects of polycystic ovary syndrome (PCOS): the Amsterdam ESHRE/ASRM-Sponsored 3rd PCOS Consensus Workshop Group. Fertil Steril. 2012;97(1): 28–38.e25.

5. Kyrou I, Randeva H, Weickert MO. Clinical problems caused by obesity. In: Weickert MO, editor. Obesity-Obesitext at Endotext.org, MDTEXT.COM, INC, S. Dartmouth; 2014. (http://www.endotext.org/section/obesity/).

6. Legro RS, Arslanian SA, Ehrmann DA, Hoeger KM, Murad MH, Pasquali R, et al.; Endocrine Society. Diagnosis and treatment of polycystic ovary syndrome: an Endocrine Society clinical practice guideline. J Clin Endocrinol Metab. 2013;98(12):4565–92.

7. Martin KA, Chang RJ, Ehrmann DA, Ibanez L, Lobo RA, Rosenfield RL, et al. Evaluation and treatment of hirsutism in premenopausal women: an endocrine society clinical practice guideline. J Clin Endocrinol Metab. 2008;93(4):1105–20.

8. Randeva HS, Tan BK, Weickert MO, Lois K, Nestler JE, Sattar N, et al. Cardiometabolic aspects of the polycystic ovary syndrome. Endocr Rev. 2012;33(5):812–41.

9. Rotterdam ESHRE/ASRM-Sponsored PCOS Consensus Workshop Group. Revised 2003 consensus on diagnostic criteria and long-term health risks related to polycystic ovary syndrome. Fertil Steril. 2004;81(1):19–25.

10. Tang T, Lord JM, Norman RJ, Yasmin E, Balen AH. Insulin-sensitising drugs (metformin, rosiglitazone, pioglitazone, D-chiro-inositol) for women with polycystic ovary syndrome, oligo amenorrhoea and subfertility. Cochrane Database Syst Rev. 2012;(5): CD003053.

11. Teede HJ, Misso ML, Deeks AA, Moran LJ, Stuckey BG, Wong JL, et al.; Guideline Development Groups. Assessment and management of polycystic ovary syndrome: summary of an evidence-based guideline. Med J Aust. 2011;195(6):S65–112.

12. Wild RA, Carmina E, Diamanti-Kandarakis E, Dokras A, Escobar-Morreale HF, Futterweit W, et al. Assessment of cardiovascular risk and prevention of cardiovascular disease in women with the polycystic ovary syndrome: a consensus statement by the Androgen Excess and Polycystic Ovary Syndrome (AE-PCOS) Society. J Clin Endocrinol Metab. 2010;95(5):2038–49.

13. Zawadski JK, Dunaif A. Diagnostic criteria for polycystic ovary syndrome: towards a rational approach. In: Dunaif A, Givens JR, Haseltine FP, Merriam GR, editors. Polycystic Ovary Syndrome. Boston: Blackwell Scientific Publications; 1992; 377–384.

14. Azziz R, Carmina E, Dewailly D, Diamanti-Kandarakis E, Escobar-Morreale HF, Futterweit W, Janssen OE, Legro RS, Norman RJ, Taylor AE, Witchel SF; Androgen Excess Society. Positions statement: criteria for defining polycystic ovary syndrome as a predominantly hyperandrogenic syndrome: an Androgen Excess Society guideline. J Clin Endocrinol Metab. 2006;91(11):4237–45.

Salt-Wasting Crisis in a Newborn

Case 14

Sabah Alvi

Abstract

A 10-day-old baby presents with failure to thrive and is found to have hyponatraemia and hyperkalaemia. In this case study the differential diagnosis is considered with a systematic approach to investigation, treatment, long-term management and complications. Current controversies are also discussed.

Keywords

Failure to thrive • Salt wasting • Congenital adrenal hyperplasia • 21-hydroxylase deficiency • Glucocorticoid • Mineralocorticoid

Case

A sick Indo-Asian baby is seen in the Accident and Emergency department. He is 10 days old and has been off his feeds. For the last 24 h he has been vomiting and has been losing weight. Initial investigations reveal the following electrolytes:

Na^+ 128 mmol/l (135–145 mmol/l)

K^+ 6.8 mmol/l (3.5–6.0 mmol/l)

Urea 8.2 mmol/l (2.5–7.5 mmol/l)

Creatinine 87 mmol/l (35–105 mmol/l)

A full sepsis screen has been performed and has shown no evidence of infection. Urine and CSF are clear, and there are no abnormalities on his chest x-ray.

> What further information would you require?

Hyponatraemia in a baby can be caused by many things. You need to know:

Prenatal history, gestation – A severely growth-retarded baby or a very bad pregnancy can cause babies to be wasted and ill.

Birth weight and mode of delivery – Traumatic births can result in some delayed effects.

Ethnicity and consanguinity – Metabolic and endocrine conditions that can cause this picture are often genetic, autosomal recessive in origin, and may occur with increased frequency in offspring of consanguineous marriages.

Any siblings and medical conditions – Again, if an inherited condition parents may already have one child with similar problems.

S. Alvi, MD, FRCPCH
Department of Paediatric Endocrinology,
Leeds Children's Hospital,
A Floor Brotherton Wing, Great George Street,
Leeds, West Yorkshire LS1 3EX, UK
e-mail: sabahalvi@nhs.net

R. Ajjan, S.M. Orme (eds.), *Endocrinology and Diabetes: Case Studies, Questions and Commentaries*,
DOI 10.1007/978-1-4471-2789-5_14, © Springer-Verlag London 2015

Any history of neonatal deaths? Many metabolic and some endocrine conditions are lethal and a past history of neonatal deaths would suggest a possible recurrence.

Family history – Same as above for inherited conditions.

Feeding history (breast, bottle, any difficulties attaching, tongue tie) – These could cause baby to feed poorly and become dehydrated.

Is the baby disinterested in feeds or hungry but not gaining weight? A baby not feeding may be unable to feed due to sepsis or other overwhelming illness, whilst a hungry baby may be feeding well but unable to retain food due to malabsorption or mechanical problems such as pyloric stenosis.

Does baby struggle to feed? Is he breathless, sweaty? Babies with congenital heart disease, or severe acidosis.

Is baby passing urine normally? A dehydrated baby may have had uncharacteristically dry nappies recently; may indicate renal problems.

What signs will you look for?

Like any patient you need to do a full examination starting with inspection.

Is the baby's colour normal?

Is the baby dehydrated? Is he failing to thrive? Early growth is highly dependent on salt, so if this baby has not been feeding and losing salt he could be quite wasted.

Is his fontanelle soft or tense, sunken (sign of dehydration) or bulging (can indicate raised intracranial pressure and is often found in meningitis)?

He needs a full systems examination to exclude any signs of cardiac disease.

Look for signs of infection, such as fever, mottled skin, petechiae, poor capillary refill. Is he irritable or very lethargic? Both are alarming signs.

Does he have any respiratory difficulties?

Is his abdomen soft? Can you feel any masses?

Does he have normal male genitalia? Are both testes in the scrotum? There may be hyperpigmentation of the genitalia, although this can be difficult to assess in a dark-skinned baby.

Summary

You are faced with a 10-day-old Asian baby with failure to thrive. He is dehydrated, listless, has a weak cry and is vomiting, but there are no dysmorphic features. His anterior fontanelle is flat. There are no petechiae/purpura and he is afebrile, but his skin is mottled. There are no abnormalities in the cardiac or respiratory systems. You cannot palpate any lumps in the abdomen. There is suggestion of some scrotal hyperpigmentation, but he has otherwise normal male genitalia, with bilaterally descended testes and a normal looking penis.

What is the differential diagnosis?

The electrolytes show hyponatraemia, hyperkalaemia and evidence of mild dehydration.

With this clinical picture, the differential diagnosis must include:

Simple failure to feed – but the hyponatraemia is too severe, and would not be associated with hyperkalaemia

Severe urinary tract infection due to urinary reflux with posterior urethral valves – but the urine is clear

Cystic dysplastic kidneys

Congenital adrenal hyperplasia

Adrenal hypoplasia congenita

Primary hypoaldosteronism

Pseudohypoaldosteronism

What further investigations will you undertake?

Immediate investigations:

Blood tests to measure 17 hydroxyprogesterone (17-OHP), plasma renin activity (PRA), aldosterone, DHEAS, androstenedione, cortisol, glucose

Capillary blood gases

Collect blood for DNA extraction for possible future +/− karyotype

Collect a sample of urine for steroid profiling

Later investigations:

Arrange an abdominal ultrasound scan

Results

Cortisol 85 nmol/l
Chloride 108 mmol/l
Bicarbonate 16 mmol/l
Glucose 3.2 mmol/l
Aldosterone, 17-OHP and plasma renin activity
   will not be available for 2 more days
USS: normal kidneys, bulky adrenal glands

What is the interpretation of these results?

The results so far suggest an adrenal problem: the cortisol is low, particularly so in the context of a sick child; the glucose is low, and there is a mild metabolic acidosis. In the newborn, adrenal glands are not readily visualised on ultrasound scanning and so if the adrenal glands are easily seen and bulky, this would support a diagnosis of congenital adrenal hyperplasia (CAH). The low cortisol, low sodium and high potassium need to be corrected. The baby is also dehydrated and as confirmatory results will not be available you must start treatment empirically.

What is the immediate management of this baby?

There is no evidence of sepsis so antibiotics are not indicated. Intravenous rehydration with dextrose saline and a bolus of hydrocortisone will deal with all the possible differentials until further results are available.

If the baby has adrenal hyperplasia or hypoplasia he will improve very rapidly with intravenous dextrose-saline and regular intravenous hydrocortisone. If there is little or no improvement, this is more likely to be hypoaldosteronism or pseudohypoaldosteronism, which will only resolve with extra sodium and bicarbonate treatment if it is pseudohypoaldosteronism, or the addition of fludrocortisone if it is primary hypoaldosteronism.

A few days later further results are available:
17OHP >300 nmol/l (normal <50)
Aldosterone 257 pmol/l (normal 1,000–6,000)
Plasma renin activity 58 nmol/l/24 h (normal <30)

What is the interpretation of this set of results?

This is strongly supportive of 21-hydroxylase deficiency congenital adrenal hyperplasia; the raised renin is appropriate in the face of hyponatraemia and confirms the severe salt-losing type. In adrenal hypoplasia or primary hypoaldosteronism, we would not see such a high 17OHP, and in pseudohypoaldosteronism the aldosterone would be very high (several tens of thousands) due to receptor insensitivity, and again, the 17OHP would not be raised.

When the baby has been stabilised and the electrolyte disturbances corrected (which may take a few days), maintenance treatment should be started with oral hydrocortisone at a dose of 15–20 mg/m²/day in four divided doses, and fludrocortisone at a dose of 25–50 mcg per day, although this may need increasing (sometimes up to as much as 300 mcg daily) within the first year or so. Sodium supplements should also be started at 5–10 mmol/kg/day as these babies need much more sodium than other babies, usually for up to a year.

What is the longer term management?

A urine steroid profile can indicate where in the pathway the block in steroid production occurs. To confirm the genetic mutation involved, DNA extraction and analysis can be undertaken-the most common cause of salt-losing congenital adrenal hyperplasia is a mutation in the gene for 21-hydroxylase. Genetic counselling and testing of parents and siblings can then be offered, with evaluation of carrier status of other family members if there is consanguinity.

The relevance of the child's ethnic background is that in some communities there is a high rate of consanguineous marriage and the risk of an autosomal recessive condition must be borne in mind.

Fludrocortisone and hydrocortisone requirements are greater in children than adults, and in babies more than in children. Adequacy of mineralocorticoid replacement is monitored by regular measurements of plasma renin activity. Hydrocortisone doses are reviewed on clinical grounds, the child's body surface area, and monitored with 17 hydroxyprogesterone profiles, either in salivary samples or blood.

As the child grows up it is important to monitor linear growth and puberty. Chronic undertreatment, either due to lack of compliance or inadequate steroid dosage, can compromise height due to the effect of excess androgens on the growth plate causing premature epiphyseal fusion. Conversely, too high a dose of steroids can also cause loss of growth.

Excess androgens can also cause priming of the pituitary gland to stimulate gonadotrophin secretion and development of central precocious puberty which may then require treatment. In young boys it is important to monitor testicular growth both clinically and radiologically as poorly controlled CAH can result in the development of testicular adrenal rest tumours, which although benign and not requiring surgical treatment, can cause discomfort and compromise fertility.

Families need educating in sick day rules, emergency treatment and the need for their child to carry a steroid card and wear a medical talisman.

Congenital Adrenal Hyperplasia

This covers a group of autosomal recessive adrenal conditions caused by genetic mutations in five main enzymes. The most common type, due to deficiency of the 21-hydroxylase enzyme, results in impaired cortisol and aldosterone synthesis and overproduction of adrenal androgens (Fig. 14.1).

Classical 21-Hydroxylase Deficiency Congenital Adrenal Hyperplasia

The incidence of congenital adrenal hyperplasia in Britain is about 1 in 18,000 [1]. Up to 95 % of cases are caused by deficiency of the 21-hydroxylase enzyme; this results from mutations in the gene encoding adrenal P450c21 and is inherited in an autosomal recessive fashion. Complete deficiency of the enzyme results in salt wasting due to inability to produce the mineralocorticoid aldosterone, and hypoglycaemia from glucocorticoid deficiency. Due to the position of 21-hydroxylase in the steroid pathway, the block causes accumulation of precursors which are diverted into the alternative pathway producing excess 17 hydroxyprogesterone, which is converted to androstenedione and thence to testosterone, both potent androgens. Females therefore present with virilisation at birth, which can vary from mild clitoromegaly to complete gender ambiguity. As they are diagnosed within the first few days of life, they rarely present with salt losing crises at diagnosis (although they are just as prone as boys with this condition to decompensate during intercurrent illnesses or other times of physical stress), but the birth of a child with genital ambiguity (disorder of sex development) is an extremely traumatic experience for the parents and great sensitivity is required in making an accurate and timely diagnosis.

Careful examination will usually show clitoromegaly, enlarged or fused labia majora, bifid or completely hypoplastic scrotum with no palpable gonads in the labioscrotal folds. Only a single perineal orifice will be seen as vagina and urethra are often fused (urogenital sinus). If faced with this situation, an urgent pelvic ultrasound should be arranged: in a girl with virilising CAH a uterus and ovaries should be visible and will immediately help to differentiate between CAH and other conditions causing disorders of sex development. A rapid karyotype will be 46 XX and biochemical confirmation can be obtained (after 48 h of age to avoid the physiological surge of maternal hormones) by checking adrenal function (17-OHP, androstenedione, cortisol, DHEAS, testosterone) and plasma renin activity. A urinary steroid profile and DNA analysis for the 21-hydroxylase gene mutation will confirm the diagnosis.

As external virilisation in boys with this condition is not a problem, boys present between 7

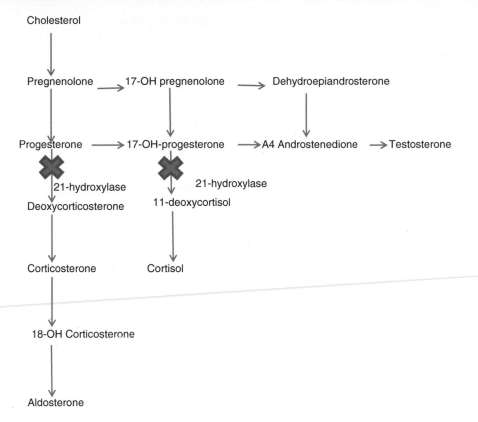

Fig. 14.1 Pathways of steroid metabolism. A block due to deficiency of 21-hydroxylase causes accumulation of precursors (17-hydroxyprogesterone, androstenedione, testosterone) and deficiency of glucocorticoids (cortisol) and mineralocorticoids (aldosterone)

and 21 days, when the baby switches from the protection of maternal hormones and relies on his own adrenal glands. Lack of mineralocorticoid precipitates salt loss which, uncorrected and in combination with glucocorticoid deficiency, precipitates an adrenal crisis. Typically this presents as poor feeding, lethargy and weight loss. Vomiting can follow with collapse if not picked up early enough. After the diagnosis has been made and the child stabilised, mutation analysis can confirm the genetic basis of the condition and allow appropriate counselling for parents, who, as this is often their first child, will want to know of recurrence risks in future pregnancies (one in four with every pregnancy). A full multidisciplinary team comprising endocrinologists, geneticists, urologists, psychologists, gynaecologists and clinical nurse specialists needs to be involved

so that the parents can be supported practically and psychologically [2]. Even after diagnosis and appropriate treatment has been instigated, infants remain very vulnerable to recurrent salt-losing crises and hospital admissions, due to their propensity to contract repeated infections, and parents must be taught how to manage illnesses at home and be given direct access to paediatric wards if their child's condition deteriorates.

In the longer term, girls with CAH will require surgery which may be minor when virilisation is not extensive, to major reconstruction with vaginoplasty/ feminising genitoplasty, sometimes followed by self-vaginal dilatation. Boys usually do not require surgery, but complications in both can include obesity, precocious puberty, short stature and subfertility, with development of polycystic ovary syndrome or adrenal rest tumours [3].

Current Controversies

Prenatal Dexamethasone Treatment

Prenatal dexamethasone has been available since the mid 1980s as an experimental treatment to prevent severe virilisation of a female fetus affected with congenital adrenal hyperplasia [4] and there is plenty of evidence to show that when started early enough (between 6 and 7 weeks of pregnancy) it can be very effective in preventing or minimising virilisation. At 10–12 weeks, a chorionic villous sample can be taken to confirm the gender of the fetus. If a male fetus is confirmed, the dexamethasone can be discontinued. For female fetuses genetic mutation analysis is undertaken, and if negative, dexamethasone treatment of the mother is discontinued. In females with a confirmed CAH gene mutation, treatment is continued to term and ceased at delivery. In this way therefore 7 out of 8 fetuses are treated with dexamethasone unnecessarily, and there are widespread concerns about the long term effects on cognition, memory and social adaptation of children who were exposed to dexamethasone in utero [5]. Maternal effects too, such as fluid retention, hypertension and striae can be very unpleasant. However, with the advent of fetal sexing from free fetal DNA in maternal plasma it is possible to identify male fetuses as early as 37 days after conception, which allows treatment to be initiated only in pregnancies with female fetuses. New et al. [6] have taken this a step further and can now analyse fetal CYP-21 status in cell-free DNA, and thereby target only affected female fetuses by 6 weeks of gestation. It is likely that this will become the standard way of offering prenatal diagnosis and treatment, but at present this non-invasive prenatal testing is not routinely available on the National Health Service.

It is therefore suggested that prenatal treatment should only be carried out in centres where there is a multidisciplinary team of experts, fully informed consent around the current uncertainties, and facilities to undertake registration and long term follow up for all treated individuals.

Neonatal Screening

In many countries including the United States all babies are screened at birth for congenital adrenal hyperplasia. Treatment can be started much earlier, and potentially fatal adrenal crises can be prevented. However, there can be a high false positive rate and screening has not been adopted in the UK at present. This policy is still under review, but a recent British study [7] does not support the hypothesis that, in an unscreened population, males affected by salt wasting CAH are dying prior to diagnosis.

Summary

Congenital adrenal hyperplasia is an autosomal recessively inherited condition which presents in the newborn with virilisation of girls or salt-losing crises in boys. It is a lifelong condition which requires treatment with glucocorticoid and mineralocorticoid replacement, and lifelong support is required with full education, first of the parents, then the individuals themselves, around the nature of the condition, illnesses and emergency steroid management, growth, puberty and pregnancy.

References

1. Khalid JM, Oerton JM, Dezateux C, Hindmarsh PC, Kelnar CJ, Knowles RL. Incidence and clinical features of congenital adrenal hyperplasia in Great Britain. Arch Dis Child. 2012;97(2):101–6.
2. Joint LWPES/ESPE CAH Working Group. Consensus statement on 21-hydroxylase deficiency from the Lawson Wilkins Pediatric Endocrine Society and the European Society for Paediatric Endocrinology. J Clin Endocrinol Metab. 2002;87:4048–53.
3. Reisch N, Arlt W, Krone N. Health problems in congenital adrenal hyperplasia due to 21-hydroxylase deficiency. Horm Res Paediatr. 2011;76(2):73–85.
4. David H, Forest MG. Prenatal treatment of congenital adrenal hyperplasia resulting from 21-hydroxylase deficiency. J Pediatr. 1984;105:799–803.
5. Hirvikoski T, Nordenstrom A, Lindholm T, Lindblad F, Ritzen EM, Wedell A, Lajic S. Cognitive functions in children at risk for congenital adrenal hyperplasia treated prenatally with dexamethasone. J Clin Endocrinol Metab. 2007;92:542–8.

6. New MI, Tong YK, Yuen T, Jiang P, Pina C, Chan KC, Khattab A, Liao GJ, Yau M, Kim SM, Chiu RW, Sun L, Zaidi M, Lo YM. Noninvasive prenatal diagnosis of congenital adrenal hyperplasia using cell-free fetal DNA in maternal plasma. J Clin Endocrinol Metab. 2014;99(6):E1022-E1030.
7. Hird BE, Tetlow L, Tobi S, Patel L, Clayton PE. No evidence of an increase in early mortality from congenital adrenal hyperplasia in the absence of screening. Arch Dis Child. 2014;99(2):158–64.

Suggested Reading

Miller W. The adrenal cortex and its disorders. In: Brook C, Clayton P, Brown R, editors. Brook's clinical pediatric endocrinology. 6th ed. Oxford, UK: Wiley-Blackwell; 2010.

Female Infertility: Diagnosis and Management

Case 15

Akwasi A. Amoako and Adam H. Balen

Abstract

Infertility is defined as failure of a couple not using any form of contraception to conceive after 12 months of regular sexual intercourse. It constitutes a major social and psychological burden amongst couples, and the prevalence is increasing. Conditions in the female partner account for the majority of cases of infertility. This chapter summarises the different etiological factors in female infertility, baseline investigative evaluation and the management options for couples presenting with female factor infertility.

Keywords

Female infertility • Hypothyroidism • Ovulatory disorders • Hyperprolactinemia • Polycystic ovary syndrome

Case

A 33-year-old woman attends the infertility clinic with her 36-year-old partner with whom she has been cohabiting for the last 10 years. She was on the combined oral contraceptive pill (COCP) for the first 7 years of their relationship but came off it 3 years ago as they wanted to start a family. They have been trying unsuccessfully to conceive in the last 3 years despite regular (3–4 times a week), unprotected sexual intercourse.

> Questions
> 1. What is the current definition of infertility?
> 2. What is the difference between primary and secondary infertility?
> 3. Which aspects of this woman's history would you further explore?
> 4. List the causes of female infertility.

Infertility is a common and major clinical, social and public health problem, and is defined

A.A. Amoako, BSc, MBChB, PhD, MRCOG (✉)
A.H. Balen, MBBS, MD, DSc, FRCOG
Leeds Centre for Reproductive Medicine,
Department of Obstetrics and Gynaecology,
Leeds Teaching Hospitals, York Road, Leeds,
West Yorkshire, UK
e-mail: a.amoako@nhs.net; a.balen@nhs.net

as the inability of a couple to achieve conception after 12 months or more of regular (3–4 times per week), unprotected sexual intercourse. Eighty-five percent of couples in their twenties having regular sexual intercourse and not using contraception will achieve conception within 12 months, although this declines with increasing female age. In the United Kingdom, it is estimated that one in seven heterosexual couples of reproductive age group have difficulty conceiving. The prevalence is similar in developed countries (10–15 %) and appears to be increasing [1]. Infertility can be classified as primary, when there is no history of pregnancy having occurred in a couple even if one partner has had a pregnancy in a previous relationship, or secondary, when inability to conceive occurs after one or more conceptions irrespective of the outcome.

There are many causes of female infertility, the commonest being damage to the fallopian tubes secondary to previous infection (e.g., Chlamydia), anovulation and endometriosis. Modifiable lifestyle factors such as obesity, diet and exercise, alcohol, smoking and use of recreational drugs contribute significantly to female infertility. Smoking is associated with reduced ovarian reserve as well as development of embryos of poorer quality. In recent years, some women delay conception until well into their mid-30s for social, professional and financial reasons and therefore experience difficulty getting pregnant as a result of the natural decline in female fertility with age and concomitant increase in the rate of miscarriage, This is due to the decline in the genetic competence of the embryo, which in turn is secondary to a failure in the mechanisms that control normal cell division contained within the oocyte. Exposure to environmental chemicals and toxins such as mercury, cadmium, volatile organic solvents, pesticides and textile dyes has also been implicated [1].

Epidemiological data from the United Kingdom show that the male partner may be solely responsible for 30 % of cases of infertility and in 40 %, both male and female factors are present. No identifiable female or male factors are

Table 15.1 Causes of female infertility

Ovulatory disorders
Hypothalamic/pituitary failure
Hypothalamic/pituitary dysfunction
Ovarian failure
Tubal damage
Previous pelvic/abdominal surgery
Past peritonitis
Past Pelvic infections
Endometriosis
Congenital abnormalities
Uterine or peritoneal disorders
Fibroids
Endometrial polyps
Endometriosis
Modifiable lifestyle factors
Advanced female age, obesity, diet and exercise, alcohol, smoking and use of recreational drugs
Environmental factors
Exposure to chemicals and toxins such as mercury, cadmium, volatile organic solvents, pesticides and textile dyes has also been implicated

found in 25 % (unexplained infertility). Genital, endocrinological, developmental and general factors in the female partner causing infertility include ovulatory disorders (25 %), tubal damage from pelvic infections or endometriosis (20 %) and uterine or peritoneal disorders such as fibroids and endometriosis (10 %) [1] (Table 15.1).

The patient is currently unemployed but previously worked as a healthcare assistant. She is fit and well and has unremarkable medical and surgical history and currently not taking any regular medication. She has not had any prior exposure to any chemotherapy or radiotherapy. She started having periods at the age of 12 years and always had regular periods with a cycle length of 28 days, which continued to be the case whilst on the COCP. She has never been pregnant. Since discontinuing the COCP 3 years ago, her periods have been very infrequent with cycle length varying between 38 and 90 days. Her period lasts from 3 and 5 days, and she describes her menstrual flow as normal, with no associated dysmenorrhoea. She had a cervical smear 2 years ago that was reported as normal.

Questions

5. This patient's menstrual history suggests anovulation as the cause of her infertility. Discuss the causes of anovulatory infertility
6. What other aspects of the patient's history are relevant to establish the cause of her anovulation?

Ovulatory dysfunction is one of the commonest causes of female infertility accounting for 20–40 % of all causes of infertility. Ovulatory dysfunction is generally manifested by irregularity of menstrual periods characterised by absence of menstruation (amenorrhoea), infrequent menstruation (oligomenorrhoea) or excessive bleeding (dysfunctional uterine bleeding). Ovulatory dysfunction can be caused by many factors; however, the majority of cases are related to female hormonal imbalances. The World Health Organisation (WHO) has provided a classification system that divides ovulatory disorders into three distinct groups based on aetiological factors [1] (Table 15.2).

WHO group 1 anovulatory infertility is caused by disorders that result in hypothalamic-pituitary-gonadal axis failure. These include hypothalamic or pituitary tumours or infection, hypothalamic or pituitary irradiation, chemotherapy, head trauma, genetic defects such as Kallmann syndrome and functional hypothalamic amenorrhoea induced by excessive exercise, lean body mass, weight loss, severe dietary restriction, anorexia or bulimia nervosa and chronic illness. Individuals with WHO group 1 ovulatory disorder have low serum concentrations of follicle stimulation hormone (FSH), luteinising hormone (LH) and oestradiol (hypogonadotrophic hypogonadism) and present with amenorrhoea, which could be primary or secondary depending on the cause [2]. Those who are underweight or over-exercise may have low-normal concentrations of FSH with an LH that is suppressed to a greater degree.

Table 15.2 Classification of ovulatory disorders

Hypothalamic/pituitary failure (WHO group 1)
Idiopathic hypogonadotrophic hypogonadism
Kallmann's syndrome
Hypothalamic pituitary damage
Tumours (craniopharyngioma)
Cranial irradiation
Head injuries
Sarcoidosis
Tuberculosis
Anorexia
Excessive aerobic exercise
Severe systemic illness
Hyperprolactinaemia
Thyroid disease
Hypopituitarism
Cushing syndrome
Hypothalamic/pituitary dysfunction (WHO group 2)
Polycystic ovary syndrome (PCOS)
Ovarian failure (WHO group 3)
Idiopathic Premature ovarian insufficiency
Genetic causes
Turner syndrome
Fragile X syndrome
Toxic causes
Chemotherapy drugs
Radiation therapy
Viral infections (such as mumps)
Autoimmune diseases

Cushing's syndrome may present with chronic anovulation due to the inhibitory effect of high levels of cortisol releasing hormone (CRH) and adrenocorticotrophic hormone (ACTH) on hypothalamic-pituitary secretion. Congenital adrenal hyperplasia is also associated with anovulation and infertility due to secondary PCOS and hyperandrogenism, which inhibit the normal hormonal cycle. Elevation in serum 17 hydroxyprogesterone (17-OHP) and androstenedione are characteristic of CAH and disturb menstrual cyclicity, cervical mucus penetration by sperm and impair endometrial maturation and implantation.

Anovulatory infertility associated with conditions classified as WHO group 2 ovulatory disorders account for 85 % of cases of ovulatory infertility and results from hypothalamic-pituitary-ovarian dysfunction. The serum hormonal profile of these individuals will usually show normal FSH, normal or elevated LH and normal or high oestradiol levels (normogonadotrophic normogonadism) [3]. Polycystic ovary syndrome (PCOS) is the commonest cause of ovulatory disorders in this group of patients, accounting for 60–85 % of cases [4]. PCOS is a complex, heterogeneous endocrine disorder. It includes a spectrum of conditions rather than a single discrete disease. Symptoms vary widely in different individuals and include irregular or absent menses and associated anovulatory infertility, hyperandrogenism (hirsutism, alopecia and acne) and associated obesity. The criteria for the diagnosis of PCOS are based on a combination of clinical, ultrasound and biochemical criteria [5].

On further questioning she admitted to acne and severe and bothersome hirsutism involving her abdomen, face, chest, buttocks, legs and back. She initially tried shaving and waxing to remove her facial hair but this regrew quickly and her doctor has suggested referring her for laser treatment of her facial hair. In the last 4 years, she has noticed a rapid increase in her weight and she is thinking of joining the gym. She smokes one pack of cigarette a day and drinks 20 units of alcohol a week on average. Her mother and two of her older sisters have type 2 diabetes, but there is no history of infertility in the family. Her partner is fit and well and has an unremarkable medical and surgical history. He is a non-smoker and drinks alcohol socially. He has 1 child aged 12 years from a previous relationship. Examination revealed an obese woman with a body mass index of 35 kg/m^2 and a normal blood pressure of 125/75 mmHg. Significant hirsutism was noted on her face, chest, legs, and back. Also noticed were brown to black, poorly defined, velvety hyperpigmented areas in the lateral folds of the neck, the armpits and groin.

Questions
7. What is the likely diagnosis based on the history and examination findings and what are the differential diagnoses?
8. What are the salient features in the history that point to the diagnosis?

The likely diagnosis is PCOS. In 2003 the European Society for Human Reproduction and Embryology (ESHRE) and the American Society of Reproductive Medicine (ASRM) held a consensus meeting in Rotterdam and proposed that the diagnosis should be made if two out of three criteria are met: namely the presence of clinical or biochemical features of hyperandrogenism, oligo-ovulation or anovulation (in other words a menstrual cycle disturbance) and/or polycystic ovaries on ultrasound, once appropriate investigations have been performed to exclude other causes of menstrual disturbance and androgen excess [6]. The aetiology of PCOS has not been fully elucidated, but it is believed to be of multifactorial origin with insulin resistance, androgen excess, abnormal gonadotrophin secretion and genetic predisposition playing important roles. Obesity occurs in 40–50 % and has been implicated in the pathogenesis of PCOS [7] secondary to the development of insulin resistance and hyperinsulinaemia, which acts directly on the ovary to amplify the hyperandrogenism, interfering with folliculogenesis and resulting in anovulation and poor-quality oocytes [5].

The differential diagnosis of PCOS includes Cushing's syndrome, virilising adrenal tumour and late onset "non-classical" congenital adrenal hyperplasia (Table 15.3). Cushing's syndrome exhibits many clinical features similar those observed in PCOS, such as obesity, low sex hormone binding protein (SHBG), increased androgens, and hirsutism and anovulation. Cushing's syndrome is rare compared with PCOS and associated with other symptoms such as easy bruising, moon facies, buffalo hump, abdominal striae, hypertension, and proximal myopathy.

Table 15.3 Differential diagnoses of polycystic ovary syndrome

Ovarian hyperthecosis
Late-onset congenital adrenal hyperplasia
Cushing's syndrome
Androgen-producing ovarian tumour
Adrenal tumour

Premature ovarian insufficiency (formerly known as "premature ovarian failure") (WHO group 3) constitutes 5 % of ovulatory disorders and results from premature exhaustion of the ovarian primordial follicular pool and is characterised by amenorrhoea in women aged <40 years. The serum hormonal profile will show evidence of high gonadotropins and low oestradiol levels (hypergonadotrophic hypogonadism). Causes of premature ovarian failure include a number of genetic conditions such as Turner's syndrome and Fragile X syndrome, previous exposure to chemotherapy and radiotherapy, and autoimmune diseases such as type 1 diabetes mellitus, systemic lupus erythematosis and Addison's disease [3].

In recent times the measurement of anti-Müllerian hormone (AMH) has been used to assess ovarian reserve or the ovarian follicle pool, with low levels indicative of declining ovarian reserve and premature ovarian insufficiency, normal levels representing normal fertility potential and elevate levels often seen in women with polycystic ovaries.

You arranged a battery of investigations including day 1–3 follicle-stimulating hormone (FSH), luteinizing hormone (LH), oestradiol, thyroid function test, prolactin, testosterone, and sex hormone binding globulin (SHBG) and obtained the following results: FSH 5.6 iu/L, LH 23.4 iu/L, oestradiol 142 pmol/L, testosterone 3.1 nmol/L, TSH 1.4 miu/L, Free T4 13.8 pmol/L. She had an ultrasound scan that reported a normal-sized anteverted uterus with homogenous myometrial echotexture. Right ovarian volume was 17.5 mL and antral follicle count of 13. Left ovarian volume was 14.4 mL and antral follicle count of 15. A hysterosalpingogram to evaluate her fallopian tubes revealed evidence of bilateral tubal patency, and her partner had a seminal fluid analysis that was reported as normozoospermia. She was immune to Rubella and genitourinary infection, screening for both couples including Hepatitis B and C, HIV, HTLV, syphilis, Chlamydia and Gonorrhoea, did not reveal any evidence of current or past infection.

Questions
10. Comment on these results and discuss the general evaluation of an infertile patient.
11. Her anovulatory infertility is due polycystic ovary syndrome (PCOS). Discuss the treatment options for this patient's infertility.

Clinical evaluation should be offered to women <35 years who fail to conceive after 12 months of regular, unprotected sexual intercourse. However, consultation, and evaluation should be offered after 6 months of frequent, unprotected intercourse in women between 35 and 40 years of age and immediately in those over 40 years of age due to the dramatic decline in fertility as a result of ovarian aging. Earlier referral and evaluation are also required for female partners with known clinical causes of infertility such as history of oligomenorrhoea/amenorrhoea, past history of pelvic infection, previous pelvic surgery, past exposure to chemotherapy or radiotherapy and endometriosis [1]. The initial evaluation of the female partner requires a focused and detailed history that may identify simple problems or solutions to improve fertility that should cover: social history, current and past medical and surgical history, menstrual history, obstetric history, sexual and contraceptive history and family history (Table 15.4).

Examination of the female partner should include assessment of body mass index (BMI), signs of hyperandrogenism (hirsutism, acne, acanthosis nigricans, and male pattern baldness), and any abnormalities of the thyroid gland. A pelvic examination is indicated to look at the

Table 15.4 Focused history of the infertile female

Social history

Age, occupation, Personal and life-style history including exercise, stress, dieting, smoking, and alcohol use, recreational drugs and caffeine consumption

Medical history

Any current associated medical illness as diabetes and/or hypertension, drug intake prescribed as non-steroidal anti-inflammatory drugs, sex steroids and previous exposure to chemotherapy or radiotherapy

Menstrual history

Age of menarche, cycle regularity, menstrual loss, average number of days of menstrual loss, pain during menstruation, intermenstrual spotting and primary or secondary amenorrhoea

Surgical history

Ovarian cystectomy, appendicectomy, laparotomy, caesarean sections, and cervical surgery

Obstetric history

Duration of infertility and results of previous evaluations and therapy, previous pregnancies and outcomes

Contraceptive and sexual history

Previous contraceptive methods, past sexually transmitted diseases, recent cervical smear, coital frequency and difficult or painful coitus

Family history

Consanguinity, diabetes mellitus, hypertension, twins delivery, early menopause

Table 15.5 Evaluation of female infertility

Baseline investigations

Rubella status

Cervical smear

Chlamydia serology

HVS for M C&S

Cervical swab and/or early morning urine sample for chlamydia and gonococcal antigens

Assessment of ovulatory function

Menstrual history

Mid luteal phase serum progesterone (days 21–23 of menstrual cycle or 7 days before expected menses)

Urinary luteinizing hormone (LH) determination

Transvaginal ultrasound follicular monitoring

Assessment of ovarian reserve

Early follicular phase FSH, LH and oestradiol E2 (days 1–3 of the menstrual cycle)

Early follicular phase antral follicle count (transvaginal USS)

Serum anti-mullerian hormone (AMH) level

Assessment of tubal patency

Hysterosalpingography (HSG)

Laparoscopy and dye test

Hysterocontrast sonography (HyCoSy)

Assessment of uterine abnormalities and peritoneal factors

Transvaginal ultrasonography

Laparoscopy

Hysteroscopy

vagina and cervix for any abnormalities and to perform an infection screen and a Pap smear if required. Bimanual examination of the uterus and adnexa will reveal uterine size, position, regularity and mobility and evidence of endometriosis or pelvic adhesions such as tenderness, fixity of the pelvic organs and nodules [1, 8].

Diagnostic Evaluation

A complete basic evaluation needs to be performed assessing ovulation, tubal patency and uterine morphology (Table 15.5). Baseline investigations should include Rubella immunity status, cervical smear in the last 3 years, genitourinary infection screening (Chlamydia serology, high vaginal swab for microscopy culture and sensitivity, cervical swab and/or early

morning urine sample for Chlamydia antigen, HIV, Hepatitis B&C and syphilis). Women with BMI $\geq$25–30 kg/m^2 should have an assessment of HbA1c or an oral glucose tolerance test, depending upon ethnicity and local policy. Semen analysis should be performed on the male partner even if he has fathered previous pregnancies [1].

Assessment of Ovulatory Function and Ovarian Reserve

Menstrual history can give valuable clues and yield the diagnosis of anovulation. A history of regular menstrual cycles (every 25–35 days) and moliminal symptoms (e.g., breast tenderness, bloating, cramping, mood changes) are compatible with ovulation in at least 95 % of women. Luteal phase serum progesterone can confirm ovulation in women with regular menstrual cycles (day 21–23 of the cycle or 7 days before expected menses). This is not necessary in women with very long and irregular cycles, as they already have evidence of ovulatory dysfunction [1, 8]. In all women with ovulatory dysfunction, TSH and prolactin assessments are indicated to exclude thyroid dysfunction and hyperprolactinaemia, respectively. Women with clinical features of anovulation, menstrual disturbances and hyperandrogenic features should have assessment of testosterone. Sex hormone binding globulin is suppressed in those who are hyperinsulinaemic and can be measured as a surrogate marker for insulin resistance as it is also a good predictor for the development of gestational DM [8].

Assessment of ovarian reserve provides prognostic information, helps to direct treatment, help to predict response to ovarian stimulation and likelihood of successful pregnancy with assisted reproductive technology especially in women at risk of diminished ovarian reserve. Serum FSH, LH and oestradiol levels provide initial assessment of ovarian reserve if performed on days 1–3 of the menstrual cycle. Transvaginal ultrasound imaging of the ovary to determine the antral follicle count (AFC) in the early follicular phase and serum antimullerian hormone (AMH) level provides additional and more accurate information on ovarian reserve [8, 9].

Assessment of Uterine Abnormalities and Fallopian Tube Patency

Hysterosalpingogram is the first-line investigation to rule out tubal occlusion in those with a short period of infertility (<2 years) and no risk factors for tubal disease such as a past history of Chlamydial infection or peritonitis and also for patients who are "at surgical or anaesthetic risk for a laparoscopy" (e.g., raised BMI, complicating medical disorders, past lower abdominal/pelvic surgery). Some patients may opt for this approach as a less invasive option, and their choice should be respected even if there are risk factors suggesting pelvic pathology. Diagnostic laparoscopy and dye test are the gold standard in assessing the pelvic anatomy and tubal patency.

It is preferable over HSG in patients with risk factors for pelvic pathology, those with a longer history of infertility, and in women over the age of 35 years. Some patients may also choose to have it as it provides a definitive diagnosis and reassurance. A diagnostic hysteroscopy should be performed at the same time to provide information about the endometrial cavity [1].

Treatment of Infertility

Treatment of female infertility depends on the cause. Women presenting with infertility should be counselled regarding the impact of lifestyle choices on fertility including smoking cessation, weight control, and avoidance of alcohol and recreational drugs. A serum rubella titre should be measured to check rubella immunity status and if non-immune a booster vaccination should be given and the patient advised to avoid pregnancy for 1 month from the last dose of vaccination. In addition, all women considering pregnancy should take folic acid to reduce the chances of having babies with neural tube defects (400 mcg daily unless obese, on anti-epileptics or past history of an affected child when the dose should be 5 mg daily) [1, 8].

Anovulatory infertility resulting from weight disorders should be addressed by weight normalisation. Hypogonadotrophic anovulation can be treated with pulsatile subcutaneous gonadotrophin releasing hormone administration, which unfortunately is no longer available in the UK or alternatively gonadotropin preparations containing FSH and LH (either human menopausal gonadotorphins [hMG] or both recombinant FSH and LH combined, as FSH alone will not be effective) [2]. Normal female anatomy, patent fallopian tubes and semen analysis should be confirmed prior to ovulation induction.

Endocrine disorders such as hyperprolactinaemia and hypothyroidism should be treated with dopamine agonists and thyroxine, respectively, and if anovulation is still persistent after normalisation of endocrine profile, then ovulation induction should be considered.

Women with PCOS who are overweight should be advised to lose weight before commencing ovulation induction. Exercise and weight loss have so far been the most physiological way to improve insulin sensitivity, and improve the metabolic abnormalities associated with the syndrome. In women with PCOS it has been demonstrated that even relatively modest weight loss improves the hormonal profile and improvement in the reproductive outcome for all forms of fertility treatment. The anti-oestrogen clomiphene citrate is the first-line agent used in ovulation induction for patients with PCOS. It is simple to administer, cheap, safe and effective in achieving ovulation. Clomiphene citrate (50–100 mg) is administered days 2–6 of a natural or artificially induced bleed. Whilst clomiphene is successful in inducing ovulation in over 80 % of women, pregnancy only occurs in about 40 %, probably due to its anti-oestrogenic effect on the endometrium [10, 11]. Ultrasound monitoring is required to confirm a response and minimise the risk of multiple pregnancy, which is approximately 10 %. The cumulative chance of conceptions is approximately 60–70 % after six cycles of treatment. Amenorrhoeic women should be given a progestogen to induce a withdrawal bleed before starting treatment.

The therapeutic options for patients with anovulatory infertility who are resistant to anti-oestrogens are either parenteral gonadotrophin therapy or laparoscopic ovarian diathermy. Because the polycystic ovary is very sensitive to stimulation by exogenous hormones, it is very important to start with very low doses of gonadotrophins, and follicular development must be carefully monitored by ultrasound scans. The advent of transvaginal ultrasonography has enabled the multiple pregnancy rate to be reduced to approximately 5 %. Cumulative conception and livebirth rates after 6 months may be 65 and 50 %, respectively, and after 12 months 75 and 60 %, respectively. Close monitoring should enable treatment to be suspended if three or more mature follicles develop, as the risk of multiple pregnancy obviously increases [10].

Laparoscopic ovarian diathermy is free of the risks of multiple pregnancy and ovarian hyperstimulation and does not require intensive ultrasound monitoring. Laparoscopic ovarian diathermy has taken the place of wedge resection of the ovaries (which resulted in extensive peri-ovarian and tubal adhesions), and it appears to be as effective as routine gonadotrophin therapy in the treatment of clomiphene-insensitive PCOS, although time to pregnancy is a little slower [10, 12].

There has been much publicity about the use of metformin for PCOS. Metformin does not appear to induce weight loss, although coincident weight loss will of course provide additional benefit. Indeed we have performed a large RCT to look at metformin versus placebo and found no benefit from metformin over 6 months with regard to either menstrual control or other symptoms [13]. Those who improved were women who lost weight whether on metformin or placebo. Two large RCTs have also demonstrated no benefit from metformin when combined with clomiphene citrate [14, 15]. Therefore, metformin does not appear to hold the promise that was initially presumed and a recent Cochrane meta-analysis confirms this to be the case [16]. We therefore only advise metformin therapy in women with impaired glucose tolerance or type 2 diabetes. The mainstay of fertility treatment for women with premature ovarian insufficiency is oocyte donation if culturally and socially acceptable [1].

In vitro fertilisation and embryo transfer (IVF-ET) should be considered in cases of unexplained infertility, tubal factors and those who fail to ovulate or achieve conception following ovulation induction. IVF can be combined with intracytoplasmic sperm injection (ICSI) where male factor infertility is present [1].

References

1. Fertility: assessment and treatment for people with fertility problems. NICE clinical guideline 156. Issued Feb 2013.
2. Yasmin E, Davies M, Conway G, Balen AH, British Fertility Society. Ovulation induction in WHO Type 1 anovulation: guidelines for practice. Hum Fertil (Camb). 2013;16(4):228–34.

3. Weiss RV, Clapauch R. Female infertility of endocrine origin. Arq Bras Endocrinol Metabol. 2014;58(2): 144–52.

4. ESHRE Capri Workshop Group. Health and fertility in World Health Organization group 2 anovulatory women. Hum Reprod Update. 2012;18(5):586–99.

5. Fauser BC, Tarlatzis BC, Rebar RW, Legro RS, Balen AH, Lobo R, Carmina E, et al. Consensus on women's health aspects of polycystic ovary syndrome (PCOS): the Amsterdam ESHRE/ASRM-Sponsored 3rd PCOS Consensus Workshop Group. Fertil Steril. 2012;97(1): 28–38.

6. Rotterdam ESHRE/ASRM-Sponsored PCOS Consensus Workshop Group. Revised 2003 consensus on diagnostic criteria and long-term health risks related to polycystic ovary syndrome. Hum Reprod. 2004;19:41–7.

7. Ben-Shlomo I, Younis JS. Basic research in PCOS: are we reaching new frontiers? Reprod Biomed Online. 2014;28(6):669–83.

8. The Practice Committee of the American Society for Reproductive Medicine. Diagnostic evaluation of the infertile female: a committee opinion. Fertil Steril. 2012;98(2):302–7.

9. Broekmans FJ, Verweij PJ, Eijkemans MJ, Mannaerts BM, Witjes H. Prognostic models for high and low ovarian responses in controlled ovarian stimulation using a GnRH antagonist protocol. Hum Reprod. 2014;29(8):1688–97.

10. Farquhar C, Brown J, Marjoribanks J. Laparoscopic drilling by diathermy or laser for ovulation induction in anovulatory polycystic ovary syndrome. Cochrane Database Syst Rev. 2012;(6):CD001122.

11. Balen AH. Ovulation induction in the management of anovulatory polycystic ovary syndrome. Mol Cell Endocrinol. 2013;373(1–2):77–82.

12. Homburg R, Hendriks ML, König TE, Anderson RA, Balen AH, Brincat M, Child T, et al. Clomifene citrate or low-dose FSH for the first-line treatment of infertile women with anovulation associated with polycystic ovary syndrome: a prospective randomized multinational study. Hum Reprod. 2012;27(2):468–73.

13. Tang T, Glanville J, Barth J, Hayden C, Balen AH. Combined lifestyle modification and metformin in obese patients with polycystic ovary syndrome. A randomised, placebo-controlled, double-blind multicentre study. Hum Reprod. 2006;21:80–9.

14. Moll E, Bossuyt PM, Korevaar JC, Lambalk CB, van der Veen F. Effect of clomifene citrate plus metformin and clomifene citrate plus placebo on induction of ovulation in women with newly diagnosed polycystic ovary syndrome: randomised double blind clinical trial. BMJ. 2006;332(7556):1485.

15. Legro RS, Barnhart HX, Schlaff WD, Carr BR, Diamond MP, Carson SA, Steinkampf MP, et al.; Cooperative Multicenter Reproductive Medicine Network. Clomiphene, metformin, or both for infertility in the polycystic ovary syndrome. N Engl J Med. 2007;356(6):551–66.

16. Tang T, Lord JM, Norman RJ, Yasmin E, Balen AH. Insulin-sensitising drugs (metformin, rosiglitazone, pioglitazone, Dchiro-inositol) for women with polycystic ovary syndrome, oligo amenorrhoea and subfertility. Cochrane Database Syst Rev. 2012;(5):CD003053. doi:10.1002/14651858.CD003053.pub5.

Diagnosis and Management of Hypocalcaemia in Adults

Afroze Abbas

Abstract

Extracellular calcium is important for the regulation of several important biological systems, particularly muscle function, intracellular signalling and coagulation. Serum calcium levels are therefore maintained in a tight physiological range, largely by parathyroid hormone (PTH) and vitamin D. Hypocalcaemia has many causes, the commonest of which are vitamin D deficiency, malabsorption, chronic kidney disease, hypoparathyroidism and acute severe illness. Acute severe hypocalcaemia is a medical emergency, and may manifest with muscle spasm, tetany, seizures or cardiac arrhythmias. In patients with hypoparathyroidism, long-term maintenance therapy with oral calcium and vitamin D metabolites is indicated. Care should be taken to restore serum calcium levels to low-normal levels, whilst avoiding hypercalciuria and the development of undesirable renal sequelae.

Keywords

Hypocalcaemia • Parathyroid hormone (PTH) • Vitamin D • Hypoparathyroidism • Pseudohypoparathyroidism • Calcitriol

Presenting History

A 65-year-old gentleman presents with a 3-month history of progressive fatigue, poor appetite, muscle cramps and spasms. He feels low in mood, and has been increasingly muddled. On direct questioning he describes paraesthesia in his fingers and numbness around his mouth. He describes having had treatment (chemotherapy, radiotherapy and operative intervention) for oesophageal cancer approximately 18 months previously.

A. Abbas, BSc (Hons), MBChB, MRCP, PhD
Leeds Centre for Diabetes & Endocrinology,
Leeds Teaching Hospitals NHS Trust,
Beckett Street, Leeds, West Yorkshire LS9 7TF, UK
e-mail: afroze.abbas@leedsth.nhs.uk

R. Ajjan, S.M. Orme (eds.), *Endocrinology and Diabetes: Case Studies, Questions and Commentaries*,
DOI 10.1007/978-1-4471-2789-5_16, © Springer-Verlag London 2015

Table 16.1 Aetiology of hypocalcaemia in adults

Low PTH	High PTH	Others
Destruction of parathyroid glands by surgery or radioactive iodine	Vitamin D deficiency or resistance	Hypomagnesaemia
Autoimmune destruction of parathyroid glands	Chronic kidney disease	Drugs
Irradiation or infiltration of parathyroid glands	PTH resistance	Spurious hypocalcaemia (assay interference)
Abnormal parathyroid gland development	Extravascular calcium deposition	
Abnormal PTH regulation	Severe sepsis or pancreatitis	
HIV infection	Tumour lysis syndrome	
Hungry bone syndrome (post parathyroidectomy)	Malabsorption	

The symptoms he describes are consistent with progressive hypocalcaemia over at least the last 3 months. Recent surgical and radiotherapy to his neck raise the possibility of acquired and worsening parathyroid gland damage.

What Are the Additional Questions to Be Asked?

The diagnostic approach to hypocalcaemia is based upon distinguishing between the numerous potential causes. Therefore, a careful history is a crucial part of this evaluation. Table 16.1 summarises the more common causes of hypocalcaemia.

Is the problem acute or chronic?

If the problem seems to be of acute onset in adult life it is more likely to be acquired. Acquired hypoparathyroidism tends to be the consequence of postsurgical or autoimmune damage. Other acute causes may be related to change in medications or recent new illness.

Is there evidence of malabsorption?

Ask specifically about symptoms of gastrointestinal disease consistent with malabsorption, lactose intolerance or a history of coeliac disease may be a predisposing factor to hypocalcaemia. Patients with gastro-oesophageal reflux disease or peptic ulcer disease tend to be on proton pump inhibitor therapy which has been associated with hypomagnesaemia, which in turn may cause hypocalcaemia.

Is there a deficiency in calcium intake?

If poor dietary intake of calcium is suspected, using a calcium calculator to calculate daily intake of calcium may be useful as part of the history. Poor calcium intake with concurrent vitamin D deficiency or coeliac disease can present with clinically significant hypocalcaemia.

Is there a history of other autoimmune conditions?

The presence of other autoimmune conditions, such as thyroid disease, adrenal insufficiency, coeliac disease, would point towards an autoimmune cause of hypocalcaemia.

What is the past medical history?

Conditions such as chronic kidney disease, cancer (particularly with bone metastases), pancreatitis, rhabdomyolysis, recent severe illness and HIV may predispose towards hypocalcaemia. Is there a history of granulomatous disorders or infiltrative disease (e.g., haemochromatosis, Wilson's disease)?

Is there a history of surgery, irradiation or cancer in head or neck?

Recent parathyroidectomy, or previous operations on thyroid or head and neck cancers in the past may have led to postsurgical parathyroid damage leading to hypocalcaemia.

Is there a family history?

A family history of hypocalcaemia may suggest a genetic cause such as an activating mutation of the calcium sensing receptor (CaSR), parathyroid hormone resistance or polyglandular autoimmune syndrome type 1. The presence of chronic mucocutaneous candidiasis and adrenal insufficiency would support a diagnosis of polyglandular autoimmune syndrome type 1.

What medication does the patient take?

Drugs associated with hypocalcaemia include, calcium chelators (citrate given during plasma exchange or large volume blood transfusion), cinacalcet, denosumab, phenytoin and bisphosphonates. Use of chemotherapy, especially cisplatin or leucovorin with 5-fluouracil is associated with hypocalcaemia. Foscarnet, an antiviral drug used in cytomegalovirus infections, may also cause symptomatic hypocalcaemia.

The patient denied any further symptoms. His chemotherapy regimen had used cisplatin, but he did not have symptoms consistent with hypocalcaemia at the time. Interestingly, he had been started on a proton pump inhibitor following oesophageal surgery. He was taking calcium carbonate supplements infrequently.

What Signs to Look Out For?

On examination the patient was of slim build with a BMI 21.3 kg/m^2. There was evidence of laryngectomy and stoma, with assisted speech. No neck masses or lymphadenopathy were evident. The patient was alert and orientated to time, place and person. Carpopedal spasm was provoked with inflation of a sphygmomanometer cuff (Trousseau's sign). Chvostek's sign was negative. There were no dental or bone abnormalities. An ECG did not show evidence of prolonged QT interval.

The symptoms and signs of hypocalcaemia are dependent on the severity, duration and rate of development of hypocalcaemia. Some patients may have no neuromuscular symptoms, and others may have non-specific symptoms such as fatigue, anxiety and low mood. A corrected calcium level of <1.9 mmol/L may lead to the acute symptoms described below.

Acute Symptoms and Signs

Acute hypocalcaemia leads to hyperexcitability of neurones and the development of tetany. Initially mild symptoms may predominate, such as peri-oral numbness, paraesthesia of the extremities and muscle spasms. Hyperventilation may result, which leads to alkalosis, which can exacerbate tetany.

More severe tetany may manifest as carpopedal spasm, seizures and laryngospasm. Carpopedal spasm involves flexion of the metacarpophalangeal joints and wrists with associated extension of the fingers and adduction of the thumb.

If the onset of hypocalcaemia is gradual, the patient is likely to have fewer symptoms.

The classical signs of hypocalcaemia are Trousseau's sign and Chvostek's sign. However, both may be negative, even in significant acute hypocalcaemia.

Trousseau's sign is the induction of carpopedal spasm by inflation of a sphygmomanometer above systolic blood pressure for 3 min.

Chvostek's sign is a contraction of facial muscles caused by tapping the facial nerve in front of the ear.

The cardiovascular system is highly sensitive to changes in calcium concentrations. Decreased cardiac output, heart failure and hypotension have all been associated with hypocalcaemia.

Table 16.2 Laboratory results in hypocalcaemia

	PTH	Corrected serum calcium	Phosphate	25-hydroxy vitamin D	Magnesium
Vitamin D deficiency	High	Low or normal	Low or normal	Low	Normal
Chronic kidney disease	High	Low	High	Low or normal	Normal
Hypoparathyroidism	Low	Low	High	Normal	Normal
Hypomagnesaemia	Low or normal	Low	Normal	Normal	Low
Activating CaSR mutation	Low or normal	Low	High	Normal	Normal
PTH resistance	High	Low	High	Normal	Normal

This impairment of myocardial function seems to be reversible with correction of hypocalcaemia. Hypocalcaemia is also associated with prolongation of the QT interval on the electrocardiograph. This may be associated with the onset of arrhythmias, particularly Torsade de Pointes.

Psychiatric symptoms such as acute confusional states, hallucinations and psychosis are rarely associated with severe hypocalcaemia.

Another sign of severe, acute hypocalcaemia is papilloedema. This again is usually reversible with correction of serum calcium concentration.

Chronic Hypocalcaemia

Chronic hypocalcaemia has multiple effects and is often specific to the underlying cause.

Dry, coarse skin, brittle nails, and sparse hair with alopecia may all be manifestations of chronic hypocalcaemia.

Longstanding hypoparathyroidism may lead to basal ganglia calcification (detectable on CT scan), which can then lead to movement disorders or Parkinsonism.

If hypocalcaemia is particularly longstanding, dental abnormalities such as dental hypoplasia and defective enamel and root formation may occur. PTH resistance is often associated with numerous developmental skeletal abnormalities.

Diffuse bone pain, muscle weakness and bone tenderness as a result of chronic hypocalcaemia secondary to osteomalacia is possible.

What Tests are Needed to Reach a Diagnosis?

Initial investigations showed that the patient had an adjusted calcium of 1.83 mmol/L (2.2–2.6 mmol/L). PTH was undetectable, total hydroxy-vitamin D

levels were low at 25 nmol/L (50–100 nmol/L), magnesium levels were also below the reference range at 0.53 mmol/L (0.7–1.0 mmol/L). Renal function and albumin were normal. Serum phosphate levels were marginally elevated.

The first step in establishing the diagnosis is to recheck calcium levels with measurement of the serum albumin concentration. Calcium is bound to proteins, mainly albumin. Therefore, total serum calcium concentrations in patients with abnormal albumin levels may not be representative of ionised (or free) calcium concentrations. Most labs will provide a corrected calcium concentration which takes this into account. Each 1 g/dL reduction in serum albumin concentration will lower total calcium concentration by approximately 0.2 mmol/L.

Repeating calcium levels will also verify that the initial measurement is correct and that we are dealing with true hypocalcaemia. Previous corrected calcium measurements, if available, should also be reviewed, as these may give an indication as to the chronicity of the problem.

Measurement of intact PTH is crucial in all cases of hypocalcaemia. Serum intact PTH measurements should be measured with simultaneous serum calcium. Serum PTH values vary according to the underlying cause of the hypocalcaemia (Table 16.2). Hypocalcaemia is a major stimulus for PTH secretion; therefore, hypocalcaemia with a low or normal serum PTH concentration is strong evidence of hypoparathyroidism.

Other tests that may help narrow the differential diagnosis include creatinine, phosphate, serum magnesium, 25 hydroxy-vitamin D, alkaline phosphatase, amylase and urinary calcium excretion.

Vitamin D

Measurement of serum 25-hydroxyvitamin D is appropriate in hypocalcaemia with high

PTH. Vitamin D deficiency leads to decreased intestinal calcium absorption, resulting in hypocalcaemia and consequent increased PTH concentration. 1,25-dihydroxyvitamin D (calcitriol) is an inhibitor of PTH production, reduced levels of calcitriol may also therefore contribute to the observed secondary hyperparathyroidism.

A low serum 25 hydroxy-vitamin D concentration in a patient with hypocalcaemia and hypophosphataemia may indicate vitamin D intake, absorption or production are impaired. Other contributory factors to vitamin D deficiency may include use of phenytoin or any condition leading to hypoproteinaemia (due to loss of vitamin D binding protein).

In chronic kidney disease 1,25-dihydroxyvitamin D concentrations are low due to impaired PTH action on the kidneys. This also results in hyperphosphataemia, due to impaired PTH action on urinary phosphate excretion. Other causes of hypocalcaemia with secondary hyperparathyroidism are usually associated with low or low-normal serum phosphate as renal PTH sensitivity remains intact.

Magnesium

Hypomagnesaemia impairs parathyroid secretory function, so may lead to hypocalcaemia by inducing PTH resistance or deficiency. Therefore, serum magnesium should be measured in patients in whom the cause of hypocalcaemia is unclear. Correction of hypomagnesaemia in these cases usually leads to quick resolution of hypocalcaemia. Patients at high risk of hypomagnesaemia include those with chronic malabsorption, alcoholism and patients on proton pump inhibitor therapy. Proton pump inhibitors reduce gastric acid secretion which leads to impaired magnesium absorption.

Parathyroid Hormone (PTH)

PTH is a potent stimulus for urinary phosphate excretion. In the absence of PTH or resistance to its action this stimulatory effect is lost, leading to hyperphosphataemia, and low fractional excretion of phosphate. Hyperphosphataemia and hypocalcaemia in the absence of chronic kidney disease, rhabdomyolysis or tumour lysis syndrome are strongly suggestive of either hypoparathyroidism or PTH resistance.

Phosphate

If serum phosphate concentrations are low with concurrent hypocalcaemia this usually implies either secondary hyperparathyroidism (e.g., vitamin D deficiency) or low dietary intake of phosphate. Serum phosphate tends to be high in hypoparathyroidism, PTH resistance or chronic kidney disease, due to reduced fractional excretion of phosphate from the kidneys.

Others

Pancreatitis may be associated with hypocalcaemia, therefore if clinically suspected, testing amylase levels may be appropriate.

Twenty-four hours urinary excretion of calcium would normally show low urinary calcium in patients with untreated hypoparathyroidism and vitamin D deficiency.

Elevated serum alkaline phosphatase (bone origin), with hypocalcaemia, is a frequent finding in osteomalacia. It may also be a finding in osteoblastic bone metastases.

Discussion of the Results and Final Diagnosis

The results obtained in our patient are consistent with hypoparathyroidism, given the undetectable PTH levels and concurrent hypocalcaemia with elevated serum phosphate. The most likely cause for this is acquired damage to parathyroid glands as a result of surgery and radiotherapy. The fact that he had only become symptomatic several months after the treatment for his oesophageal cancer suggests that progressive damage from the radiotherapy may be the most likely aetiology in combination with poor compliance with calcium carbonate therapy. However, infiltrative disease was excluded with further cross-sectional imaging of the neck. Further tests for other causes of hypocalcaemia were negative. The hypocalcaemia may have been exacerbated by his low vitamin D status, and this was corrected with colecalciferol. The low magnesium levels were corrected and proton pump inhibitor discontinued, but this was not felt to be a significant causative factor in this case given the continued absence of any parathyroid hormone secretion. Once calcium levels were stabilised with intravenous calcium therapy, maintenance therapy with oral calcium carbonate and calcitriol was initiated with the restoration of a low-normal serum calcium level and alleviation of symptoms as the main goal of therapy. Long-term follow-up in the metabolic bone clinic is underway, with particular emphasis on monitoring urinary calcium excretion and development of nephrocalcinosis or renal failure.

Treatment of Hypocalcaemia

The treatment of hypocalcaemia may be divided into the management of acute, symptomatic hypocalcaemia versus the treatment of largely asymptomatic or chronic hypocalcaemia. The optimal treatment also depends in large part on the underlying cause for hypocalcaemia.

Treatment of Acute Hypocalcaemia

In the acute setting when confronted with a patient who has had an acute fall in calcium levels, and is symptomatic, the immediate goal of therapy is to rapidly elevate calcium levels back towards the normal reference range. There is a lack of randomised controlled trial evidence for the optimal treatment algorithms to do this, however most institutions would advocate the use of IV calcium for symptomatic patients (carpopedal spasm, bradycardia, seizures, etc.), patients with prolonged QT on ECG or asymptomatic patients with an acute decrease in calcium levels <1.9 mmol/L.

Initially 10 ml intravenous calcium gluconate 10 % or calcium chloride 10 % may be infused over 15–20 min with cardiac monitoring. Rapid administration of IV calcium solutions may provoke cardiac dysfunction, so should be undertaken with caution. The half-life of intravenous calcium infusions is short (2–3 h), so further therapy is likely to be required.

Following this, if necessary, a prolonged calcium gluconate infusion may be given aiming to deliver between 0.5 and 1.5 mg/kg of calcium per hour depending on patient requirements and response to therapy. If a prolonged calcium infusion is required, this is usually best delivered via a large peripheral vein or central vein, as calcium solutions are highly irritant to veins. Calcium gluconate is usually dissolved in either a dextrose solution or saline. They should never be given in the same IV line as bicarbonate or phosphate due to the risk of precipitation of calcium salts.

For those patients with milder symptoms, or calcium concentrations >1.9 mmol/L oral calcium supplementation should be used, at a dose of between 1,500 and 2,000 mg of elemental calcium daily.

Treating the Cause of Hypocalcaemia

Hypoparathyroidism
Hypoparathyroidism occurs if there is destruction of the parathyroid glands, abnormal parathyroid gland development or altered PTH action/secretion. Most patients with hypoparathyroidism require lifelong calcium and vitamin D supplementation. The aim of therapy in this scenario is to relieve symptoms of hypocalcaemia, by raising calcium levels to the low-normal range, without causing significant hypercalciuria.

If the underlying cause of hypocalcaemia is vitamin D deficiency or hypoparathyroidism, concurrent use of vitamin D or its metabolites is advocated. PTH is required for the renal conversion of calcidiol (25-hydroxyvitamin D) to the active metabolite calcitriol (1,25-dihydroxyvitamin D), so patients with hypoparathyroidism or chronic kidney disease are usually treated with calcitriol. This is used at a starting dose of 0.25–0.5 mcg twice daily in these scenarios, due to its rapid onset of action. The biological half-life of calcitriol is 4–6 h. Vitamin D requirements vary from person to person and the correct amount is arrived at by careful monitoring of response (initially weekly) and adjustment of doses until desired stable calcium and phosphate levels are reached.

Hypercalcaemia and hypercalciuria are potential consequences of inappropriate therapy with vitamin D metabolites. Hypercalciuria occurs as patients with hypoparathyroidism lack the usual stimulatory effect of PTH on renal calcium reabsorption. This can lead to renal calculi formation, nephrocalcinosis and renal failure. Patients on long-term therapy with vitamin D metabolites should be regularly monitored for the development of these complications. Once levels are stable serum and urinary calcium levels should be checked at least annually. If hypercalciuria is problematic, a thiazide diuretic may be used to reduce urinary calcium excretion.

Recombinant human PTH is currently being investigated as a treatment for hypoparathyroidism, but is not yet approved for this indication.

Vitamin D Deficiency

Vitamin D deficiency (vitamin D <20 nmol/L) is usually treated with dietary and lifestyle (sun exposure) advice in conjunction with oral colecalciferol (vitamin D3). Several different regimens are available for correction of vitamin D with colecalciferol. Most involve the administration of approximately 300,000 units of vitamin D3 over a 6-week period. Once vitamin D levels have been restored (total vitamin D 50–100 nmol/L), maintenance therapy is often required. Calcium levels should be monitored whilst loading with colecalciferol, as rarely hypercalcaemia can be an issue.

Hypomagnesaemia

If magnesium concentrations are found to be low, this is best corrected concurrently with correction of hypocalcaemia. Hypocalcaemia is likely to be resistant until magnesium concentrations have been rectified. Intravenous magnesium replacement should be considered in patients with magnesium levels <0.4 mmol/L. Local guidelines for magnesium replacement should be adhered to. Persistent hypomagnesaemia (as sometimes seen with malabsorption) should be treated with long-term oral magnesium (usually 300–400 mg magnesium daily in divided doses).

Autosomal Dominant Hypocalcaemia

This is a rare disorder where an activating mutation in the CaSR (calcium-sensing receptor) leads to inappropriately high urinary calcium excretion in the context of hypocalcaemia. Increasing serum calcium in this situation increases urinary calcium excretion further and predisposes the patient to nephrocalcinosis and renal failure. In this condition, treatment is aimed at alleviating any symptoms, therefore restoration of serum calcium levels to normal may not be necessary. In the future, novel therapies such as recombinant PTH therapy or calcilytics (which inhibit CaSR function) may be able to normalise serum calcium levels without causing increased urinary calcium excretion.

Pseudohypoparathyroidism

End-organ resistance to the actions of PTH presents with hypocalcaemia, hyperphosphataemia and elevated PTH levels. This group of disorders is treated in a similar manner to hypoparathyroidism (see above). However, this group of patients are less likely to develop significant hypercalciuria with maintenance calcium and vitamin D therapy, compared to those with hypoparathyroidism. As such the goal of therapy is to normalise calcium levels. Patients with pseudohypoparathyroidism may also have other endocrine conditions, so assessment of gonadal and thyroid function is warranted.

Suggested Reading

Cooper MS, Gittoes NJ. Diagnosis and management of hypocalcaemia. BMJ. 2008;336:1298.

Hannan FM, Thakker RV. Investigating hypocalcaemia. BMJ. 2013;346:2213.

Kurokawa K. Calcium-regulating hormones and the kidney. Kidney Int. 1987;136:52.

Mantovani G. Clinical review: pseudohypoparathyroidism: diagnosis and treatment. J Clin Endocrinol Metab. 2011;96:3020.

Riccardi D, Brown EM. Physiology and pathophysiology of the calcium-sensing receptor in the kidney. Am J Physiol Renal Physiol. 2010;298:485.

Rubin MR, Levine MA. Hypoparathyroidism and pseudohypoparathyroidism, Chapter 75. In: Primer on the metabolic bone diseases and disorders of mineral metabolism. 7th ed. Washington, DC: American Society of Bone and Mineral Research; 2014. p. 354.

Shoback D. Clinical practice. Hypoparathyroidism. N Engl J Med. 2008;359:391.

Shoback D. Hypocalcaemia: definition, etiology, pathogenesis, diagnosis and management, Chapter 68. In: Primer on the metabolic bone diseases and disorders of mineral metabolism. 7th ed. Washington, DC: American Society of Bone and Mineral Research; 2014. p. 313.

Tohme JF, Bilezikan JP. Hypocalcaemic emergencies. Endocrinol Metab Clin North Am. 1993;22:363.

Hypoglycaemia Case Study

Case 17

Nicola N. Zammitt and Brian M. Frier

Abstract

The case of a 38-year-old woman with Addison's disease, diabetes and recurrent severe hypoglycaemia is described. After some initial diagnostic uncertainty, it was confirmed that she had autoimmune diabetes. She subsequently developed recurrent episodes of severe hypoglycaemia with few or no warning symptoms. The options for managing this scenario are discussed, including increased blood glucose monitoring, carbohydrate counting, education on insulin adjustment, insulin pump therapy and islet cell transplants.

Keywords

Hypoglycaemia • Addison's disease • Impaired awareness of hypoglycaemia • Islet cell transplant

Case

A 38-year-old female nursery schoolteacher was referred urgently to the diabetes out-patient department by her GP, with a 4-week history of polydipsia, polyuria, lethargy and unintentional

N.N. Zammitt, BSc (Med Sci), MBChB, MD, FRCPE (✉)
Department of Diabetes,
Royal Infirmary of Edinburgh,
51, Little France Crescent, Edinburgh, Lothian
EH16 4SA, Scotland, UK
e-mail: nzammitt@doctors.org.uk

B.M. Frier, BSc (Hons), MD, FRCPE, FRCPG
BHF Centre for Cardiovascular Science,
The Queen's Medical Research Institute,
University of Edinburgh, Edinburgh, Lothian,
Scotland, UK
e-mail: brian.frier@ed.ac.uk

weight loss of 3 kg. She had developed Addison's disease 7 years earlier but had no other past medical history. Her medications at presentation were:

Hydrocortisone 20 mg mane; 10 mg afternoon
Fludrocortisone 100 mcg mane

She had a family history of autoimmune disease. Her father had Addison's disease and autoimmune hypothyroidism secondary to Hashimoto's thyroiditis and also had type 2 diabetes treated with metformin. A maternal aunt had Hashimoto's thyroiditis. The patient was single, lived alone and was a non-smoker who consumed occasional alcohol. She held an ordinary (Group 1) driving licence.

On examination, her BP was 92/59 mmHg and she appeared well hydrated with no obvious pigmentation. She had a normal body habitus with

R. Ajjan, S.M. Orme (eds.), *Endocrinology and Diabetes: Case Studies, Questions and Commentaries*,
DOI 10.1007/978-1-4471-2789-5_17, © Springer-Verlag London 2015

body mass index (BMI) of 23.8 kg/m^2 (weight 71.9 kg).

Initial investigations showed:

Random blood glucose: 14.5 mmol/l and 13.6 mmol/l

HbA1c 73 mmol/mol (9 %)

Urinalysis: negative for ketones

Questions
1. What type of diabetes do you think this lady has? Consider which of her presenting features are typical of type 1 diabetes and type 2 diabetes respectively.
2. How would you approach her initial clinical management?

In view of this lady's family history of type 2 diabetes and the absence of ketonuria, she was given a trial of a sulfonylurea, gliclazide 80 mg bd. She was taught home blood glucose monitoring with a glucose meter that also allowed measurement of capilary ketones. Her weight loss and normal BMI of 23.8 kg.m^2 was suggestive of a diagnosis of type 1 diabetes, which was consistent with her personal and family history of autoimmune disease. Islet cell autoantibodies and GAD (glutamic acid decarboxylase) antibodies were requested.

Subsequent Course

She developed symptomatic hypoglycaemia after commencing gliclazide 80 mg bd so the dose was reduced to 80 mg daily and metformin was commenced at a dose of 500 mg bd. Gliclazide was subsequently discontinued and metformin was increased to 1 g bd, resulting in capillary blood glucose readings between 4 and 8 mmol/l. Within 2 months of diagnosis, her HbA1c had declined to 44 mmol/mol (6.2 %)

However, within 6 months of commencing these oral medications, she was recording low fasting blood glucose readings (between 3 and 4 mmol/l) while by late evening her capillary readings were rising to values in the teens, despite preprandial readings of 6.7 mmol/l or less. Given

the previous problems with sulfonylurea-induced hypoglycaemia, repaglinide 500 mg was prescribed with her evening meal. This also caused hypoglycaemia, as did subsequent treatment with glimepiride.

Question
3. What was the rationale behind the trials of repaglinide and glimepiride?

A meta-analysis of treatment with sulfonylureas calculated relative risks of hypoglycaemia of 2.23–3.58 for gliclazide, 2.96 for glipizide and 1.42–1.24 for glimepiride [1]. The meglitinides (repaglinide and nateglinide) are rapid-acting insulin secretagogues with a more rapid onset and shorter duration of action than the sulfonylureas [2, 3]. However, despite their shorter duration of action, the meglitinides also have a potential risk of inducing hypoglycaemia, both as monotherapy [2] and in combination with metformin [2–4].

Questions
4. Does her sensitivity to sulfonylureas suggest that she may have another type of diabetes?
5. How would you investigate this possibility?

The family history of diabetes in a first-degree relative, the pattern of adult onset diabetes on a background of a normal body habitus and the sensitivity to sulfonylurea therapy raised the possibility of having a type of monogenic diabetes, such as the types caused by HNF1α and HNF4α mutations [5]. This possibility could be tested by arranging DNA analysis. However, by this stage, her GAD antibody results had been reported to be strongly positive at 64 U/ml (normal reference range 0–1 U/ml).

To characterise her hypoglycaemia with greater precision, a period of continuous glucose monitoring (CGM) was arranged which confirmed post-prandial hyperglycaemia with readings of up to 22 mmol/l, co-existing with episodic nocturnal hypoglycaemia. Her HbA1c was 49 mmol/mol (6.6 %).

Thirteen months after diagnosis, oral antidiabetes agents were discontinued and she commenced 2 units of a rapid-acting insulin analogue, taken with lunch and the evening meal. In view of the nocturnal hypoglycaemia demonstrated with CGM, she was not commenced on basal insulin. Risks of hypoglycaemia related to driving were discussed.

> Question
> 6. What advice should she be given regarding insulin and driving?

She was told to inform the British driving licensing authority, the Driving and Vehicle Licensing Agency (DVLA), that her diabetes was now being treated with insulin and was informed that her driving licence would be changed to a period-restricted licence. She was advised to test blood glucose before driving on every occasion and at 2 hourly intervals on long journeys. An information leaflet was provided reinforcing the recommendation to keep carbohydrate for emergency use and blood glucose testing equipment in the car. She was also informed that if she had an episode of hypoglycaemia behind the wheel, she should stop the vehicle as soon as safely possible, leave the driving seat, treat the low blood glucose and wait for 45 min after the restoration of euglycaemia before recommencing driving. Full recovery of some aspects of cognitive function, such as reaction time, can lag behind normalisation of blood glucose levels by 40–75 min [6].

Two months after commencing prandial insulin, her fasting blood glucose began to rise so she commenced 6 units of a basal, long-acting insulin analogue and her prandial insulin doses were increased to 4 units at lunch and 5 units before her evening meal. An education session on carbohydrate counting was arranged 18 months after diagnosis. Her insulin requirements were still low at 1 unit of insulin for 30 g of carbohydrate and a correction dose of 1 unit of insulin to reduce her blood glucose by 6 mmol/l. At review she expressed concern about ongoing weight loss.

Her weight had declined to 62 kg (compared with 71.9 kg at diagnosis)

> Question
> 7. What possible reasons should be considered to explain her continuing weight loss?

Coeliac serology and thyroid function were both normal. Her glucocorticoid and mineralocorticoid replacement for her Addison's disease were considered to be more than adequate. It was therefore thought that her weight loss reflected under-treatment with insulin. She was asked to take 1 unit of insulin for 25 g of carbohydrate and was reviewed by the diabetes specialist nurses. HbA1c was 61 mmol/mol (7.7 %)

In March 2009, she had her first episode of severe hypoglycaemia (defined as an episode requiring external assistance for recovery). She collapsed at work without warning and was witnessed to have a generalised tonic-clonic seizure. A CT brain scan did not reveal any abnormality. This episode followed exercise in the form of swimming undertaken during the previous evening, without any adjustment to her insulin dose. At this time, her insulin requirements had risen and she was using 1 unit of insulin for 10 g of carbohydrate. She was advised to reduce her insulin by 30–50 % around the time of exercise and instructed to inform the DVLA of this episode.

She was reviewed in the diabetes clinic 2 weeks later and an inpatient admission was arranged to investigate any potential precipitants for the unexpected episode of severe hypoglycaemia. A cortisol day curve on 20 + 10 mg of hydrocortisone suggested that she was slightly over-replaced, with cortisol peaking at 1,391 nmol/l, declining to 130 nmol/l by mid-afternoon and peaking at 600 nmol/l in the early evening before becoming undetectable at 02.00 h (Fig. 17.1). It was suggested that she reduce hydrocortisone to 10 mg with breakfast and 5 mg with her evening meal with the prospect that a reduction in the peak cortisol levels should improve her glucose profiles and lower her insulin requirements. Faecal elastase measurement (360 μg/g; normal

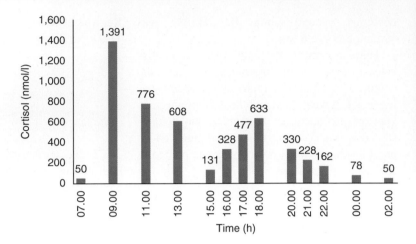

Fig. 17.1 Cortisol day curve performed after first episode of severe hypoglycaemia

reference range 200–1,000) and routine blood tests, including coeliac serology, did not suggest any evidence of malabsorption. She denied non-adherence to medications. She was discharged on lower doses of insulin glargine and of hydrocortisone, as described.

Unfortunately, 6 months later she experienced a further episode of severe hypoglycaemia at work, involving a further blackout and collapse, again associated with a generalised tonic-clonic seizure. Her capillary blood glucose, measured immediately after the seizure, was 11 mmol/l but it had fallen to 3.2 mmol/l by the time she arrived at hospital. It was presumed that this seizure had also been precipitated by hypoglycaemia with no preceding warning symptoms. Neuroradiological investigation with CT and MRI scans of the brain, showed no abnormalities and review by a neurologist supported the presumption that this had been another hypoglycaemia-induced seizure. The patient informed the DVLA of this second severe hypoglycaemia episode and her driving licence was revoked.

She was reviewed within 2 weeks in the diabetes clinic and was noted to have a capillary blood glucose of 2.8 mmol/l without any symptoms of hypoglycaemia being experienced. Her insulin to carbohydrate ratio was reduced to 1 unit for 12 g. The patient had restored her hydrocortisone dose to 20+10 mg as she was concerned that the previous reduction in steroid replacement therapy may have contributed to the further episode of severe hypoglycaemia. As her

insulin requirements had increased, her weight had stabilised and she now weighed 66.5 kg. She was considered to have developed impaired awareness of hypoglycaemia.

> **Question**
> 8. How can you assess awareness of hypo-glycaemia in an individual patient?

Various methods can be used to assess awareness of hypoglycaemia [7, 8]. The method by Clarke et al. [8] consists of eight questions to document the individual's exposure to hypoglycaemia along with their glycaemic threshold for the development of hypoglycaemic symptoms and the nature of these symptoms, with a score of 4 or above suggesting impaired awareness of hypoglycaemia. The method by Gold and colleagues [7] poses the question "do you know when your hypos are commencing?" The subject gives their answer on a 7-point Likert scale where 1 represents "always aware" and 7 represents "never aware." A score of 4 or above suggests impaired awareness of hypoglycaemia. In a 1-year prospective study utilising this method, the incidence of hypoglycaemia in 29 patients with impaired awareness was 2.8 episodes per person per year with a prevalence of 66 %. By contrast, the incidence in the normal awareness group (n=31) was only 0.5 episodes per person per year with a prevalence of 26 % [7]. This heightened risk of severe hypoglycaemia highlights the importance of identifying impaired awareness of hypoglycaemia.

Very good concordance has been found between the Clarke and Gold methods [9]. The prevalence of impaired awareness of hypoglycaemia in that study [9] using the Clarke and Gold methods was similar to the prevalence observed in previous population studies, indicating a prevalence of 20–27 % in unselected individuals with insulin-treated diabetes [10–13].

After a further 6 months the patient sustained another episode of severe hypoglycaemia with no warning during a short walk. Specialist review confirmed that she had little understanding of carbohydrate counting and had been adopting a reactive approach to her diabetes by taking corrective doses in response to hyperglycaemia rather than pre-empting the dose required according to carbohydrate intake and exercise. Consequently, significant swings were noted in her blood glucose readings. The diabetes nurse specialists attempted re-education but she maintained that she could not comprehend carbohydrate counting and attempting to pursue this made her feel very anxious. Her weight had now almost reached her premorbid baseline at 70 kg and HbA1c was 72 mmol/mol (8.9 %). Because of her past experience of nocturnal hypoglycaemia she had reduced her basal insulin analogue dose to just 6 units. Consequently, fasting blood glucose readings were consistently in double figures and she was compensating by taking large doses of rapid-acting analogue with her breakfast, which frequently resulted in hypoglycaemia by late morning. A programme of diabetes nurse follow-up was instigated to titrate the dose of her basal insulin and reduce the large doses of rapid-acting insulin being injected at breakfast. The availability of glucagon at home was discussed but as she lived alone she felt that this would not be useful. The possibility that over-treatment with hydrocortisone might be contributing to some of the hyperglycaemic spikes was met with resistance by the patient, who said that she was terrified of reducing her hydrocortisone again in case this provoked another episode of severe hypoglycaemia.

Despite these measures and despite frequent blood glucose monitoring, she continued to suffer episodic severe hypoglycaemia without warning symptoms. A hypoglycaemia-induced seizure in a supermarket just before lunch required the previous proposal to reduce her breakfast rapid-acting insulin analogue to be reiterated, with a further reduction in her morning dose. About 6 months later she had a blackout and collapsed in a theatre despite having eaten beforehand. She was treated with glucagon by emergency paramedical staff. One year later she suffered a further episode of severe hypoglycaemia causing loss of consciousness in the cinema. Despite her mealtime insulin doses having been reduced, she had taken 20 units of rapid-acting analogue for a meal that contained much less than 200 g of carbohydrate. It was apparent that attempts at re-education had not been successful.

Question
9. What other options could be considered to reduce the frequency of her recurrent severe hypoglycaemia?

The possibility of an insulin pump was considered but discarded. While insulin pumps can significantly reduce the frequency of severe hypoglycaemia in individuals [14], this option was felt to be impractical given her inability (or reluctance) to understand and utilise carbohydrate counting. Having had six episodes of severe hypoglycaemia requiring emergency medical treatment, an islet cell transplant was discussed. The National Institute for Health and Clinical Excellence recommends islet cell transplantation as an option for patients with impaired awareness of hypoglycaemia in recognition of the fact that the procedure can significantly lower the risk of hypoglycaemia and may help to restore awareness of hypoglycaemia [15].

After some consideration, the patient agreed to referral and was reviewed for islet cell transplantation, at which time her HbA1c was 77 mmol/mol (9.2 %). In view of the initial diagnostic uncertainty, blood was taken for autoantibodies and C-peptide. These investigations

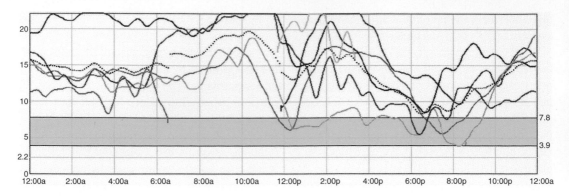

Fig. 17.2 CGM prior to islet cell transplant

Fig. 17.3 (**a**) CGM readings taken 1 week after first islet transplant. (**b**) CGM readings taken 2 weeks after second islet transplant

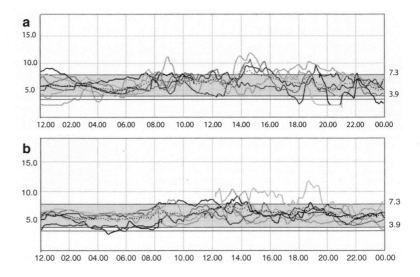

confirmed insulin deficiency (C-peptide 68 pmol/l; normal reference range 600–800) secondary to autoimmune type 1 diabetes (GAD titre >2,000 U/ml; normal reference range 0–5 U/ml). Repeat coeliac serology and thyroid function tests were normal. A further period of CGM demonstrated significant swings in blood glucose levels, with avoidance of hypoglycaemia resulting in repeated episodes of hyperglycaemia (Fig. 17.2). She confirmed that her life was "completely governed by blood glucose readings" and that she had an "extreme fear" of hypoglycaemia. The option of carbohydrate counting, with or without an insulin pump, was revisited. She reiterated her previous view that she became "extremely stressed" when trying to undertake and apply carbohydrate counting and felt that her

glycaemic control was worse when she attempted this. She agreed to join the waiting list for an islet cell transplant.

After a 5 month wait, she received her first islet cell transplant in November 2011 with a second transplant in March 2012. Repeat CGM studies showed a substantial reduction in glucose variability (Fig. 17.3) and her insulin requirement dropped markedly so that she was only taking 30 % of her previous total daily dose. HbA1c had fallen to 58 mmol/mol while her hypoglycaemia awareness score [7] had improved (from 6 to 2) with C-peptide rising to 515 pmol/l. She regained confidence to the degree that she has recommenced swimming. After being free of severe hypoglycaemia for a year she was able to apply to have her driving licence restored.

References

1. Gangji AS, Cukierman T, Gerstein HC, Goldsmith CH, Clase CM. A systematic review and meta-analysis of hypoglycemia and cardiovascular events: a comparison of glyburide with other insulin secretagogues and with insulin. Diabetes Care. 2007;30:389–94.

2. Marbury T, Huang W, Strange P, Lebovitz H. Repaglinide versus glyburide: a one-year comparison trial. Diabetes Res Clin Pract. 1999;43(3):155–66.

3. Ristic S, Collober-Maugeais C, Cressier F, Tang P, Pecher E, Ristic S, Collober-Maugeais C, Cressier F, et al. Nateglinide or gliclazide in combination with metformin for treatment of patients with type 2 diabetes mellitus inadequately controlled on maximum doses of metformin alone: 1-year trial results. Diabetes Obes Metab. 2007;9(4):506–11.

4. Ristic S, Collober-Maugeais C, Pecher E, Cressier F. Comparison of nateglinide and gliclazide in combination with metformin, for treatment of patients with type 2 diabetes mellitus inadequately controlled on maximum doses of metformin alone. Diabet Med. 2006;23(7):757–62.

5. Murphy R, Ellard S, Hattersley AT. Clinical implications of a molecular genetic classification of monogenic beta-cell diabetes. Nat Clin Pract Endocrinol Metab. 2008;4:200–13.

6. Zammitt NN, Warren RE, Deary IJ, Frier BM. Delayed recovery of cognitive function following hypoglycemia in adults with type 1 diabetes. Effect of impaired awareness of hypoglycemia. Diabetes. 2008;57:732–6.

7. Gold AE, MacLeod KM, Frier BM. Frequency of severe hypoglycemia in patients with type 1 diabetes with impaired awareness of hypoglycemia. Diabetes Care. 1994;17:697–703.

8. Clarke WL, Cox DJ, Gonder-Frederick L, Julian D, Schlundt D, Polonsky W. Reduced awareness of hypoglycemia in adults with IDDM. A prospective study of hypoglycemic frequency and associated symptoms. Diabetes Care. 1995;18:517–22.

9. Geddes J, Wright RJ, Zammitt NN, Deary IJ, Frier BM. Evaluation of methods of assessing impaired awareness of hypoglycemia in type 1 diabetes. Diabetes Care. 2007;30(7):1868–70.

10. Pramming S, Thorsteinsson B, Bendtson I, Binder C. Symptomatic hypoglycaemia in 411 type 1 diabetic patients. Diabet Med. 1991;8:217–22.

11. Geddes J, Schopman JE, Zammitt NN, Frier BM. Prevalence of impaired awareness of hypoglycaemia in adults with Type 1 diabetes. Diabet Med. 2008; 25:501–4.

12. Mühlhauser I, Heinemann L, Fritsche E, von Lennep K, Berger M. Hypoglycemic symptoms and frequency of severe hypoglycemia in patients treated with human and animal insulin preparations. Diabetes Care. 1991;14:745–9.

13. Orchard TJ, Maser RE, Becker DJ, Dorman JS, Drash AL. Human insulin use and hypoglycaemia: insights from the Pittsburgh Epidemiology of Diabetes Complications Study. Diabet Med. 1991;8:469–74.

14. National Institute for Health and Clinical Excellence. Continuous subcutaneous insulin infusion for the treatment of diabetes mellitus. NICE technology appraisal guidance 151; 2008. Ref Type: Online Source, London.

15. National Institute for Health and Clinical Excellence. Allogeneic pancreatic islet cell transplantation for type 1 diabetes mellitus. Interventional procedure guidance 257; 2008. Ref Type: Online Source, London.

Spontaneous Hypoglycaemia

Case 18

Mark W.J. Strachan

Abstract

Spontaneous hypoglycaemia has a very wide differential diagnosis that depends in a large part on clinical context. A hypoglycaemic disorder should only be confirmed if all three parts of Whipple's Triad are met. In the context of a patient presenting to an out-patient department with suspected hypoglycaemia, confirmation will usually require prolonged fasting. If a hypoglycaemic disorder is confirmed, measurement of serum insulin and c-peptide concentrations at the time of biochemical hypoglycaemia will help to refine the diagnostic possibilities. Non-islet cell tumour hypoglycaemia (NICTH) is a rare cause of spontaneous hypoglycaemia, which occurs usually in the context of malignant sarcomas with significant tumour bulk. Hypoglycaemia is associated with high serum levels of an abnormal IGF-2 protein. Treatment of NICTH is difficult, especially if the tumour cannot be successfully resected or debulked, and usually revolves around systemic glucocorticoid therapy in high dose.

Keywords

Hypoglycaemia • Whipple's triad • Insulinoma • Non-islet cell tumour hypoglycaemia

Case

Presentation

A 74-year-old woman is referred to the endocrinology clinic with a 6-month history of "funny turns." These episodes have been occurring with increasing frequency and now are happening every other day. The patient reports that during a typical episode, she notices her

M.W.J. Strachan, BSc, MBChB, MD, FRCP
Metabolic Unit, Western General Hospital,
Crewe Road, Edinburgh, Midlothian
EH4 2XU, UK
e-mail: mark.strachan@nhs.net

R. Ajjan, S.M. Orme (eds.), *Endocrinology and Diabetes: Case Studies, Questions and Commentaries*,
DOI 10.1007/978-1-4471-2789-5_18, © Springer-Verlag London 2015

vision becoming blurred and she feels nauseous. She is aware of her heart thumping and feels very hungry, but the symptoms usually pass when she has something to eat. On some instances she has undoubtedly become muddled and on one occasion recently, her husband had to call an ambulance because he could not rouse her from sleep. The ambulance crew had found her capillary blood glucose to be "low" and had administered some intra-muscular glucagon. She had recovered quickly following the injection and was not taken to hospital.

What are the questions to be asked?

You do not have to be a rocket scientist, or indeed an even an astute endocrinologist, to realise that this lady potentially has a significant hypoglycaemic disorder. She is describing symptoms suggestive of hypoglycaemia, recovery following ingestion of food and there is even a potential diagnostic blood test. This means we are tantalisingly close to having met all three of the essential criteria for making a diagnosis of a hypoglycaemic disorder, i.e., Whipple's triad. However, we cannot yet be certain, because we do not know what her blood glucose levels were and, of course, capillary blood glucose test strips are notoriously inaccurate in the hypoglycaemic range.

The first question to ask when assessing someone with potential hypoglycaemia is "*When do your symptoms occur?*" and to follow that up with "*How do they relate to meals and exercise?*" Spontaneous hypoglycaemia is conventionally divided into two broad categories – "fasting" and "post-prandial." "Fasting hypoglycaemia," or that occurring following a missed meal or vigorous exercise, is generally associated with organic pathology. "Post-prandial hypoglycaemia," i.e., symptoms of hypoglycaemia occurring a few hours after food, is commonly regarded as having a functional basis and indeed not to be true hypoglycaemia at all. The diagnosis of post-prandial hypoglycaemia was traditionally made on the basis of a "prolonged glucose tolerance test." It is normal during the course of this test for *venous* blood glucose to fall into the "hypoglycaemic"

Table 18.1 Symptoms of hypoglycaemia

Autonomic	Neuroglycopenic
Sweating	Dizziness
Trembling	Confusion
Warmness	Tiredness
Anxiety	Difficulty with speaking
Hunger	Headache
Pounding heart	Blurred vision
	Weakness
	Difficulty in concentrating

range, particularly in healthy young women. This fact was not appreciated by clinicians performing this test in the 1970s and 1980s and such falls in venous blood glucose were ascribed as the cause of post-prandial symptomatology, despite little or no correlation of these symptoms with the symptoms that actually occurred when the venous blood glucose levels were low. However, while fasting symptoms are undoubtedly more discriminatory for organic pathology, post-prandial hypoglycaemia is now increasingly recognised to occur in organic disorders, such as insulinoma and following bariatric surgery; there are even very rare cases of glucagon-like peptide 1 secreting tumours causing post-prandial hypoglycaemia.

Establishing the symptom profile is also important and patients should be asked to describe these in detail. Symptoms of hypoglycaemia can be divided into two broad categories – autonomic and neuroglycopenic (Table 18.1). Autonomic symptoms normally occur at higher plasma glucose levels than neuroglycopenic symptoms and so act as an early warning for the individual to treat hypoglycaemia before "brain failure" occurs. The fact that this lady is describing symptoms from both groups is significant, because it implies a degree of cerebral adaptation, i.e., her brain has started to get used to low blood glucose levels and so now autonomic symptoms are occurring either at the same time or after the onset of neuroglycopenia. This is significant for three reasons. First, it substantially increases the likelihood of this being a true hypoglycaemic disorder – autonomic symptoms on their own are invariably not due to true hypoglycaemia. Second, it implies a chronicity to the hypoglycaemia, because such cerebral adaptation takes time and repeated episodes

Table 18.2 Differential diagnosis of spontaneous hypoglycaemia according to insulin and C-peptide levels

High insulin and high c-peptide
Insulinoma
Sulfonylureas
Pentamidine
Hyperinsulinaemia of infancy
High insulin and low c-peptide
Exogenous insulin
Low insulin and low c-peptide
Alcohol
Drugs, e.g., quinine, quinidine
Critical illness, e.g., septicaemia, liver failure, renal failure, falciparum malaria
Hypopituitarism (rare)
Adrenocortical failure, especially in children
Non-islet tumour hypoglycaemia
Inborn errors of metabolism

of hypoglycaemia to develop. Third, it increases the likelihood that she will have an episode of severe hypoglycaemia (an event requiring assistance from a third party). If her brain is not working properly when she first gets symptoms, she is much more likely not to treat the hypoglycaemia properly.

The next group of questions relates to possible underlying causes of hypoglycaemia and in that regard a detailed previous medical history and systematic enquiry are crucial. The most important question to ask is *What medication are you taking?*" Clearly the most common cause of hypoglycaemia is insulin or sulfonylurea therapy for diabetes, but even in people without diabetes, drug therapy is a very important precipitating factor (Table 18.2). The other potential causes of hypoglycaemia relate to the context of the patient. The differential diagnosis is completely different in a hospitalised patient, where liver disease and sepsis predominate, compared with an out-patient setting. Moreover, there are definite geographical variations in the aetiology of hypoglycaemia – falciparum malaria and consumption of unripe ackee fruit are common causes in some parts of the world.

In this case, the patient reports that she has noticed a change in her symptom profile. She does not sweat as nearly as much now during episodes as she did when they first started happening. She does not take any regular medication.

The only previous history of note is that 4 years previously she had developed lower abdominal pain and was found to have a "growth" in her pelvis that was successfully removed. On systems enquiry, she does say that she has lost about 6 kg in weight over the last 6 months and that she has been experiencing some discomfort in the right upper quadrant of her abdomen.

What are the signs to look for?

This history is becoming increasingly worrying. Patients with insulinomas invariably present with weight gain, because they have been eating more than normal to avoid hypoglycaemia. Weight loss, in the context of a previous tumour, is not good news. It is unlikely that she will be hypoglycaemic at the time you see her in clinic. Usually clinical examination of a patient with suspected spontaneous hypoglycaemia is remarkably unrewarding, but in this situation we need to look for signs of potential malignant disease.

Examination of the lady's abdomen, reveals 4 cm of palpable hepatomegaly with a worryingly coarse feel to the liver.

Summary of Symptoms and Signs

This lady has presented with symptoms consistent with a hypoglycaemic disorder and signs of a metastatic cancer. We need to find out urgently what the nature was of the tumour removed 4 years ago; we need to confirm the occurrence of hypoglycaemia and we need to establish its aetiology. She could have a malignant insulinoma, but that would mean the previous tumour is unrelated. Alternatively, she could have significant hepatic impairment, secondary to cancer, with hypoglycaemia a consequence of depleted glucagon reserves. However, one would expect her to be more unwell in this situation and possibly even jaundiced. Finally, she could have non-islet cell tumour hypoglycaemia.

What diagnostic tests are required?

In reality, with a patient of this sort, investigations would happen in parallel rather than in series. However, for the sake of clarity, they will be presented in a logical sequence.

Liver function tests showed only marginal elevation of alkaline phosphatase and gamma GT. Bilirubin was not elevated and albumin was 34 g/dl. This makes hypoglycaemia secondary to loss of hepatic reserve unlikely.

Confirming the Presence of a Hypoglycaemic Disorder

Unless you are lucky enough to have the patient present to a hospital emergency department in a hypoglycaemic state, it is likely that you will have to try an induce an episode of hypoglycaemia in a controlled fashion. Even, if she does present to an emergency department with symptomatic hypoglycaemia, the chances are small that the treating doctor will know that 'additional' blood tests would be helpful in establishing an underlying diagnosis; chances are even smaller that this doctor will know what these blood tests are!!

It will therefore fall on the endocrine team to arrange the further investigations. The key diagnostic test is the 72-h fast. In this case, it is highly likely that only a short period of fasting will be required before the patient becomes hypoglycaemic. Some endocrine departments ask patients to come in fasting from 10 pm the night before, but that might be quite risky in this patient and she should be asked simply to avoid breakfast and attend at 8 am. The location for performing a 72-h fast is important. If you do not have the luxury of an in-patient investigation facility, it may have to be a medical ward. Whatever the location, it is crucial that there is a formal written protocol and that staff adhere to it. There needs to be regular monitoring and recording of patient's symptoms and blood glucose levels (capillary and venous). There needs to be clear instructions on when to stop the fast – there is nothing more annoying than a patient having fasted for 48 h and for the test to be stopped when a capillary blood glucose reads 3.5 mmol/l, only for the formal cotemporaneous laboratory venous glucose to return at 4.2 mmol/l. There also needs to be clear instructions on when, how and what 'addiitonal' bloods are taken. Usually these will be bloods for insulin and c-peptide, and possibly bloods for sulfonylurea activity, pro-insulin and beta-hydroxybutyrate. In this case, measurement of IGF-2 and IGF-1 levels during hypoglycaemia will be crucial.

Establishing the Aetiology of Hypoglycaemia

The first aim of the prolonged fast will be to establish that the patient has a hypoglycaemic disorder, by meeting the criteria of Whipple's triad. There is no level of blood glucose which is diagnostic of hypoglycaemia, but the lower the glucose levels is below 3.5 mmol/l, the more likely it is to have pathological significance.

As is shown in Table 18.2, interpretation of insulin and c-peptide levels during the episode of hypoglycaemia then helps to refine the diagnosis. Strictly speaking, insulin and c-peptide should be interpreted in the context of the prevailing blood glucose levels, using a validated nomogram [1], because in normal individuals, the lower the blood glucose, the lower the insulin and c-peptide levels should be. As a rough rule of thumb though, an insulinoma is likely if venous glucose is <3.0 mmol/l, plasma insulin >18 pmol/l, and c-peptide >0.2 nmol/l [2]. When insulin and c-peptide levels are both elevated, sulfonylurea activity should be measured even in non-diabetic individuals, as there are well-described instances of factitious or felonious administration of these drugs [3].

Examination of the case records revealed that the patient had a neurofibrosarcoma resected 4 years previously. The resection margins were clear, but there was evidence of vascular invasion. CT scanning confirmed significant, bulky malignant disease in the liver (Fig. 18.1), and also low-volume pulmonary metastases. A liver biopsy confirmed that the tumour deposits were metastatic neurofibrosarcoma. During the prolonged fast, the patient became symptomatically hypoglycaemic with a formal laboratory glucose of 2.6 mmol/l and her symptoms resolved completely following ingestion of Lucozade. Insulin

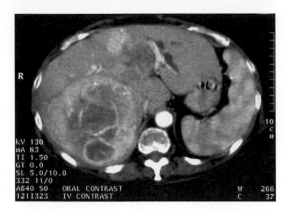

Fig. 18.1 CT scan of liver showing bulky hepatic metastases

and c-peptide levels were undetectable (0.5 pmol/l and <0.05 nmol/l respectively), but IGF-2 levels were substantially elevated at 75.1 nmol/l (normal range 35–70 nmol/l). IGF-2:IGF-1 ratio was also elevated at 39.5 (normal <10).

What is the final diagnosis?

This lady had metastatic neurofibrosarcoma. The elevated IGF-2 result was pathognomonic of non-islet cell tumour hypoglycaemia (NICTH). This classically occurs in the context of malignant sarcomas, often later in the course of the disease when there is bulky local or distant disease [4]. NICTH can also occur with other tumour types, including hepatocellular carcinoma, hemangiopericytoma and mesothelioma. The tumour secretes an abnormal IGF-2 protein, which binds to insulin receptors causing hypoglycaemia.

How would you manage this lady?

The ideal scenario in NICTH is to resect or debulk the tumour. Most often though, as in this case, that is not possible because of the extensive nature of local or metastatic disease. Sarcomas tend to respond less well to conventional chemotherapy and radiotherapy. Embolisation therapies can be tried for liver metastases that are causing recurrent hypoglycaemia.

The endocrinology team is then left with the difficult task of reducing or preventing hypoglycaemia. The patient should be counselled about the risks of hypoglycaemia and the potential for a further change or loss of warning symptoms. She should be taught how to monitor capillary blood glucose and should undertake this at least four times daily and do additional tests if there are any unusual symptoms. She should be given dietary advice on the treatment and prevention of hypoglycaemia. Nocturnal hypoglycaemia is of particular concern, and pre-bed testing is mandatory. She should be advised to consume a low glycaemic index snack before bed, such as porridge, and never to go to bed with a blood glucose below 6 mmol/l. Particular care and advice will also need to be given with regards to driving – testing blood glucose beforehand will be imperative.

Pharmacological prevention of hypoglycaemia is often of limited efficacy. Diazoxide has no role, because this is an insulin-independent form of hypoglycaemia. Somatostatin analogues can be tried, but often are ineffective, presumably because of lack of coupling of IGF-2 secretion to somatostatin receptors at a cellular level. Human growth hormone therapy has been advocated by some to raise levels of IGF-2 binding proteins, but is a flawed strategy (see below). In most instances, the most effective pharmacological therapy is high dose glucocorticoid therapy. In effect, the object of therapy here is to induce insulin resistance. The treatment does work, though as the tumour progresses, it tends to become less effective and the patient becomes increasingly Cushingoid.

NICTH has a poor prognosis. As the patient's disease progresses, his or her life revolves around an increasingly futile battle to avoid hypoglycaemia. It is sometimes necessary to consider overnight nasogastric feeding, but often by this stage palliation of symptoms is the best option.

In this case, the patient was treated with dexamethasone 4 mg twice daily. This was effective in abolishing hypoglycaemia for many months and it was possible to wean down the dose of steroid. She became very Cushingoid and that caused her and her family distress. Growth hormone and octreotide were ineffective. She was followed up on a monthly basis in the endocrine clinic and, in between times, the patient and her family remained in e-mail and telephone contact with the endocrine nurse specialists.

As her disease progressed, the hypoglycaemia returned and her husband would routinely set his alarm for 2 and 4 am so he could check his wife's blood glucose and administer oral carbohydrate as necessary. She declined an overnight nasogastric tube and died peacefully through the night, almost 1 year to the day following her initial attendance at the endocrinology clinic.

Commentary

This was a classic case of NICTH. IGF-2 is an important growth factor in utero, but it appears to have little role following delivery. As with IGF-1,

IGF-2 is bound in plasma primarily to IGFBP-3 and is inactive in this bound state. Stable binding requires the presence of a third protein, called acid-labile subunit (ALS). As with many hormones, IGF-2 is secreted as a pre-pro-hormone that undergoes post-translational glycosylation and cleavage to release IGF-2. In NICTH, there is a failure of normal glycosylation in tumour cells, which means that the IGF-2 is not cleaved at the appropriate sites, resulting in the secretion of big-IGF-2. This protein cannot bind to ALS and, as a consequence, levels of free IGF-2 rise and hypoglycaemia occurs when it binds to insulin receptors (Fig. 18.2). Raising levels of the binding proteins with agents such as growth hormone is, therefore, not likely to be an effective strategy to reduce hypoglycaemia, although growth hormone could help hypoglycaemia by increasing insulin resistance.

It is not clear why NICTH occurs late in the disease course of malignant sarcomas. There is

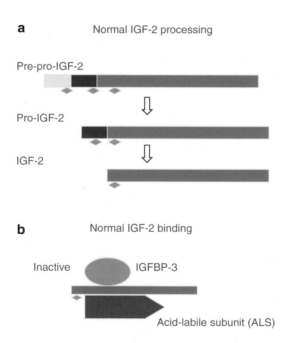

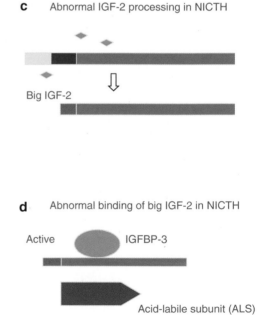

Fig. 18.2 Normal and abnormal processing of IGF-2. Pre-pro-IGF-2 undergoes post-translational glycosylation (represented by *green diamonds*). This allows cleavage to release IGF-2 (**a**) and subsequent binding in plasma to IGFBP3 and ALS (**b**). In NICTH, normal glycosylation does not occur, resulting in abnormal cleavage and release of Big IGF-2 (**c**), which cannot bind to ALS. This results in increased levels of metabolically active free protein (**d**)

clearly a critical mass effect, but also presumably different oncogenes become activated, as the disease progresses, that result in abnormal IGF-2 processing.

NICTH rarely causes diagnostic difficulty. The extent of tumour burden may already be known and the hypoglycaemia is not subtle. It adds an additional burden to patients and family, over and above that of the cancer, and negatively impacts on quality of life. Often patients will die as a consequence of the hypoglycaemia, rather than from a mass effect of the tumour.

References

1. Service FJ. Hypoglycemic disorders. N Engl J Med. 1995;332:1144–52.
2. Cryer PE, Axelrod L, Grossman AB, Heller SR, Montori VM, Seaquist ER, Service FJ. Evaluation and management of adult hypoglycemic disorders: an endocrine Society Clinical Practice Guideline. J Clin Endocrinol Metab. 2009;94:709–28.
3. Marks V, Teale JD. Hypoglycemia: factitious and felonious. Endocrinol Metab Clin North Am. 1999;28: 579–601.
4. Teale JD, Wark G. The effectiveness of different treatment options for non-islet cell tumour hypoglycaemia. Clin Endocrinol (Oxf). 2004;60:457–60.

Thyroid Nodule in a Child (MEN 2)

Case 19

Roly Squire

Abstract

MEN 2 syndromes are associated with an almost certain risk for the development of medullary thyroid carcinoma (MTC), which results in a high mortality. Prophylactic thyroidectomy in childhood, prior to the development of MTC is the best way to mitigate this risk. Identification of children with MEN at an early age requires vigilance: vigilance to identify a kindred with the MEN 2A gene from a single family member (index case) who presents with MTC in later life; vigilance to pick up MEN 2B in infancy from associated clinical features such as intractable constipation and phenotypic appearance. Only by identifying MEN 2 children before they present with their thyroid lump can we significantly improve their clinical outcome.

Keywords

Multiple endocrine neoplasia syndromes • Multiple endocrine neoplasia type 2a • Medullary thyroid carcinoma • Thyroidectomy • Child • Adolescent

Clinical History

A 12-year-old boy was being seen regularly by a paediatrician for the management of intractable constipation, and at the planned follow-up appointment his mother drew the paediatrician's attention to a swelling in the left side of the neck.

R. Squire, MBBS, FRCS (Paed)
Paediatric Surgery, Leeds Children's Hospital,
Leeds General Infirmary,
Leeds, West Yorkshire LS1 3EX, UK
e-mail: r.squire@nhs.net

On examination the paediatrician found a 2-cm thyroid nodule. The boy was clinically euthyroid, and the lump was aymptomatic. On direct questioning the boy said that he had first noticed the swelling about 6 months previously, but had not told anyone about it.

The only relevant past medical history was that the boy had been constipated since birth, with a poor response to oral laxative regimes. A rectal biopsy was carried out when he was 6 months old, which ruled out Hirschprung's disease. The pathology report had commented on the presence of transmural rectal ganglioneuromas, of uncertain significance.

R. Ajjan, S.M. Orme (eds.), *Endocrinology and Diabetes: Case Studies, Questions and Commentaries*,
DOI 10.1007/978-1-4471-2789-5_19, © Springer-Verlag London 2015

Recently the boy had told his mother that he had an annoying lump on the side of his tongue.

> What was the likely pathological diagnosis of the thyroid nodule, and what was the underlying condition?

> What are the typical clinical features of this condition?

The thyroid nodule was caused by medullary thyroid carcinoma (MTC). Transmural ganglioneuromatosis of the rectal submucosa is diagnostic for MEN 2B syndrome [1], a genetic condition which typically has the following clinical features: intestinal dysmotility and constipation secondary to the abnormal intestinal innervation; typical facial phenotype with swollen lips and eyelids; Marfanoid appearance; oro-glossal neuromas; skeletal problems such as kyphoscoliosis [2]. This boy should have been picked up as having MEN 2B in infancy because of the intestinal pathology, which could have alerted clinicians to the probability of an underlying genetic abnormality. MEN 2B could then have been confirmed by a geneticist on phenotypic parameters, even prior to genetic testing.

> What investigations should be carried out?

The diagnosis of MTC should be confirmed by measurement of the serum calcitonin.

Ultrasound of the neck is recommended primarily to identify pathological lymph nodes, but also to identify multiple primary tumours. This can be supported by MRI or CT scan if there is any evidence of significant extra-thyroid disease.

Genetic testing should be carried out to confirm the genetic abnormality; 99 % of MEN 2B have a germline abnormilty of the RET oncogene in codon 918 [3, 4]. Nearly all MEN 2B patients are new mutations, but a careful family history will quickly reveal evidence of an inherited abnormality. Referral to a geneticist will be required at some stage, but may be best delayed until after treatment of the primary pathology, since counselling relates predominantly to advice about the risk of MEN 2B in future children. In the rare circumstance, probably less than 5 %, where a new presentation of MEN 2B brings a family history to attention which suggests a previously unsuspected inherited germline abnormality a more urgent genetics referral is indicated to ensure that other members of the family can be investigated without delay.

In older children it is wise to arrange a 24 h urine collection for urinary fractionated metanephrines prior to any surgical interventions, to rule out simultaneous development of a phaeochromocytoma [5]. There is an approximately 50 % risk of a patient with MEN 2B developing a phaeo, but this is not likely to happen before 10 years of age. If a patient has both a phaeo and MTC the phaeo should be treated first to reduce the risk to the patient.

> What treatment should be carried out?

All cases of MEN 2B should undergo total thyroidectomy at the earliest opportunity [6]. In this boy, who has established MTC, the aim is to completely excise all the disease, and so there should be careful preoperative assessment and planning to decide on the extent of associated lymph node dissection. Surgical planning and management should be carried out in a specialist centre with experience of MTC, and with the support to manage thyroid surgery in childhood. There is no advantage to carrying out a preoperative fine-needle aspiration (FNA) in this situation: the diagnosis is already strongly suspected from the clinical presentation, and is confirmed by elevated serum calcitonin. In the unlikely circumstance that the calcitonin level is not elevated then FNA may be considered, but in this age group may require anaesthesia, and so many specialists proceed direct to resection, carrying out a lobectomy for frozen section histology, expecting to complete the thyroidectomy at the same operation. If there are abnormal lymph nodes one of these can be sent for frozen section analysis at the start of the procedure to speed up the process. The role of lymph node dissection is controversial: it is not recommended for prophylactic thyroidectomies in MEN syndromes when carried out at an age when MTC is unlikely to have developed. Lymph node dissection is recommended if the adjacent lymph nodes are abnormal in a child like this with a thyroid nodule. The value of lymph node dissection in late prohylactic thyroidectomy is not clear [7].

The preparation for total thyroidectomy should follow the standard procedure appropriate for all age groups. The patient and parents/guardians should be warned of the risk of damage to the recurrent laryngeal nerves, and of postoperative hypocalcaemia as a result of damage to the parathyroid glands. For the experienced surgeon the risk to the recurrent laryngeal nerves is low in children, who tend to have clean tissue planes in thinner necks without invasive disease. It is good practice to carry out pre-operative cord assessment in older children and adolescents, but this should not delay the surgery. The risk of postoperative hypocalcaemia is greater in children than in adults, possibly because the blood supply to the parathyroid in this age group is less well developed [8]. Baseline calcium measurement can be carried out immediately preoperatively, after induction of anaesthesia, in order to minimise preoperative interventions and distress. It is wise to ask the anaesthetist to insert two substantial cannulae to assist with postoperative management, keeping one for blood sampling. Regular postoperative calcium levels should be measured for at least 48 h, longer if the calcium level is not stable. Children are poor at reporting symptoms of hypocalcaemia, and so it is preferable to rely upon blood levels, using symptom reporting as an adjunct, rather than the opposite.

> What is the post-operative management?

Following total thyroidectomy he will need thyroid replacement therapy under the supervision of a paediatric endocrinologist. Since there is no role for radioactive iodine in the management of MTC it is usual to start with levothyroxine (T4) in the immediate postoperative period.

This boy will need lifelong follow-up to screen for progression or recurrence of his MTC, and also to screen for development of phaeochromocytoma. This will involve regular measurement of calcitonin and 24-h urinary metadrenaline and normetadrenaline levels. It is not unusual for the serum calcitonin level to remain elevated following thyroidectomy, signifying residual MTC [9]. If the postoperative calcitonin does not return to normal, or if there is a subsequent recurrence of elevated calcitonin, reinvestgation can be carried out with cross-sectional imaging and selective venous sampling to guide reoperation in an attempt to achieve a surgical cure.

The boy and his family should be referred for genetic counselling.

General Discussion

MEN syndromes include MEN1, 2A and 2B. It is rare for children to develop features of MEN1, which does not involve the thyroid gland and is not discussed further in this chapter.

The clinical features and risks for MEN 2A and 2B are listed in Table 19.1.

MEN 2 syndromes are autosomal dominant, although with variable penetrance particularly in MEN 2A. This can mean that the age of developing MTC in untreated family members who have the RET mutation can vary widely. Autosomal dominance means that statistically 50 % of children of a family member with the RET mutation will also have MEN 2.

MEN2A is more prevalent than MEN2B, and in children almost exclusively presents as a genetic diagnosis following investigation of the kindred of an adult *index* case of MTC. More recently children are also being identified by screening children with Hirschprung's disease, since Hirschprung's is sometimes be caused by the same the RET mutation as MEN 2A [10, 11]. Ninety seven percent of individuals with MEN2A have a germline mutation of the RET oncogene [12, 13]. Historically families were screened for the development of early MTC using calcitonin screening, but this is unreliable [14], and outcome studies have shown that this approach results in late diagnosis and

Table 19.1 Typical clinical features and risks (%) for subjects with genetically confirmed MEN 2 syndromes

MEN 2A	MEN 2B
MTC (100 %)	MTC (100 %)
Phaeochromocytoma (50 %)	Phaeochromocytoma (50 %)
Parathyroid adenoma (25 %)	Mucosal neuromas: tongue/lips (95 %)
	Typical facies: swollen lips/thick eyelids (90 %)
	Intestinal motility disorders (90 %)
	Marfanoid habitus
	Musculoskeletal abnormalities: spinal deformity/ hypotonia/ slipped epiphyses/pes cavus/talipes equinovarus

ineffective prophylactic thyroidectomy. With appropiate genetic testing of children identified as being at risk within an MEN 2A family it is possible to select children with the RET mutation who will have more-or-less a 100 % future risk of MTC development [15]. Current advice is that these children should undergo prophylactic total thyroidectomy before the fifth birthday, since pathological specimens after this age sometimes show that small foci of MTC have already developed. Even by age 5 most show significant C-cell hyperplasia. Rarely MEN2A children have been reported as developing MTC as early as age 3, and it is increasingly possible to stratify patients by genotype to select children who are at risk of earlier MTC development [16]. These children should be offered earlier thyroidectomy. There is still no unequivocal evidence to show that prophylactic thyroidectomy confers a survival advantage in MEN2A, but since complete resection is the only curative option for MTC it is impossible to argue against the logic of carrying out prophylactic surgery before MTC has developed, at least until there is evidence to the contrary.

Children with MEN2B develop MTC much earlier, often by age 1 year [6]. However only 5 % are identified as a result of kindred testing. The typical facies assist in early identification of affected individuals, and in these children neonatal testing and prophylactic thyroidectomy under the age of 6 months is recommended. The presence of transmural ganglioneuromatosis in 90 % of MEN 2B individuals can fortuitously lead to identification of affected children as a result of intestinal biopsy to investigate possible Hirschprung's. As should have happened in the boy described in this case study, intestinal ganglioneuromatosis should alert pathologists and clinicians to the possibility of underlying genetic conditions, which include MEN2B and neurofibromatosis. In MEN2B the ganglioneuromas are transmural. Early identification of a child with a new MEN2B mutation can allow prophylactic thyroidectomy to be carried out at an age where it is most likely to be effective.

Following prophylactic thyroidectomy all MEN 2 children will need regular long-term follow up with screening not just for development of MTC despite the thyroidectomy, but also for phaeochromocytoma in both MEN 2A and 2B, and parathyroid overactivity in MEN 2A. Most centres will screen for phaeochromocytoma with 6 monthly urinary fractionated metanephrines from 5 years of age, although in reality development of a phaeo in MEN is unlikely before the age of 10 years. Fortunately, parathyroid adenomas do not generally appear until late adolescence at the earliest.

References

1. Carney JA, Go VL, Sizemore GW, Hayles AB. Alimentary tract ganglioneuromatosis. A major component of the syndrome of multiple endocrine neoplasia type 2b. N Engl J Med. 1976;295:1287–91.
2. Gorlin RJ, Sedano HO, Vickers RA, Cervenka J. Multiple mucosal neuromas, phaeochromocytoma and medullary carcinoma of the thyroid- syndrome. Cancer. 1968;22:293–9.
3. Eng C, Clayton D, Schuffenecker I, Lenoir G, Cote G, Gagel RF, et al. The relationship between specific RET proto-oncogene mutations and disease phenotype in multiple endocrine neoplasia type 2: International RET mutation Consortium analysis. JAMA. 1996;276:1575–9.

4. Gimm O, Marsh DJ, Andrew SD, Frilling A, Dahia PL, Mulligan LM, et al. Germline dinucleotide mutation in codon 883 of the RET proto-oncogene in multiple endocrine neoplasia type 2DB without codon 918 mutation. J Clin Endocrinol Metab. 1997;82:3902–4.

5. Ilias I, Pacak K. Diagnosis, localisation and treatment of phaeochromocytoma in MEN 2 syndrome. Endocr Regul. 2009;43:89–93.

6. Leboulleux S, Travagli JP, Caillou B, Laplanche A, Bidart JM, Schlumberger M, et al. Medullary thyroid carcinoma a part of a multiple endocrine meoplasia type 2 B syndrome: influence of stage on the clinical course. Cancer. 2002;94:44–50.

7. Skinner MA, Moley JA, Dilley WG, Owzar K, Debendetti MK, Wells JR. Prophylactic thyroidectomy in multiple endocrine neoplasia type 2A. N Engl J Med. 2005;353:1105–13.

8. Sosa JA, Tuggle CT, Wang TS, Thomas DC, Boudourakis L, Rivkees S, et al. Clinical and economic outcomes of thyroid and parathyroid surgery in children. J Clin Endocrinol Metab. 2008;93:3058–65.

9. Marchens A, Niccoli-Sire P, Hoegel J, Frank-Raue K, van Vroonhoven TJ, Roeher HD, et al.; European Multiple Endocrine Neoplasia (EUROMEN) Study Group. Early malignant progression of hereditary medullary thyroid cancer. N Engl J Med. 2003;349:1517–25.

10. Decker RA, Peacock ML, Watson P. Hirschprung disease in MEN 2A: increased spectrum of RET exon 10 genotypes and strong genotype-phenotype correlation. Hum Mol Genet. 1998;7:129–34.

11. Borrego S, Eng C, Sanchez B, Saez M, Navarro E, Antinolo G. Molecular analysis of the RET and GDNF genes in a family with multiple endocrine neoplasia type 2A and Hirschsprung disease. J Clin Endocrinol Metab. 1998;83:3361–4.

12. Carling T. Multiple endocrine neoplasia syndrome: genetic basis for clinical management. Curr Opin Oncol. 2005;17:7–12.

13. Mulligan LM, Kwok JB, Healey CS, Elsdon MJ, Gardner E, Love DR, et al. Germ-line mutations of the RET proto-oncogene in multiple endocrine neoplasia type 2A. Nature. 1993;363:458–60.

14. Marsh DJ, McDowell D, Hyland VJ, Andrew SD, Schnitzler M, Gaskin EL, et al. The identification of false positive responses to the pentagastrin stimulation test in RET mutation negative members of MEN 2A families. Clin Endocrinol (Oxf). 1996;44:213–20.

15. Gagel RF, Cote GJ, Martins Bugalho MJG, Boyd III AE, Cummings T, Goepfert H, et al. Clinical use of molecular information in the management of multiple endocrine neoplasia type 2A. J Intern Med. 1995;238:333–41.

16. Yip L, Cote GJ, Shapiro SE, Ayers GD, Herzog CE, Sellin RV, et al. Multiple endocrine neoplasia type 2: evaluation of the genotype-phenotype relationship. Arch Surg. 2003;138:409–16.

Suggested Reading

Brandi ML, Gagel RF, Angeli A, et al. Consensus guidelines for diagnosis and therapy of MEN Type 1 and Type 2. J Clin Endocrinol Metab. 2001;86:5658–71.

Kloos RT, Eng C, Evans DB, Francis GL, Gagel RF, Gharib H, et al. Medullary thyroid cancer: management guidelines of the American Thyroid Association. Thyroid. 2009;19:565–612.

Moline J, Eng C. Multiple Endocrine neoplasia type 2: an overview. Genet Med. 2011;13:755–64.

What Kind of Diabetes?

Case 20

Katharine R. Owen

Abstract

This patient was diagnosed with assumed type 1 diabetes at the age of 20. She had several years of poor control and gained weight on insulin. Six years post-diagnosis a strong family history was revealed when her brother developed young-onset type 2 diabetes and it was also noted that her mother had diabetes. A C-peptide in the normal range showed that she continued to make endogenous insulin, which would be unusual in type 1 diabetes post-honeymoon period. Molecular genetic testing showed that the patient and her affected family members had maturity-onset diabetes of the young (MODY) due to a hepatocyte nuclear factor 1 alpha (*HNF1A*) mutation. Following this diagnosis she stopped basal-bolus insulin and her diabetes was managed on 40 mg gliclazide with improved HbA1c.

Keywords

Maturity-onset diabetes of the young • MODY • Monogenic diabetes • Young adult diabetes • HNF1A-MODY

Case

Jennifer was found to have raised blood glucose at the age of 20 whilst suffering from an intercurrent illness. She had a random blood glucose of 27 mmol/L and urine ketones +++. Her weight was 60 kg (BMI 22.5 kg/m²). There was no history of osmotic symptoms or weight loss.

K.R. Owen, MD, MRCP
Oxford Centre for Diabetes, Endocrinology and Metabolism (OCDEM), University of Oxford, Churchill Hospital, Oxford, Oxon OX3 7LJ, UK
e-mail: Katharine.owen@drl.ox.ac.uk

What is your preliminary diagnosis?

Despite the high blood glucose she did not complain of previous symptoms of hyperglycaemia. A diagnosis of type 1 diabetes was made and she was commenced on human soluble and isophane insulins, later changed to basal bolus analogue insulin.

She was followed up in the young adult diabetes clinic, but was depressed by having diabetes and poorly engaged with the clinic, frequently missing appointments. Insulin treatment (1 unit/kg) lead to weight gain of 20 kg over the years

R. Ajjan, S.M. Orme (eds.), *Endocrinology and Diabetes: Case Studies, Questions and Commentaries*, DOI 10.1007/978-1-4471-2789-5_20, © Springer-Verlag London 2015

Fig. 20.1 Family pedigree

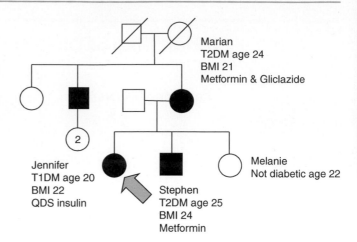

Marian
T2DM age 24
BMI 21
Metformin & Gliclazide

2

Jennifer
T1DM age 20
BMI 22
QDS insulin

Stephen
T2DM age 25
BMI 24
Metformin

Melanie
Not diabetic age 22

(BMI 30 kg/m^2) and she maintained a moderate HbA1c of 65–80 mmol/mol (8.1–9.5 %).

Six years after her diagnosis, the Specialist nurse team were contacted by a local GP surgery asking for telephone advice because Jennifer's brother had been diagnosed with type 2 diabetes at the age of 25. He was apparently lean and asymptomatic. The surgery commenced metformin treatment but chose not to refer to secondary care.

Is this relevant to our original case?

The appearance of two different types of young-onset diabetes in the same sibship made us reconsider the aetiology of the diabetes. With an assumed diagnosis of type 1 diabetes, Jennifer would be expected to have positive β-cell antibodies and an absence of endogenous insulin secretion post-honeymoon period. GAD antibodies were negative and a random plasma C-peptide was found to be 0.49 nmol/L (fasting reference range 0.27–1.28 nmol/L) with a paired glucose of 7.8 mmol/L. Further collateral history revealed that Jennifer's mother had been diagnosed with type 2 diabetes during pregnancy aged 24 and was currently treated with oral agents (Fig. 20.1).

What is your diagnosis now?

Evidence now suggested that Jennifer did not have type 1 diabetes. We then considered whether she had evidence for type 2 diabetes. This seemed unlikely as she was lean at onset and had no other features of insulin resistance (i.e., was normotensive, no dyslipidaemia or symptoms of polycystic ovarian syndrome). The clinical picture of familial young-onset diabetes with negative β-cell antibodies, C-peptide positivity several years after diagnosis and no signs of insulin resistance was very suggestive of a diagnosis of MODY (Table 20.1).

A mutation in the gene hepatocyte nuclear factor 1-alpha (HNF1A), the commonest form of MODY in adults [1, 2], was confirmed in Jennifer, her brother and her mother. All three were reviewed in the genetic diabetes clinic and the diagnosis explained.

Would you change the treatment of this patient?

Those with HNF1A-MODY have been shown in an RCT [3] to be very sensitive to low-dose sulphonylurea (SU) treatment and this is the first line recommended treatment for diabetes due to *HNF1A* (and *HNF4A*) mutations [4]. Patients treated with insulin from diagnosis (on the assumption that they have type 1 diabetes) have successfully transferred to SU even many years after diagnosis [5].

Table 20.1   Characteristics of MODY compared to type 1 and type 2 diabetes

	HNF1A- and HNF4A MODY	GCK-MODY	Type 1 diabetes	Type 2 diabetes
Typical age of onset	Second-fourth decade	Lifelong fasting hyperglycaemia	First-third decade	>25 years
Beta-cell antibodies	Usually negative	Usually negative	Usually positive	Negative
Diabetic ketoacidosis	Rare	Rare	Common	Rare
Presence of metabolic syndrome	Unusual	Unusual	Unusual	Common
Family history of diabetes	Parent usually affected, but not always reported	Usually fasting hyperglycaemia in one parent, but may be missed	10–15 %	Common
C-peptide	Normal	Normal	Low or undetectable (post-honeymoon)	Normal/high
CRP	HNF1A-MODY Very low HNF4A-MODY Normal	Normal	Normal	Frequently chronically elevated
First-line treatment	Low-dose sulphonylurea	Nil	Insulin	Metformin

Jennifer agreed to a trial of SU. Her basal bolus insulin was stopped and gliclazide 40 mg commenced (see http://www.diabetesgenes.org/content/guidance-transferring-hnf1a-or-hnf4a-patients-insulin-sulphonylureas for advice on how to do this). Stopping insulin can cause great anxiety in those previously told they have type 1 diabetes, so daily contact with our local Genetic Diabetes Nurse [6] was offered during the transition period. Happily she was able to transfer to gliclazide with no problems. Over the next few months Jennifer lost all the weight she had gained on insulin and her HbA1c fell to 40 mmol/mol (5.8 %). She reported very infrequent hypoglycaemia.

> What about treatment of Jennifer's brother and mother?

Jennifer's brother, Stephen, had been commenced on metformin shortly after diagnosis in the assumption that he had type 2 diabetes. He had a suboptimal HbA1c on metformin treatment (60 mmol/mol, 7.6 %) and his GP had then added gliclazide 80 mg daily. This had caused severe hypoglycaemic episodes and the gliclazide had been stopped. When he was diagnosed with HNF1A-MODY, we suggested stopping metformin and commencing a very low dose of gliclazide (20 mg increasing to 40 mg). This had the effect of controlling his diabetes without hypoglycaemia and HbA1c improved to 48 mmol/mol, 6.5 %.

Their mother, Marian, was already treated with metformin 1 g and gliclazide 40 mg daily with a good HbA1c (45 mmol/mol, 6 %), so no treatment changes were suggested.

> Jennifer and Stephen have a younger sister, Melanie, who is healthy, and Jennifer wants to know whether she requires screening. What advice would you give her?

Melanie is at 50 % risk of inheriting the *HNF1A* mutation from her mother. Melanie did not have diabetes, so we also discussed the pros and cons of predictive genetic testing with her. Predictive testing is a diagnostic genetic test in someone who has not yet inherited the disease. An informed decision should be made to have predictive test: clinical genetic services can be involved if necessary and we always recommend this for those under age 18. Melanie decided to go ahead with predictive testing to inform her risk of developing diabetes in the future. She was not found to carry the mutation and so her lifetime risk of developing diabetes is the same as the general population.

In non-diabetic family members who either carry the mutation or do not know their mutation status, we recommend annual screening for diabetes using either oral glucose tolerance test (OGTT; this tends to become abnormal first in HNF1A-MODY) or a combination of fasting blood glucose (FPG) and HbA1c.

Marian's brother also has diabetes, diagnosed in his late 40s. He declined further investigation.

Five years later, Jennifer remains on gliclazide 40 mg, with no deterioration in HbA1c. She married recently and attended the diabetes clinic for pre-conception advice. She was anxious about the prospect of restarting insulin for pregnancy.

> What advice would you give the patient?

There are no studies of pregnancy outcomes in those with HNF1A-MODY, or specific advice in national guidelines, so advice was given based on evidence in type 1 and type 2 diabetes and expert opinion. Glibenclamide is considered safe in pregnancy in type 2 diabetes, although it is not currently recommended by NICE guidelines. Given that Jennifer had maintained much better control on low dose gliclazide than she did on insulin, we were happy to advise that the benefits of transferring to glibenclamide pre-conceptionally, and for as long as good control was maintained during pregnancy, would outweigh any risks associated with glibenclamide treatment. This needs to be an informed decision, made on a one to one basis with patients with HNF1A (and HNF4A-MODY), until definite outcome data is available. Jennifer remained on a low dose of glibenclamide until week 16 of her pregnancy, when her blood glucoses were rising and she agreed to go back onto basal bolus insulin. She delivered a healthy baby boy at 38 weeks and returned to low-dose gliclazide treatment.

Clinical Features of HNF1A-MODY

HNF1A is a transcription factor controlling regulation of genes in the liver, gut and kidney as well as the pancreas. Patients are normoglycaemic in childhood, but develop progressive β-cell dysfunction and diabetes in their second-fourth decade. Diabetes complications frequently develop if diabetes control is suboptimal.

The expression of *HNF1A* in other tissues leads to some extra-pancreatic features that are unique to HNF1A-MODY. There is decreased expression of the high affinity low capacity sodium-glucose transporter-2 (SGLT2) in the proximal renal tubule. Therefore *HNF1A* mutations result in decreased glucose reabsorption and a low renal threshold for glucose in HNF1A-MODY leading to glycosuria inappropriate for the blood glucose levels [7]. This feature is used in clinical practice to identify non-diabetic mutation carriers who are developing hyperglycaemia [8]. A number of secreted liver proteins are altered in HNF1A-MODY. Apolipoprotein M [9] and C-reactive protein [10] both have lower serum levels than healthy controls and there is interest in CRP as a potential clinical biomarker for selecting those in the clinic at high risk of having an *HNF1A* mutation [11, 12].

Other Aspects of Management of HNF1A-MODY

As already discussed, those with HNF1A-MODY are exquisitely sensitive to SU treatment, but with time secondary SU failure usually occurs. At that point other oral medication or insulin can be used: there is no particular evidence to recommend one treatment above another. There is little data available on cardiovascular outcomes, but generally CV risk factors are managed in the same way as type 1 diabetes, with statin treatment recommended in those who have had diabetes for a number of years or who have other risk factors. Features of the metabolic syndrome are less commonly seen than in type 2 diabetes [13].

Differential Diagnosis of Diabetes Arising in Young Adults

Most of the monogenic causes of diabetes present in the young-adult age range. Clinical features overlap between the various subtypes of monogenic diabetes and type 1 and type 2 diabetes. This can make clinical diagnosis of aetiology very challenging.

There are two major forms of MODY seen in practice. HNF1A-MODY accounts for about 50 % of cases in the UK [1] and shares many clinical features with HNF4A-MODY (10 % of UK cases), including SU sensitivity. One important difference is that *HNF4A* mutations are associated with fetal hyperinsulinaemia, macrosomia and neonatal hypoglycaemia [14]. This remits after a variable period and re-presents as diabetes some years later. The cause is unknown. Low renal glucose threshold and reduced CRP are not observed in HNF4A-MODY.

Glucokinase (GCK) mutations are the commonest cause of MODY in children and account for 30 % of UK MODY cases [1]. GCK-MODY has a phenotype of mild, lifelong, fasting hyperglycaemia (range 6–8 mmol/L) caused by a resetting of the normal threshold for glucose-stimulated insulin secretion. Insulin secretion remains regulated, but blood glucose remains around 2 mmol/L higher than normal. The increment of post-carbohydrate glucose rise is similar to that seen in the non-diabetic population [15], meaning that post-prandial excursions are not marked and HbA1c is only mildly elevated ($\leq$60 mmol/mol, 7.6 %). Treatment is not indicated and is probably ineffective. Observational studies in patients suggest they do not develop significant microvascular complications [16].

HNF1B mutations account for about a further 10 % of MODY cases, and are associated with a distinct phenotype of renal cystic disease and other developmental anomalies of the GU tract. Diabetes rarely occurs alone. Insulin treatment is usually required.

Mutations in the mitochondrial genome also commonly cause diabetes. This is usually accompanied by neurological manifestations, particularly deafness as in the maternally inherited diabetes and deafness (MIDD) syndrome. Myopathy, retinal dystrophy, renal disease and a number of other complications are also seen with mitochondrial disease [17]. The clinical picture is complicated by the variable content of the abnormal mitochondria in different tissues and it is recommended that specialist mitochondrial

services are involved. Metformin is relatively contra-indicated due to risk of lactic-acidosis and early progression to insulin requirement often occurs.

Severe insulin resistance syndromes and lipodystophies present a contrasting clinical phenotype to MODY. The commonest mutations are in the genes *LMNA* and *PPARG*, associated with early onset metabolic syndrome and body fat distribution abnormalities [18]. BMI may not be elevated, but patients have marked central obesity.

Investigations in Young Adult-Onset Diabetes

Diagnostic molecular genetic testing is available in the UK for all the monogenic causes of diabetes described above. Prior to requesting genetic testing, standard laboratory biochemical and immunological tests can be performed to identify those at high risk of having monogenic diabetes. Negative β-cell antibodies (e.g., GAD, IA2 and ICA) and presence of C-peptide are suggestive of a non-type 1 diabetes aetiology. C-peptide can be measured in blood or urine and a random or post-prandial sample (with a paired glucose sample if measuring in blood) is recommended to show presence of endogenous insulin secretion. Dyslipidaemia and a C-peptide above the normal range are suggestive of insulin resistance, which could indicate young type 2 diabetes or monogenic severe insulin resistance depending on other clinical features. The MODY probability calculator (http://www.diabetesgenes.org/content/mody-probability-calculator) can also be used to help judge the probability that your patient has MODY according to clinical features.

Summary

Assessment of aetiology should be included in care pathways for newly-diagnosed diabetes to allow patients to benefit from molecular advances in diagnostics and personalised medicine. Identifying the correct aetiology in young adults with diabetes allows for optimal treatment decisions, e.g., sulphonylureas in HNF1A/HNF4A-MODY, diet treatment in GCK-MODY, insulin in Type 1 diabetes and mitochondrial diabetes, and insulin sensitisers in type 2 diabetes and severe insulin resistance. Additionally information about treatment course and prognosis can be shared with patients and family members can be followed up appropriately.

Key Points

- Monogenic diabetes is often misdiagnosed as type 1 or type 2 diabetes. It's always worth revisiting the diagnosis if new information suggests the wrong aetiology has been assigned.
- Family history of apparently mixed forms of young-onset diabetes could have a unifying diagnosis of MODY
- Presence of C-peptide indicating endogenous insulin secretion in those with a clinical label of type 1 diabetes post honeymoon period is unusual and should prompt consideration of a different aetiology.
- Apparent type 2 diabetes in young, lean adults is unusual and should prompt consideration of a different aetiology
- Patients with HNF1A/HNF4A -MODY are sensitive to low-dose SU and experience hypoglycaemia on standard doses; SUs are the first-line treatment and can often be substituted for insulin.

References

1. Shields BM, Hicks S, Shepherd MH, Colclough K, Hattersley AT, Ellard S. Maturity-onset diabetes of the young (MODY): how many cases are we missing? Diabetologia. 2010;53(12):2504–8.
2. Thanabalasingham G, Owen KR. Diagnosis and management of maturity onset diabetes of the young (MODY). BMJ. 2011;343:d6044.
3. Pearson ER, Starkey BJ, Powell RJ, Gribble FM, Clark PM, Hattersley AT. Genetic cause of hyperglycaemia and response to treatment in diabetes. Lancet. 2003;362:1275–81.
4. Ellard S, Bellanne-Chantelot C, Hattersley AT. Best practice guidelines for the molecular genetic diagnosis of maturity-onset diabetes of the young. Diabetologia. 2008;51:546–53.
5. Shepherd M, Shields B, Ellard S, Rubio-Cabezas O, Hattersley AT. A genetic diagnosis of HNF1A diabetes alters treatment and improves glycaemic control in the majority of insulin-treated patients. Diabet Med. 2009;26:437–41.
6. Genetic types of diabetes. http://www.projects.ex.ac.uk/diabetesgenes/.
7. Menzel R, Kaisaki PJ, Rjasanowski I, Heinke P, Kerner W, Menzel S. A low renal threshold for glucose in diabetic patients with a mutation in the hepatocyte nuclear factor-1alpha (HNF-1alpha) gene. Diabet Med. 1998;15:816–20.
8. Stride A, Ellard S, Clark P, Shakespeare L, Salzmann M, Shepherd M, et al. Beta-cell dysfunction, insulin sensitivity, and glycosuria precede diabetes in hepatocyte nuclear factor-1alpha mutation carriers. Diabetes Care. 2005;28:1751–6.
9. Richter S, Shih DQ, Pearson ER, Wolfrum C, Fajans SS, Hattersley AT, et al. Regulation of apolipoprotein M gene expression by MODY3 gene hepatocyte nuclear factor-1alpha: haploinsufficiency is associated with reduced serum apolipoprotein M levels. Diabetes. 2003;52:2989–95.
10. Owen KR, Thanabalasingham G, James TJ, Karpe F, Farmer AJ, McCarthy MI, et al. Assessment of high-sensitivity C-reactive protein levels as diagnostic discriminator of maturity-onset diabetes of the young due to HNF1A mutations. Diabetes Care. 2010;33:1919–24.
11. McDonald TJ, Shields BM, Lawry J, Owen KR, Gloyn AL, Ellard S, et al. High-sensitivity CRP discriminates HNF1A-MODY from other subtypes of diabetes. Diabetes Care. 2011;34:1860–2.
12. Thanabalasingham G, Shah N, Vaxillaire M, Hansen T, Tuomi T, Gasperikova D, et al. A large multi-centre European study validates high-sensitivity C-reactive protein (hsCRP) as a clinical biomarker for the diagnosis of diabetes subtypes. Diabetologia. 2011;54:2801–10.
13. Owen KR, Shepherd M, Stride A, Ellard S, Hattersley AT. Heterogeneity in young adult onset diabetes: aetiology alters clinical characteristics. Diabet Med. 2002;19:758–61.
14. Pearson ER, Boj SF, Steele AM, Barrett T, Stals K, Shield JP, et al. Macrosomia and hyperinsulinaemic hypoglycaemia in patients with heterozygous mutations in the HNF4A gene. PLoS Med. 2007;4:e118.

15. Stride A, Vaxillaire M, Tuomi T, Barbetti F, Njolstad PR, Hansen T, et al. The genetic abnormality in the beta cell determines the response to an oral glucose load. Diabetologia. 2002;45:427–35.

16. Steele AM, Shields BM, Wensley KJ, Colclough K, Ellard S, Hattersley AT. Prevalence of vascular complications among patients with glucokinase mutations and prolonged, mild hyperglycemia. JAMA. 2014; 311(3):279–86. PubMed PMID: 24430320.

17. Murphy R, Turnbull DM, Walker M, Hattersley AT. Clinical features, diagnosis and management of maternally inherited diabetes and deafness (MIDD) associated with the 3243A>G mitochondrial point mutation. Diabet Med. 2008;25: 383–99.

18. Parker VE, Savage DB, O'Rahilly S, Semple RK. Mechanistic insights into insulin resistance in the genetic era. Diabet Med. 2011;28:1476–86.

Managing Diabetes in Pregnancy

Case 21

Eberta J.H. Tan and Eleanor M. Scott

Abstract

We discuss a case of diabetes in pregnancy that illustrates the thought processes and strategies for managing a patient with diabetes in pregnancy. It is certain that treating hyperglycemia in pregnancy translates to significant clinical benefit in terms of obstetric outcomes and fetal health benefits. However, there are still controversies on how best to conduct screening for gestational diabetes mellitus, the optimal dietary recommendations, and uncertainty over whether oral hypoglycemic agents should be given a larger role to play in the treatment of diabetes in pregnancy. The continued presence of large for gestational age (LGA) babies in women with seemingly excellent control of blood glucose during pregnancy also begs the question of whether there are other contributing factors we are not yet adequately addressing. We will be addressing these pertinent questions in the clinical update section as trainees should also be aware of these clinical controversies.

Keywords

Diabetes • Pregnancy • Case studies • Ketosis-prone • Diagnosis • Management

E.J.H. Tan, MBBS, MRCP (UK)
Endocrinology, Changi General Hospital, Singapore, Singapore

E.M. Scott, BM, BS, BMedSci, MD, FRCP (✉)
Leeds Institute of Genetics Health and Therapeutics, University of Leeds, Clarendon Way, Leeds, West Yorkshire LS2 9JT, UK
e-mail: e.m.scott@leeds.ac.uk

Case

A 35-year-old African lady with no apparent past medical history of diabetes mellitus attended at the end of the day to the diabetes clinic after being referred by her General Practitioner for a high capillary blood glucose reading at his practice. She spoke little English and had only recently moved to the area. She had attended her General Practitioner as she suspected that she was pregnant due to her

R. Ajjan, S.M. Orme (eds.), *Endocrinology and Diabetes: Case Studies, Questions and Commentaries*,
DOI 10.1007/978-1-4471-2789-5_21, © Springer-Verlag London 2015

increasing abdominal girth and missed periods. She was unsure of the date of her last menstrual period but looked like she was into her third trimester of pregnancy. She had no hand-held notes and had no evidence of having undergone an oral glucose tolerance test. Her capillary glucose performed in the diabetes clinic was 28 mmol/L, and a urine dipstick revealed glucose of 4+ and was negative for ketones. Her BMI was 36 kg/m^2, her blood pressure normal, hydration status was good, physical examination was unremarkable apart from a palpable gravid uterus and she looked well.

> What further history and examination findings would you, as the managing diabetologist at the clinic, like to know?

It is likely that this lady has diabetes mellitus and is into the third trimester of her pregnancy. We are unsure if she has developed gestational diabetes or has pre-existing diabetes mellitus, as the severity of hyperglycemia does not reliably differentiate between gestational or pre-existing diabetes mellitus.

An obstetric history, in particular of any miscarriages, fetal abnormalities, fetal macrosomia, previous gestational diabetes mellitus and a family history of type 2 diabetes mellitus would suggest the possibility of pre-existing type 2 diabetes mellitus that was previously not detected. Previous fetal macrosomia and a family history of type 2 diabetes mellitus or a previous pregnancy complicated with gestational diabetes mellitus could suggest gestational diabetes mellitus (GDM). A family history of type 1 diabetes mellitus could also be present, although less frequently than in type 2 diabetes mellitus, if this lady has type 1 diabetes mellitus.

Her BMI of 36 kg/m^2 does suggest the presence of a degree of insulin resistance and the possibility of GDM or type 2 diabetes mellitus, although concurrent insulin resistance can occur in overweight or obese patients with type 1 diabetes mellitus. Other clues on physical examination that suggest insulin resistance would be the presence of acan-

thosis nigricans. Features of any other autoimmune disease would on the other hand suggest the possible diagnosis of type 1 diabetes mellitus.

> What are the important clinical issues in this lady?

In view of her significantly high capillary blood glucose, the clinical concern would be whether she was in diabetic ketoacidosis, although the fact she had urine that was negative for ketones, makes this unlikely. As she might have had pre-existing diabetes mellitus and hence hyperglycemia during conception and the first two trimesters of pregnancy, another concern would be whether there are any diabetes related fetal complications like organ malformations, macrosomia or stillbirth.

> What would be your management plan for her at this point?

The first priority is to ensure that this lady is not in diabetic ketoacidosis or progressing towards this serious complication.

Thereafter, normalising her blood glucose levels for the rest of the pregnancy and arranging for a fetal ultrasound to assess fetal gestational age, well-being and size would be pertinent to plan further management.

As she was well with no apparent osmotic symptoms and no ketones in her urine, she was commenced on self-monitored capillary blood glucose testing and basal-bolus subcutaneous insulin and reviewed by the diabetes specialist nurse (DSN) the following morning. Her fasting capillary blood glucose in the morning was 20 mmol/L and the decision was made to admit her to the antenatal ward to optimize blood glucose control and to expedite the assessment of the fetus. She was still feeling well then and inpatient investigations (including urinary ketones and blood gases for pH) again excluded diabetic ketoacidosis. Fetal ultrasound revealed that she was 34 weeks pregnant but that the pregnancy was non-viable as there was no fetal heartbeat or movement. Induction of labour was performed and she delivered a stillborn macrosomic male infant. Immediately following delivery, her venous blood glucose level was 4.2 mmol/L. Her HbA1c came back at 9.6 %. Her 6 week postnatal oral glucose tolerance test revealed a fasting glucose of 4.3 mmol/L and 2 h glucose of 5.6 mmol/L. Her anti-GAD and islet cell antibodies were negative.

> What does the patient's progress suggest about the diagnosis?

After delivery of the infant, this patient's OGTT revealed normoglycaemia, confirming the diagnosis of gestational diabetes mellitus.

> What would your treatment plan be from this stage?

Gestational diabetes mellitus resolves after delivery as the hormones responsible for its appearance relinquish to their normal non-pregnant levels after the placenta is delivered. Hence, no medical therapy is required at this stage. However, vigilance must be kept as these patients are at high risk of developing type 2 diabetes mellitus in future (50 % within 5 years) or gestational diabetes mellitus during any future pregnancies and advice should be given to these patients to help them delay the onset of type 2 diabetes mellitus, including the importance of healthy weight loss and exercise. In addition it is advised that they are screened yearly for diabetes with a fasting glucose or HbA1c.

As this patient was keen to plan for another pregnancy an appointment was made for her for the diabetes pre-conception clinic. She continued having normal capillary blood glucose readings and conceived 3 months later. Capillary blood glucose readings remained normal during the first trimester of pregnancy and an OGTT done at

14 weeks of gestation was normal (0-h glucose of 4.1 mmol/L and 2-h glucose of 6.5 mmol/L). A repeat OGTT at 26 weeks of gestation revealed a 0-h glucose of 6.4 mmol/L and 2-h glucose of 10.9 mmol/L.

> What is the diagnosis and how would you manage this lady?

She has developed gestational diabetes mellitus again in this pregnancy. She should be managed with dietary advice, and if necessary, medical therapy and regular fetal ultrasound scans to monitor fetal growth.

She was started on subcutaneous insulin 1 week later as her capillary blood glucose readings were still not optimal with lifestyle modification. Serial fetal ultrasound scans revealed normal fetal growth and she delivered a healthy male infant of 3.5 kg at 38 weeks of gestation. Her 6-week postnatal OGTT had a 0-h glucose of 4.4 mmol/L and 2-h glucose of 6.5 mmol/L.

She had a further pregnancy, during which she similarly developed gestational diabetes mellitus in the second trimester, was managed with insulin and delivered a healthy female infant. Six-week postnatal OGTT remained normal. She was not planning a further pregnancy and understood the importance of preconception care having received it previously. She was henceforth discharged to her general practitioner, with advice to lose weight, have her venous blood glucose checked yearly by her GP, earlier if planning a further pregnancy and was informed of the need to have an early OGTT if she became pregnant in future.

She telephoned the diabetes clinic a year later, informing the team that she was 6 weeks pregnant. She gave a history of 3 weeks of thirst and polyuria. Capillary blood glucose in clinic was high. A venous blood glucose was performed and came back at 32 mmol/L, she had urine ketones of 4+. She was admitted immediately and was found to have a metabolic acidosis and managed for diabetic ketoacidosis. Her HbA1c done at that point was 9.8 %. She chose to terminate the pregnancy.

Capillary blood glucose readings remained elevated postnatally at 8–10 mmol/L. Her anti-GAD and islet cell antibodies were again negative and she was diagnosed with ketosis prone type 2 diabetes mellitus and commenced on metformin 500 mg three times a day. HbA1c improved to 6.2 % with metformin and dietary and lifestyle modification. She remained in contact with the diabetes team and a year later planned a subsequent pregnancy after receiving multidisciplinary diabetes preconception care.

In her subsequent planned pregnancy, she was managed with metformin and insulin and delivered a healthy female infant. She underwent sterilization and was henceforth discharged to the GP on metformin.

> What are the possibilities behind this lady with features of type 2 diabetes mellitus presenting with diabetic ketoacidosis in pregnancy?

Patients with type 2 diabetes mellitus can present with diabetic ketoacidosis. However, these patients are often in the advanced stage of the disease and insulin deficient. This lady's diabetes had been adequately controlled with metformin and lifestyle modification and was not insulin-dependent. A presentation with diabetic ketoacidosis without any precipitating cause except perhaps the stress of pregnancy would be clinically unusual. The consideration of the diagnosis of possible ketosis-prone diabetes should be made, because of the unusual presentation of this lady in a decompensated state of DKA without an obvious precipitant, compounded with the fact that she is of African descent.

The understanding of atypical forms of diabetes in particular ketosis prone diabetes has advanced considerably over the years. Ketosis-prone diabetes is being increasingly recognized, initially in African persons and in African-American individuals in the United States [1], and now also in Native-Americans, Japanese, Chinese, Hispanic and white populations [2]. Patients often present initially with DKA or unprovoked ketosis despite lacking the classic phenotype of autoimmune type 1 diabetes, and the majority (76 %) eventually can attain insulin-independence within weeks to months despite presenting in DKA, in contrast to "classic" auto-immune type 1 diabetes. They have been referred to as having diabetes type 1B, idiopathic type 1 diabetes, atypical diabetes, Flatbush diabetes, type 1.5 diabetes, and more recently, ketosis-prone type 2 diabetes [2].

DKA is known to recur during periods of stress or infection or even without precipitating cause in ketosis prone diabetes and hence patients should be educated about this possibility and taught to check for ketones if ill and having deterioration in glycemic control, and seek medical help if unwell.

Clinical Update

Although it is certain that treating hyperglycemia in pregnancy translates to significant clinical benefit in terms of obstetric outcomes and fetal health benefits, there is still controversy over how best to conduct screening for gestational diabetes mellitus, the optimal dietary recommendations, and uncertainty over whether oral hypoglycemic agents should be given a larger role to play in the treatment of diabetes in pregnancy. The continued presence of large for gestational age (LGA) babies in women with seemingly excellent control of blood glucose during pregnancy also begs the question of whether there are other contributing factors we are not yet adequately addressing. We will be addressing these clinical questions in the discussion below.

> Which screening test should be done for gestational diabetes mellitus, and when?

Internationally, there are at least six different criteria for the diagnosis of gestational diabetes (Table 21.1) These include the 50 g 1-h oral glucose challenge test (50 g 1-h OGCT) without regard to timing of last meal, with a glucose threshold of 7.2 mmol/L, 7.8 mmol/L, 8.0 mmol/L or 10.3 mmol/L, the 2-h 75 g oral glucose tolerance

Table 21.1 Screening tests for diabetes mellitus in pregnancy

Test	Number of abnormal values	Threshold (equal or greater than) in mmol/L				Organisation
		0 h	1 h	2 h	3 h	
50 g OGCT	1	–	7.2	–	–	CC, IWC
	1	–	7.2 or 7.8	–	–	ACOG
	1	–	7.8 or 8.0	–	–	ADIPS
	1	–	7.8 or 10.3	–	–	CDA
75 g OGTT	1 or more	5.1	10.0	8.5	–	IADPSG/ADA
	1	6.1 for IGT 7.0 for DM	–	7.8 for IGT 11.1 for DM	–	WHO
	1	5.5	–	8.0 or 9.0	–	ADIPS
	2 or more	5.3	10.6	8.9	–	CDA
100 g OGTT	2 or more	5.3	10.0	8.6	7.8	CC & IWC
	2 or more	5.8	10.5	9.1	8.0	NDDG

test (2 h 75 g-OGTT) taking either the 0-h or 2-h glucose or 0-, 1- or 2-h glucose levels, and 3-h 100 g OGTT with different cut-off values for diagnosis depending on criteria. The most commonly used test is the 2-h 75 g OGTT used by the WHO (World Health Organisation) taking a 0 h glucose cut-off of 7.0 mmol/L or 2-h glucose cut-off of 7.8 mmol/L for diagnosis of impaired glucose tolerance (IGT) in pregnancy, and the IADPSG (International Association of Diabetes and Pregnancy Study Group) and ADA (American Diabetes Association), who use a cut-off of either a fasting glucose more than 5.1 mmol/L, 1-h glucose of more than 10.0 mmol/L or 2-h glucose of more than 8.5 mmol/L [3]. The WHO, in its latest recommendation in August 2013 has also adopted the same diagnostic criteria recommended by the IADPSG [4]. This latest recommendation by the IADPSG and ADA was based on the largest prospective trial to date – the HAPO (Hyperglycemia and Adverse Pregnancy Outcomes) Study Cooperative Research Group [5]. The IADPSG-recommended diagnostic thresholds are the average glucose values at which odds for birth weight, cord C-peptide, and percent body fat, each >90th percentile reached 1.75 times the estimated odds of these outcomes at mean fasting, 1-h, and 2-h OGTT glucose values, based on fully adjusted logistic regression models. It is also important to know that the HAPO study showed that the associations of glucose values and outcomes are continuous

and linear. Women who have slightly raised glucose levels but not beyond the thresholds also have an increased risk of a high birth weight, cord C-peptide and percent body fat compared to women who are normoglycaemic and according to good clinical practice, should be given dietary and lifestyle advice to normalize glucose levels as much as possible to achieve good pregnancy outcomes. HbA1c is not recommended for diagnosing diabetes during pregnancy.

The second controversy would be over whether universal or selective screening should be done. The selective principle means that the screening model would be limited only in the selected group of pregnant women with various risk factors for GDM that existed before pregnancy or are developed during pregnancy. It has been shown that a consequence of risk factor screening is that a significant number of women with impaired carbohydrate metabolism would remain unrecognized and at risk of perinatal complications [6, 7]. There is no properly conducted randomized control trial with a sufficient number of patients examined for the benefit of selective or universal screening for GDM compared with no screening. Moreover, performances of screening would also vary according to the population studied, frequency of risk factors and the thresholds used. Most publications show that between 3 and 10 % of women with GDM are not diagnosed by selective screening but this can go to as high as 30–50 % in some series.

Currently, the ACOG, SOGC and NICE recommend routine risk-factor-based screening, whereas the USPSTF, ADA, IADPSG, ADIPS, CDA and ATLANTIC DIP network recommend universal screening in asymptomatic pregnant women at 24–28 weeks of gestation, followed by definitive testing only in those women who are labeled as high-risk population.

Timing of screening most commonly mentioned in the literature is between 24 and 28 weeks, but it has to be emphasized that this recommendation specifically refers to healthy women without anamnestic risk factors. GDM classically occurs in the third trimester of pregnancy (from 24 weeks) due to physiopathological changes in glucose metabolism during pregnancy, including progressive insulin resistance caused by increased placental secretion of diabetogenic hormones growth hormone (GH), corticotropin releasing hormone (CRH) which drives release of adrenocorticotrophic hormone (ACTH) and cortisol, human placental lactogen and progesterone and a postreceptor defect. It is not logical to screen after 28 weeks of pregnancy because the initial phase of fetal growth acceleration has already begun.

Early GDM accounts for between 15 and 20 % of cases, although a high proportion of early GDM cases are probably undiagnosed type 2 diabetes mellitus. Screening for overt diabetes not diagnosed before pregnancy before 20 weeks of gestation is in general consensus recommended for populations at high risk for type 2 diabetes mellitus. These include women with a previous diagnosis of gestational diabetes, a first-degree relative with diabetes, a family origin with a high prevalence of diabetes, polycystic ovarian syndrome (PCOS), a previous large for gestational age baby and severe obesity. The NICE guidelines recommend screening for women with a previous diagnosis of GDM at 16–18 weeks [8]. Other guidelines by the ADA recommend screening either fasting or random glucose levels, 2-h glucose post OGTT or the HbA1c in such populations at first booking [9].

What type of dietary recommendations should we make to women with gestational diabetes mellitus, existent type 1 diabetes mellitus and type 2 diabetes mellitus?

For healthy pregnant women, energy needs are no higher than the estimated energy requirement for nonpregnant women until the second trimester [10]. The extra energy need is 340 kcal in the second and 450 kcal in the third trimester. Prepregnancy body mass index, rate of weight gain, maternal age, and appetite must be considered when tailoring this recommendation to the individual. Moreover, for obese women with GDM, caloric restriction of 30 % may improve glycemic control without increasing ketonuria.

There is scant level 1 evidence to support most aspects of nutritional prescription for GDM. However, it does make clinical sense that the goals of medical nutritional therapy should be to achieve normoglycaemia, prevent ketosis, provide adequate weight gain based on their body mass index and contribute to fetal well-being. Nutrition therapy has been shown to improve glycemic control for people living with overt diabetes and for women with gestational diabetes [11]. Hence, nutritional therapy is widely recommended as an integral part of the treatment of women with gestational diabetes mellitus.

Is carbohydrate restriction necessary?

The acceptable macronutrient distribution ranges for consumption of carbohydrates, protein and fat as a percentage of total energy intakes for healthy pregnant women are estimated to be 45–65 % for carbohydrate, 10–35 % for protein and 20–35 % for fat.

The conventional diet approach to gestational diabetes mellitus (GDM) advocates carbohydrate restriction (35–40 % of total calories) [12–14], with carbohydrate intake distributed across meals and snacks in order to blunt postprandial glucose and mitigate glucose-mediated fetal macrosomia.

For women with type 1 diabetes, a lower proportion of carbohydrate during pregnancy such as 40 % of energy (moderate-low carbohydrate diet) has also been suggested to result in normoglycaemia and excellent pregnancy outcome [15].

Few studies have been done in pregnant women with type 2 diabetes mellitus with regards to which dietary treatment would give the best outcome for mother and fetus. A low carbohydrate diet with 35 % of the calories as carbohydrates was described to reduce the incidence of hyperglycemia in women with type 2 diabetes mellitus during pregnancy, with a reduced need for insulin treatment and a significant reduction in the incidence of macrosomia [16]. Nonetheless, the same principles of avoiding excessive weight gain and controlling postprandial glucose levels apply, as in gestational diabetes mellitus and type 1 diabetes mellitus, and again, the long term fetal and maternal outcomes of these interventions are not yet conclusively known.

It is worth noting that although carbohydrate restriction is often useful in the management of diabetes in pregnancy, it should not be done excessively. The IOM (Institute of Medicine) clinical guidelines recommend a minimum intake of 175 g carbohydrate/day to ensure sufficient supplementation of glucose to the mother and fetus including 33 g/day for the fetal brain and avoid the possibility of low carbohydrate diet induced ketogenesis that may be associated with a decrease in intelligence and fine motor skills in the offspring [17].

On the other hand, perhaps carbohydrate restriction is not the only component in the equation when working towards better glycemic control in women with diabetes in pregnancy. Carbohydrate restriction often results in higher fat intake, given that protein intake is remarkably constant at 15–20 %. Outside of pregnancy, a high-fat diet typically increases serum free fatty acids, promoting insulin resistance. In nonhuman primates and in some human studies, a maternal high-fat diet increases fetal fat accretion and infant adiposity, promotes hepatic steatosis, increases inflammation and oxidative stress, and impairs skeletal muscle glucose uptake. This might explain why in a recent randomized controlled trial of carbohydrate restriction to 40 % (with 40 % fat) versus 55 % (with 25 % fat) in women with gestational diabetes, there was no significance difference in the need for insulin treatment or pregnancy outcomes [18]. Perhaps, also, the choice of carbohydrate, in particular the glycemic index of carbohydrate, plays an equally important role in attaining good glycemic control.

Is low glycaemic index diet helpful?

Several studies have revealed that a diet that is high in carbohydrates of low glycaemic index improves overall glucose control and reduces postprandial glucose excursions in pregnant women with no diabetes [19], gestational diabetes mellitus [20], nonpregnant individuals with type 1 diabetes mellitus and type 2 diabetes mellitus [21, 22] and reduces the need for insulin in gestational diabetes [23]. However, evidence for obstetric and fetal advantages are still lacking. Currently, only three published randomized controlled trials have studied fetal and obstetric outcomes between pregnant women with gestational diabetes treated with a diet with low-moderate glycaemic index and controls on moderate-high glycaemic index carbohydrates. These have shown no significant differences in rates of macrosomia, large for gestational age infants, caesarean section, operative vaginal birth and normal vaginal birth [23–25]. The ROLO study of 800 women without diabetes but with a previous infant weighing greater than 4 kg showed that a low glycaemic index diet in pregnancy did not reduce the incidence of large for gestational age infants, but did have a significant positive effect on gestational weight gain and maternal glucose tolerance [26]. At this moment, there are no studies or data with regards to long-term fetal and maternal health outcome data in women with gestational diabetes prescribed a pregnancy diet high in carbohydrates of low glycaemic index.

What about carbohydrate counting?

Carbohydrate counting is a very essential strategy for the improvement of glycemic control in non-pregnant patients with type 1 diabetes and is frequently used together with insulin pump treatment for pregnant as well as for non-pregnant patients. Although data on the effect in pregnancy are lacking, it makes clinical sense for the continuation of accurate carbohydrate counting with intensive reviews of these patient's postprandial glucose levels as these will intuitively impact on macrosomia.

Is metformin recommended for use in gestational diabetes mellitus and pre-existing type 1 and type 2 diabetes mellitus in pregnancy?

Regular insulin, the rapid-acting insulin analogues aspart and lispro, the long-acting insulin analogue levemir and human insulin are licensed for use in gestational diabetes mellitus and pre-existing diabetes mellitus in pregnancy. Metformin is not licensed for use in gestational diabetes mellitus and pre-existing diabetes mellitus in pregnancy but certain national institutes like the England and Wales National Institute for Health and Clinical Excellence included metformin and glyburide as GDM and type 2 diabetes in pregnancy treatment options, with the proviso that it is not licensed for these indications and that there should be informed consent on the use of metformin or glyburide if the managing diabetologist would like to use it due to strong evidence for its effectiveness and safety so far [8].

The lure of using metformin in pregnancy is its low cost, easy administration without need for much patient training (unlike insulin), low risk of hypoglycaemia, especially when used as monotherapy, and potential for prevention of excessive weight gain, a useful advantage when used in

patients requiring insulin, or if used instead of insulin for glycaemic control. Its disadvantage would be its failure rate of about 40–50 % of patients (the proportion being dependent on the population studied), and the lack of long-term safety data.

The use of metformin in early pregnancy in several randomized controlled trials of pregnant women with polycystic ovary syndrome has revealed no increased risk of major congenital malformations and in fact showed reduction in adverse pregnancy outcomes, reduction in the incidence of gestational diabetes and higher pregnancy and live birth rates [27–30].

The non-inferiority in terms of effectiveness and safety of metformin compared to insulin in the treatment of gestational diabetes was also proven in the Metformin in Gestational Diabetes (MiG) trial [31]. In this randomized control trial of 751 women with gestational diabetes randomly allocated to open-label treatment with metformin (1,000–2,000 mg daily) or to insulin alone, there was no significant difference in the primary outcome (composite of neonatal complications including hypoglycaemia, respiratory distress, phototherapy, birth trauma, low APGAR and prematurity). In fact, severe neonatal hypoglycaemia occurred more commonly in the insulin group than in the metformin group. There were no differences in the number of congenital abnormalities between groups. There was also less maternal weight gain (metformin 0.4 vs. insulin 2.0 kg, p=0.001) and more treatment satisfaction in favour of metformin. Seven more recent but smaller trials have also largely confirmed the safety and efficacy of metformin in gestational diabetes compared to insulin [32–35].

There also seems to be potential in the addition of metformin to insulin therapy in women with type 2 diabetes mellitus with pregnancy. A recent randomized controlled trial on 90 women with either gestational or pre-existing diabetes mellitus having poor glycaemic control at a daily dose of insulin of ≥1.12 units/kg (defined as having insulin resistance in this study) showed that adding metformin to insulin therapy in these women achieved good glycemic control in 75 % of without needing an increased insulin dose [36]. Addition of metformin was also associated with a reduction in hospital stay, maternal hypoglycemia, neonatal hypoglycemia, NICU admission and neonatal respiratory distress syndrome. We await the results of the Metformin in Women with Type 2 Diabetes in Pregnancy (MiTy) trial of 500 pregnant women with type 2 diabetes recruited from 25 centres in Canada who will be randomized to receive metformin or placebo in addition to their usual regimen of insulin. This study will clarify whether adding metformin to insulin in women with type 2 diabetes will be beneficial to the mothers and infants (Clinical Trials Registry No; NCT 01353391).

The long-term follow-up of the MiG study will also provide important insights into the long-term consequences including potential benefits on the offspring of mothers with diabetes mellitus exposed to metformin in utero. The first follow-up of infants of women with GDM randomized to receive either metformin or insulin during pregnancy has been done at 2 years of age [37]. Offspring exposed to metformin in utero had increased subscapular and biceps skinfolds when compared with the unexposed infants, while total body fat was similar. The hypothesis is that this represents a possible benefit as this may signal a healthier fat distribution. Longer term studies will examine this question of whether children exposed to metformin will indeed develop less visceral fat and ben more insulin sensitive.

> What should be our glucose targets in GDM and pregnant women with pre-existing type 1 or type 2 diabetes mellitus?

The glucose level at which the benefits of initiating insulin therapy outweigh its disadvantages has not been definitively determined and there is little consensus in the literature. The American Diabetes Association (ADA) [9] and the American College of Obstetricians and Gynecologists (ACOG) [38] recommend the following upper limits for glucose levels, with insulin therapy initiated if they are exceeded:

- Fasting blood glucose concentration ≤5.3 mmol/L
- One-hour postprandial blood glucose concentration ≤7.8 mmol/L
- Two-hour postprandial glucose concentration ≤6.7 mmol/L

These targets represent the upper limit of desirable glucose concentration, well above the mean glucose values in nondiabetic pregnant women described in a 2011 literature review of studies of the normal 24-h glycemic profile of pregnant women [39]. If two standard deviations are added to the means of these nondiabetic pregnant women, the upper limit of normal fasting glucose would be 4.8 mmol/L, 1-h postprandial value 7.5 mmol/L and 2-h value 6.6 mmol/L.

The NICE guidelines recommend that if it is safely achievable, women with diabetes should aim to keep fasting blood glucose between 3.5 and 5.9 mmol/L and 1-h postprandial blood glucose below 7.8 mmol/L during pregnancy [8]. These recommendations were based on studies that examined the relationship between birth weight, respiratory distress, congenital malformations, stillbirth and neonatal death and blood glucose control during pregnancy that revealed that postprandial blood glucose levels have a stronger association with incidence of macrosomia than HbA1c during the second and third trimesters and monitoring of postprandial blood glucose produced better outcomes than preprandial monitoring.

The HAPO study showed a continuous relationship between maternal glucose and adverse outcomes, with a fasting plasma glucose level of 5.6–5.8 mmol/L associated with a risk of macrosomia five-fold greater than that with a fasting glucose level less than 4.2 mmol/L [5]. Whether there would be benefit to lowering the targets for initiating therapy in GDM in an effort to further lower the increased prevalence of large for gestational age infants is a hypothesis which could be tested, bearing in mind that there is evidence that overly tight metabolic control in GDM with insulin (i.e., average blood glucose levels ≤4.8 mmol/L) can result in an increase in small for gestational age offspring [40]. Nonetheless, from the preliminary good results from dietary interventions in this group of women, it will be good clinical practice to institute dietary changes and exercise as this has been shown increasingly to improve both maternal and fetal outcomes.

> What are the aims of preconception care in women with diabetes mellitus?

It is important for healthcare professionals and women with diabetes to realize that complications associated with diabetes in pregnancy can be avoided and the risks reduced down to that seen in the background population by receiving structured multidisciplinary preconception care. The key aim of this is to achieve tight glycemic control (HbA1c <6.1 %; 43 mmol/mol), where safely achievable, prior to conception.

Other aims of preconception care are to assess and address pre-existing complications of diabetes mellitus, including addressing any diabetic retinopathy and nephropathy and complications of treatment like hypoglycemia, which can prove even more problematic in pregnancy due to the reduced hypoglycemic awareness, especially in the first trimester. Indeed screening for retinopathy is recommended in each trimester throughout pregnancy.

Medications that the patient is currently on should also be reviewed and potential teratogenic agents should be stopped at the point of consultation if unnecessary or switched to other medications more suitable for pregnancy if required for control of the patient's medical conditions.

Women with diabetes are known to have an increased risk of having a baby with a neural tube defect. Studies in women with a previous poor pregnancy outcome have shown that being on folic acid supplementation prior to pregnancy was associated with a reduced risk of poor pregnancy outcomes. Although these studies were not done exclusively in women with diabetes in pregnancy, it is recommended that folate should be supplemented at a higher dose of 5 mg per day until organogenesis is complete (12 weeks gestation) [8].

A point that should not be overlooked is the management of obesity before conception, with a continuing aim to control overt weight gain during pregnancy. The body mass index (BMI) of the mother affects baby's outcome significantly. Over time with better glucose control of women with diabetes mellitus, the risk for congenital malformations has decreased but not the risk for large for gestational age (LGA) [41]. Obesity is also associated with increased rates of gestational hypertension, preeclampsia, GDM and retained weight postpartum [42–44]. A retrospective analysis of the records of 9.835 women has shown that obese GDM women had a 5.5-fold increased risk of LGA, whereas obesity alone or GDM alone had a 1.7 or 2.0-fold increased risk of LGA, respectively, similar to the HAPO report [45]. Overall, however, obesity and overweight accounted for 21.6 % of LGA and when GDM was added to obesity or overweight the combination accounted for a total of 23.3 % of LGA. Most LGA occurs independently of obesity and hyperglycemia and it remains to be seen what other factors contribute to LGA. Preconception BMI influences the incidence of LGA more so than weight gain during pregnancy and so the role of public awareness of the adverse consequences of obesity for the baby and the role of the diabetologist in optimizing the mother's starting body weight before conception is important. Providing advancing maternal age or other time-related pressures are not an issue it is well worth helping women to lose weight as part of their preconception care. This has the added benefit of helping improve their glycemic control reducing the need for drugs in pregnancy. In women with type 2 diabetes who have suboptimal glycemic control on metformin the only safe option to optimize glycemic control preconception is to add in insulin. However, this almost inevitably leads to significant weight gain in these women which can negatively impact on their chances of pregnancy particularly if they are requiring fertility treatment. In these situations it is worth trying GLP-1 agonists in preference to insulin, provided the woman is counselled not to become pregnant whilst using it and use of adequate contraception is discussed. The benefits are that over a 6 month period, there is a chance of significant weight loss, together with tighter glycemic control. The GLP-1 agonist is then stopped electively prior to actively trying for pregnancy and the woman with type 2 diabetes has a far healthier pre pregnancy baseline with regard to weight, glycemic control and unnecessary medications.

Last but not least, although it may seem counterintuitive, contraception is an important component of diabetes preconception care It needs discussing regularly with all women with diabetes of child bearing age including those who have not yet achieved tight enough glycaemic control or a healthy weight before attempting conception, and women with diabetes who have just had a baby, in order to prevent an unplanned pregnancy whilst their glucose control is suboptimal.

References

1. Mauvais-Jarvis F, Sobngwi E, Porcher R, Riveline J-P, Kevorkian J-P, Vaisse C, et al. Ketosis-prone type 2 diabetes in patients of sub-Saharan African origin: clinical pathophysiology and natural history of beta-cell dysfunction and insulin resistance. Diabetes. 2004;53(3):645–53.
2. Umpierrez GE, Smiley D, Kitabchi AE. Narrative review: ketosis-prone type 2 diabetes mellitus. Ann Intern Med. 2006;144(5):350–7.
3. International Association of Diabetes and Pregnancy Study Groups Consensus Panel, Metzger BE, Gabbe SG, Persson B, Buchanan TA, Catalano PA, et al. International association of diabetes and pregnancy study groups recommendations on the diagnosis and classification of hyperglycemia in pregnancy. Diabetes Care. 2010;33(3):676–82.
4. Diagnostic criteria and classification of hyperglycaemia first detected in pregnancy [Internet]. Geneva: World Health Organization; 2013 [cited 2014 Apr 4]. Available from: http://www.ncbi.nlm.nih.gov/books/NBK169024/.
5. HAPO Study Cooperative Research Group, Metzger BE, Lowe LP, Dyer AR, Trimble ER, Chaovarindr U, et al. Hyperglycemia and adverse pregnancy outcomes. N Engl J Med. 2008;358(19):1991–2002.
6. Cosson E, Benbara A, Pharisien I, Nguyen MT, Revaux A, Lormeau B, et al. Diagnostic and prognostic performances over 9 years of a selective screening strategy for gestational diabetes mellitus in a cohort of 18,775 subjects. Diabetes Care. 2013;36(3):598–603.
7. Ostlund I, Hanson U. Occurrence of gestational diabetes mellitus and the value of different screening indicators for the oral glucose tolerance test. Acta Obstet Gynecol Scand. 2003;82(2):103–8.
8. Walker JD. NICE guidance on diabetes in pregnancy: management of diabetes and its complications from preconception to the postnatal period. NICE clinical guideline 63. London, March 2008. Diabet Med. 2008;25(9):1025–7.
9. American Diabetes Association. Standards of medical care in diabetes – 2014. Diabetes Care. 2014;37 Suppl 1:S14–80.
10. Kaiser L, Allen LH, American Dietetic Association. Position of the American Dietetic Association: nutrition and lifestyle for a healthy pregnancy outcome. J Am Diet Assoc. 2008;108(3):553–61.
11. Reader D, Splett P, Gunderson EP, Diabetes Care and Education Dietetic Practice Group. Impact of gestational diabetes mellitus nutrition practice guidelines implemented by registered dietitians on pregnancy outcomes. J Am Diet Assoc. 2006;106(9):1426–33.
12. Peterson CM, Jovanovic-Peterson L. Percentage of carbohydrate and glycemic response to breakfast, lunch, and dinner in women with gestational diabetes. Diabetes. 1991;40 Suppl 2:172–4.
13. Clapp 3rd JF. Effect of dietary carbohydrate on the glucose and insulin response to mixed caloric intake and exercise in both nonpregnant and pregnant women. Diabetes Care. 1998;21 Suppl 2:B107–12.
14. Jovanovic L. Achieving euglycaemia in women with gestational diabetes mellitus: current options for screening, diagnosis and treatment. Drugs. 2004;64(13):1401–17.
15. Jovanovic L, Peterson CM. Management of the pregnant, insulin-dependent diabetic woman. Diabetes Care. 1980;3(1):63–8.
16. Hone J, Jovanovic L. Approach to the patient with diabetes during pregnancy. J Clin Endocrinol Metab. 2010;95(8):3578–85.
17. Institute of Medicine (US) and National Research Council (US) Committee to Reexamine IOM Pregnancy Weight Guidelines. Weight gain during pregnancy: reexamining the guidelines [Internet]. Rasmussen KM, Yaktine AL, editors. Washington, DC: National Academies Press; 2009 [cited 2014 Apr 10]. Available from: http://www.ncbi.nlm.nih.gov/books/NBK32813/.
18. Moreno-Castilla C, Hernandez M, Bergua M, Alvarez MC, Arce MA, Rodriguez K, et al. Low-carbohydrate diet for the treatment of gestational diabetes mellitus: a randomized controlled trial. Diabetes Care. 2013;36(8):2233–8.
19. Clapp 3rd JF. Maternal carbohydrate intake and pregnancy outcome. Proc Nutr Soc. 2002;61(1):45–50.

20. Nolan CJ. Improved glucose tolerance in gestational diabetic women on a low fat, high unrefined carbohydrate diet. Aust N Z J Obstet Gynaecol. 1984;24(3):174–7.

21. Ludwig DS. The glycemic index: physiological mechanisms relating to obesity, diabetes, and cardiovascular disease. JAMA. 2002;287(18):2414–23.

22. Burani J, Longo PJ. Low-glycemic index carbohydrates: an effective behavioral change for glycemic control and weight management in patients with type 1 and 2 diabetes. Diabetes Educ. 2006;32(1):78–88.

23. Moses RG, Barker M, Winter M, Petocz P, Brand-Miller JC. Can a low-glycemic index diet reduce the need for insulin in gestational diabetes mellitus? A randomized trial. Diabetes Care. 2009;32(6):996–1000.

24. Balas-Nakash M, Rodríguez-Cano A, Muñoz-Manrique C, Vásquez-Peña P, Perichart-Perera O. Adherence to a medical nutrition therapy program in pregnant women with diabetes, measured by three methods, and its association with glycemic control. Rev Invest Clin. 2010;62(3):235–43.

25. Grant SM, Wolever TMS, O'Connor DL, Nisenbaum R, Josse RG. Effect of a low glycaemic index diet on blood glucose in women with gestational hyperglycaemia. Diabetes Res Clin Pract. 2011;91(1):15–22.

26. Walsh JM, McGowan CA, Mahony R, Foley ME, McAuliffe FM. Low glycaemic index diet in pregnancy to prevent macrosomia (ROLO study): randomised control trial. BMJ. 2012;345:e5605.

27. Vanky E, Salvesen KA, Heimstad R, Fougner KJ, Romundstad P, Carlsen SM. Metformin reduces pregnancy complications without affecting androgen levels in pregnant polycystic ovary syndrome women: results of a randomized study. Hum Reprod. 2004;19(8):1734–40.

28. Vanky E, Stridsklev S, Heimstad R, Romundstad P, Skogøy K, Kleggetveit O, et al. Metformin versus placebo from first trimester to delivery in polycystic ovary syndrome: a randomized, controlled multicenter study. J Clin Endocrinol Metab. 2010;95(12): E448–55.

29. Begum MR, Khanam NN, Quadir E, Ferdous J, Begum MS, Khan F, et al. Prevention of gestational diabetes mellitus by continuing metformin therapy throughout pregnancy in women with polycystic ovary syndrome. J Obstet Gynaecol Res. 2009;35(2): 282–6.

30. Morin-Papunen L, Rantala AS, Unkila-Kallio L, Tiitinen A, Hippeläinen M, Perheentupa A, et al. Metformin improves pregnancy and live-birth rates in women with polycystic ovary syndrome (PCOS): a multicenter, double-blind, placebo-controlled randomized trial. J Clin Endocrinol Metab. 2012;97(5):1492–500.

31. Rowan JA, Hague WM, Gao W, Battin MR, Moore MP, MiG Trial Investigators. Metformin versus insulin for the treatment of gestational diabetes. N Engl J Med. 2008;358(19):2003–15.

32. Ijäs H, Vääräsmäki M, Morin-Papunen L, Keravuo R, Ebeling T, Saarela T, et al. Metformin should be considered in the treatment of gestational diabetes: a prospective randomised study. BJOG. 2011;118(7):880–5.

33. Niromanesh S, Alavi A, Sharbaf FR, Amjadi N, Moosavi S, Akbari S. Metformin compared with insulin in the management of gestational diabetes mellitus: a randomized clinical trial. Diabetes Res Clin Pract. 2012;98(3):422–9.

34. Spaulonci CP, Bernardes LS, Trindade TC, Zugaib M, Francisco RPV. Randomized trial of metformin vs insulin in the management of gestational diabetes. Am J Obstet Gynecol. 2013;209(1):34.e1–7.

35. Tertti K, Ekblad U, Koskinen P, Vahlberg T, Rönnemaa T. Metformin vs. insulin in gestational diabetes. A randomized study characterizing metformin patients needing additional insulin. Diabetes Obes Metab. 2013;15(3):246–51.

36. Ibrahim MI, Hamdy A, Shafik A, Taha S, Anwar M, Faris M. The role of adding metformin in insulin-resistant diabetic pregnant women: a randomized controlled trial. Arch Gynecol Obstet. 2014;289(5):959–65.

37. Rowan JA, Rush EC, Obolonkin V, Battin M, Wouldes T, Hague WM. Metformin in gestational diabetes: the offspring follow-up (MiG TOFU): body composition at 2 years of age. Diabetes Care. 2011;34(10): 2279–84.

38. Committee on Practice Bulletins – Obstetrics. Practice Bulletin No. 137: Gestational diabetes mellitus. Obstet Gynecol. 2013;122(2 Pt 1):406–16.

39. Harmon KA, Gerard L, Jensen DR, Kealey EH, Hernandez TL, Reece MS, et al. Continuous glucose profiles in obese and normal-weight pregnant women on a controlled diet: metabolic determinants of fetal growth. Diabetes Care. 2011;34(10):2198–204.

40. Langer O, Levy J, Brustman L, Anyaegbunam A, Merkatz R, Divon M. Glycemic control in gestational diabetes mellitus–how tight is tight enough: small for gestational age versus large for gestational age? Am J Obstet Gynecol. 1989;161(3):646–53.

41. Johnstone FD, Lindsay RS, Steel J. Type 1 diabetes and pregnancy: trends in birth weight over 40 years at a single clinic. Obstet Gynecol. 2006;107(6): 1297–302.

42. Nohr EA, Vaeth M, Baker JL, Sørensen TI, Olsen J, Rasmussen KM. Combined associations of prepregnancy body mass index and gestational weight gain with the outcome of pregnancy. Am J Clin Nutr. 2008;87(6):1750–9.

43. Ludwig DS, Currie J. The association between pregnancy weight gain and birthweight: a within-family comparison. Lancet. 2010;376(9745):984–90.

44. Cheng YW, Chung JH, Kurbisch-Block I, Inturrisi M, Shafer S, Caughey AB. Gestational weight gain and gestational diabetes mellitus: perinatal outcomes. Obstet Gynecol. 2008;112(5):1015–22.

45. Black MH, Sacks DA, Xiang AH, Lawrence JM. The relative contribution of prepregnancy overweight and obesity, gestational weight gain, and IADPSG-defined gestational diabetes mellitus to fetal overgrowth. Diabetes Care. 2013;36(1):56–62.

Inability to Lose Weight

Case 22

Katarina Kos

Abstract

More than a quarter of adults in the UK are obese and whilst previously endocrinologists may have seen the occasional case of unexplained weight gain, weight management clinics have become increasingly common place. Even without working in an obesity clinic many clinicians will be dealing with weight related complications. For this purpose the current chapter is not only aimed to help understanding of the principles of weight management but gives an overview of the issues faced when managing subjects with weight problems. This includes patients' concerns and worries which may influence outcome and enable holistic management. Furthermore, in line with current NICE guidance, there is a discussion of surgical practise and postoperative care. Keeping endocrinology in mind, there is also a review of typical hormonal changes with obesity especially the interpretation of some laboratory findings which may become a challenge.

Keywords

Obesity • Weight management • Lifestyle change • Bariatric surgery • Obesity complications

Case

A 67-year-old woman presents to the endocrine clinic with inability to lose weight. She is referred from the orthopaedic department. A hip replacement is being deferred until she manages to lose sufficient weight. Her mobility has decreased especially in the last year. She is frustrated as she feels that she has no life or future unless you can help her. She feels she had done everything she could to lose weight, has attended weight loss organisations, tried several diets and lately also used meal replacements. Latter helped in achieving her biggest weight loss of two stones. Since then her weight crept up and she is

K. Kos, MD, PhD
Diabetes and Obesity Research, University of Exeter, Barrack Road, Exeter, Devon EX2 5DW, UK
e-mail: k.kos@exeter.ac.uk

R. Ajjan, S.M. Orme (eds.), *Endocrinology and Diabetes: Case Studies, Questions and Commentaries*,
DOI 10.1007/978-1-4471-2789-5_22, © Springer-Verlag London 2015

heavier than ever before. At consultation her weight is recorded as 148 kg (23 st 4 lb) and the body mass index (BMI: calculated as weight/height^2) BMI 49.5 kg/m^2.

> Which questions will help to establish the cause of her weight problem?

Information is required about the duration of the weight problem, a list of current and past medications which will not only reveal her medical history but may contain drugs which are making weight loss difficult such as steroids, tricyclic antidepressants and atypical antipsychotics. A history of dietary shortfalls which include food preferences and drink history (not just alcohol) will help to guide in individualised diet and behavioural intervention planning. A non-judgemental question on what makes the patient eat will help explore potential emotionally triggered disordered eating behaviours and should include attention to loss of control over eating, a feature of binge eating. A history of depression, anxiety, mental illness and psychological trauma or abuse will elicit the need of an individual psychology and/or psychiatric assessment prior surgery. The smoking history is important as smoking can be used for weight control and smoking cessation can lead to considerable weight gain (see SIGN guidelines [1]). Current alcohol and substance abuse are contraindications to weight loss surgery (see below).

> Which medical conditions would you like to exclude? Which tests do you consider?

The risk of diabetes exponentially increases with every single increment in BMI. Obesity accounts for 80–85 % of the overall risk for developing Type 2 diabetes. Obstructive sleep apnoea should be excluded, e.g., by screening with the Epworth questionnaires which establishes the degree of tiredness and if scoring high, the diagnosis established with sleep studies such as pulse oxymetry. Treatment of this condition with continuous positive airway pressure (CPAP) devices can improve physical activity of affected subjects by improving their day time tiredness. Other conditions which should be considered are

liver steatosis by assessment of liver function. Women with menstrual disturbances should be screened for polycystic ovary disease, infertility and/or hirsutism. In presence of cushingoid features, e.g., purple stretch marks, bruising and stretch marks, screen for Cushing's disease with 24-h urine collections or an overnight dexamethasone suppression tests. Hypothyroidism needs to be excluded, however, is rarely the cause of morbid obesity per se. Many obese subjects suffer from depression and anxiety and a simple questionnaire may help to establish yet undiagnosed problems.

> Which hormones may be abnormal as a result of her obesity?

Several studies have shown an association with lower SHBG and free testosterone levels with increased fat mass and their improvement after bariatric surgery. Adipose tissue increases aromatisation of androgens to oestradiol and oestrogen levels can be higher than in normal weight women. Obesity can cause relative hypogonadism with low LH and FSH levels even when classical signs of PCOS and hyperandrogenism are lacking and many morbidly obese women have amenorrhea which can normalise after weight loss. In men, low levels of testosterone with low/normal FSH and LH are commonly seen. Cortisol levels can be elevated as result of obesity but the circadian rhythm of cortisol remains normal in subjects with obesity. Vitamin D levels are typically lower in obesity, however there is currently no specific guidance in replacing low Vitamin D levels in obesity whilst replacement especially after malabsorptive bariatric surgery is recommended [1, 2].

> You have excluded a medical condition as cause of obesity and suggest a lifestyle programme. She feels that she is unable to engage due to her joint problems. She feels that she had already done all she could to lose weight. She strongly emphasises that you are her last hope as she no longer could lose weight herself. How would you proceed?

Your consultation skills are being challenged and it is worthwhile to consider motivational interviewing techniques. Motivational interviewing is a person centred approach in which the motivation of change is elaborated, a change plan negotiated and commitment consolidated by use of specific interviewing techniques. It incorporates careful expectation management and empowerment of the patient by working on the readiness of change and increasing the confidence in making required changes. A past history of successful weight loss may be a useful stepping stone to help building confidence in the ability to lose weight. A demonstration of commitment towards lifestyle changes before referring for surgery evidenced by some weight loss is a requirement in most specialists medical obesity services (see below). Most weight management services work with a dedicated dietetic and psychologist team who can help identify and break down emotional barriers to healthy eating. Involving family and partners in consultations as well as peer support gained in weight management group sessions can offer additional help.

> She is wondering about bariatric surgery and whether she is too old for surgery? What are the NICE criteria for funding of bariatric surgery?

The National Institue of Clinical Excellence (NICE) does not limit bariatric surgery to an age target. Provided that she does not have any particular anaesthetic risk and there is no local funding limitation her age does not disqualify her from surgery. The BMI criteria for surgery according to NICE are equal or more than 35 kg/m^2 in patients and other significant disease (see below) or equal or more than 40 kg/m^2 in subjects with no co-morbidities, but there may be regional variations due to funding issues. Her osteoarthritis will, in some centres, be considered as significant co-morbidity [3].

> She would like to have gastric banding, can you think of any contraindications?

There are no clear contraindications other than the typical anaesthetic risk, however, subjects with sugar cravings and disordered eating traits are prone to develop complications such as gastric pouch dilatation leading to band slippage and erosions; as such a greater compliance is required to reduced calorie than with a gastric bypass. Contraindications to surgery are current drug and alcohol abuse and resistant psychiatric illness as well as lack of commitment to a healthy lifestyle change (see below).

In ladies of child bearing age a gastric band may be chosen in preference in order to avoid the possibility of malabsorption and foetal malnutrition during pregnancy. Many patients prefer a gastric band as a less invasive and reversible procedure. They may be unaware of the need of prolonged follow up for band refills and a lower net weight loss than with gastric band. A surgical revision of band to bypass is possible however not routinely funded by the NHS unless this is due to technical failure of the band itself. Currently there is a tendency of bariatric surgeons preferring recommendation of gastric bypass and gastric sleeve procedures.

> Blood results confirm that she has diabetes, would that change your management?

You may want to consider the addition of glucagon like peptide-1 (GLP-1) analogues in the medical management of diabetes to aid weight loss, in case her first line hypoglycaeamic therapy fails to control glucose levels. This should not overshadow the need to establish sustainable lifestyle changes. GLP-1 analogues are gaining license for use in weight management in patients without diabetes. Gastric bypass has been shown to be more successful in remission of Type 2 diabetes which has been reported to range from 40–80 % depending on the duration of diabetes and definition of remission [4]. The mechanism is in part due to caloric/energy restriction which improves hepatic insulin sensitivity and improved β cell function by exaggerated GLP-1 secretion [4]. Updated NHS guidelines recommend an expedited referral to bariatric surgery in subjects with diabetes of less than ten years duration and consideration of weight loss surgery from a BMI of 30 kg/m².

> Two years have passed; she underwent a laparoscopic gastric bypass operation 4 months ago and was admitted with a collapse to the A&E department. What are the likely diagnoses and what would be your management plan?

She may have experienced a hypoglycaemic episode after energy dense carbohydrate intake known as late Dumping syndrome characterised by postprandial reactive hypoglycaemia. Hypoglycaemic episodes can be common in the first few months after surgery and in most cases cease after dietary adjustments and can occur in bariatric patients with or without previous diabetes. The diagnosis can be confirmed by recording of hypoglycaemia in a prolonged oral glucose tolerance test typically up to at least 4 h. Hypoglycaemia is thought to be a result of the increased GLP-1 production and subsequent inappropriate high insulin levels. If symptoms persist and dietary changes are insufficient to resolve symptoms acarbose, diazoxide and calcium channel antagonists can be tried and in resistant cases somatostatin analogues may be helpful [5]. In refractory cases subjects may need further surgery for introduction of a restriction or reconstruction of gastrointestinal continuity. In few subjects with extensive hypertrophy of islets and development of nesidioblastosis (insulinoma like symptoms with excessive islet cell hyperplasia of the pancreas) partial or total pancreatic resections have been used which should remain the last treatment option [6].

Summary

Obesity is defined by a BMI above 30 kg/m². Most weight management clinics accept referral of patients with a BMI equal or above 40 kg/m² or equal or above 35 kg/m² with co-morbidities as suggested by NICE guidelines [3]. However due to funding implications there are wide regional variations especially in the definition of co-morbidites though typically include Type 2 diabetes and uncontrolled hypertension.

Monogenetic disorders (leptin mutation causing leptin deficiency, melanocortin receptor four mutation) or pleiotropic genetic syndromes as causes of obesity are rare and usually present in childhood. People with extreme obesity from early childhood, learning difficulties and insatiable hunger are potential candidates for screening of genetic disorders as well as, for Prader-Willi syndrome and Bardet-Biedl syndrome.

Obesity is typically acquired by prolonged energy surplus by inappropriate high dietary intake and inadequate physical activity. Food intake is typically underreported and commercials imply a bigger need of energy as what is typically required for a sedentary lifestyle which frequently blurs the estimates of what is a normal portion and meal size. This is not helped by the fact that being overweight has become the norm (more than 60 % of UK adults are overweight or obese). As we tend to compare our portion size with others, the acknowledgement that a man's daily energy need is up to a third higher than that of a woman of the same age and weight is frequently lost. The decreased energy need with age is not adjusted for. In addition, most people nowadays work in sedentary jobs and the requirement not adjusted from when people were younger and more physically active.

Frequently people with obesity eat because of emotional needs such as comfort, boredom, loneliness and feeling low. Stress without adequate time for eating contributes to the modern "obesogenic" lifestyle. Increasingly people rely on meal deals, ready-made meals and have no peace to eat undisturbed without distraction such as watching TV or working on the computer whilst consuming their meals. Subjects who suffer from extreme obesity have frequently suffered traumatic life events or abuse which may not have been sufficiently emotionally resolved and need attention before being able to commit to sustained lifestyle changes. Obesity commonly coexists in several family members and engaging the whole family in the treatment is recommended.

At diagnosis and clinical assessment it is important to keep in mind the above mentioned endocrine disorders and beside an occasional new diagnosis of diabetes in the weight management clinic the screening for Cushing's disease can be limited to those with unexplained weight gain, a suggestive body composition and appearance and purple stretch marks.

The term obesity or being called obese can be perceived as insulting and some patients feel embarrassed about attending an obesity clinic or let others know about it. Care has also to be taken when obtaining a family history of obesity and when dealing with family members.

The objective of weight management clinics is to target on sustainable life style changes rather than to provide extreme diets after which the weight loss may not be possible to be maintained. Both NICE and the SIGN guidelines recommend a 600 kcal deficit diet that is tailored to individual preference; this by reducing the intake of energy dense foods, by minimizing the consumption of fast foods and alcohol intake and introduction of a balanced diet [1].

Setting realistic goals and clear weight targets with every visit will aid success. This will typically be no more than 0.5–1 kg per week leading to a weight loss of 5–10 % in a year. Behaviour interventions and physical activity alongside dietetic guidance will help in this process. For further information on food composition and behaviour intervention see the SIGN guidance [1].

There is a lack of approved pharmaceutical treatment for obesity and Orlistat is the only agent currently licensed in the UK. This should only be prescribed after adequate concomitant advice on fat intake reduction and counselling to its side effects to ensure adequate adherence. GLP-1 analogues which substitute the reduced levels of the gut hormone glucagon like peptide-1 in obesity and diabetes can help to promote weight loss by their action on stomach emptying and central inhibition of appetite in subjects with diabetes. Currently these agents are soon going to be available for weight reduction in non-diabetic individuals clinical trials suggest that they may be an effective adjunct to weight management.

In adult patients with a BMI equal or above 40 or 35 kg/m^2 with significant co-morbidities such as Type 2 diabetes in whom appropriate non surgical measures were unsuccessful are according to NICE recommended to have surgery with the exception of subjects with a BMI more than 50 kg/m^2 in whom surgery is recommended as a first-line option [4]. Weight loss prior surgery and improvement of glycaemia in subjects with diabetes improves surgical outcomes. The recently updated NICE guideline advises to expedite subjects with recent diagnosis of diabetes of less than 10 years duration to surgery and already consider surgery if the BMI is less than 30kg/m^2.

Contraindications to surgery are current drug and alcohol abuse and resistant psychiatric illness as well as lack of commitment to a healthy lifestyle change. A commitment to follow up and lifelong follow up post bariatric surgery should be established not only to ensure commitment to adequate mineral and vitamin supplementation but also to be able to intervene early to slips in the newly developed eating habits to prevent surgical failure, weight regain and complications. Depression, binge eating disorders and past history of substance abuse are not an absolute contraindication to surgery [1]. There is however an increased risk of suicide, self-harm and divorce after bariatric surgery and issues with body image may either not resolve or may become worse due to remaining skin flaps after bariatric surgery. Bariatric surgery should not be used for the treatment of body image issues associated with obesity and depending on presurgical BMI not all patients can expect to be able to reach their ideal body weight with bariatric surgery. The risk of postsurgical alcohol abuse is increased after bypass surgery and alcohol tolerance reduced.

Even if during the medical weight management a certain amount of weight has been lost, surgeons commonly subject patients to a low calorie diet known to most as the "liver shrinkage diet" in an attempt to reduce the size of the liver before surgery by reducing its glycogen stores, consequently helping to enhance safety of the surgical procedure.

Most common **bariatric surgical procedures** are laparoscopic adjustable banding or laparoscopic

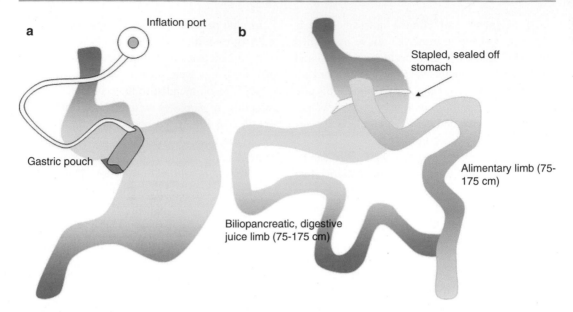

Fig. 22.1 The two most common surgical procedures. (**a**) Adjustable gastric banding. (**b**) Roux en Y gastric bypass

Table 22.1 Comparison of the characteristics of the two most common surgical interventions

Characteristics	Laparoscopic adjustable gastric banding- LAGB	Laparoscopic Roux en Y gastric bypass- RYGB
Estimated cost	Circa £7,000 with band fills	£8,000–15,000
Principle technique	Reversible and restrictive	Irreversible, restrictive and malabsorptive
Weight loss	About 50 % EWL at 1 year	About 70 % EWL at 1 year
Type 2 diabetes	Higher than with diet but less than RYGB	Improvement or remission shortly after surgery (40–80 %)
After care	Repeated follow up requirement for band adjustments	Lifelong mineral and vitamin supplementation
Common complications	Band erosions, ulceration, band slippage, pouch dilation, wound infections	Anastomotic leaks, internal hernias, pulmonary embolus, sepsis, wound infections
Side effects	Nausea, vomiting, dyspepsia	Nausea, vomiting, dumping syndrome, vitamin deficiencies, malnutrition
Surgical mortality	0.05 %	0.5 % with higher risk of intra-operative complications
Revision	Required in 10–25 %, this typically to RYGB	Less common and technically difficult

Roux-en-Y gastric bypass (RYGB; see Fig. 22.1 and Table 22.1) which till recently used to make up more than 90 % of the surgical bariatric interventions. RYGB has gained increasing popularity in recent years. Figure 22.1 demonstrates the anatomic changes of the surgical bypass procedures. Extremely obese subjects sometimes start with a gastric balloon which is fitted endoscopically before it is inflated to float freely in the stomach. This is used in subjects in whom other types of surgery are unsafe or technically not possible. The balloon will be kept in place till sufficient weight is lost (but not longer than 6 months) to enable a safe operation and proceed with another procedure. A gastric sleeve is an alternative for heavier subjects, e.g., above a BMI of 50 kg/m^2 and is typically part of a two-stage procedure followed by a malabsorptive procedure after a year or 2. However, if good weight loss results are achieved a second operation may not be needed. At the time of writing this article, the gastric sleeve is gaining popularity in the

USA as a stand alone procedure. The surgical risk is lowest with a gastric band, but also requires more patient self discipline and dietary adherence in order to be successful in weight loss and the follow up without complications. The table below compares the characteristics of the two most common types of surgery. Rapid weight loss and with this any bariatric surgery also increases the risk of gall stones and cholelecystitis especially in men and also predisposes to gout. Patients with frequent attacks of gout may benefit from prophylactic medication to avoid an acute attack after bariatric surgery.

Postsurgically, the patient will undergo a gradual change from fluid to solid food intake important in restrictive surgery to minimise symptoms like vomiting which can lead to reflux and increase the danger of rupture of surgical anastomoses. Adequate protein content is necessary as patients do not only lose adipose tissue but also lose lean body mass with surgery especially after malabsorptive procedures.

Nutritional reinforcement of healthy eating behaviour and food composition with exclusion of carbohydrate dense meals and drinks is necessary also after RYGB to avoid or reduce gastrointestinal symptoms such as Dumping syndrome including abdominal pain, nausea, diarrhoea, cramps, flushing, light-headedness and syncope ([2]; see also above).

Lifelong mineral and vitamin supplementation after bariatric surgery is necessary which includes supplementation of calcium and vitamin D to ensure adequate bone health [1]. About 30–40 % of patients will develop vitamin B12 deficiency after RYGB. Iron deficiency is common in women with menorrhagia or heavy menstrual bleeding. Adequate blood tests should be repeated 6 monthly.

Figure 22.2 shows the typical weight loss trajectory after bariatric surgery. Weight regain after bariatric surgery may necessitate revision in 10–25 % of subjects after gastric banding, which is typically a conversion to RYGB. Failure of RYGB is less common, revision is technically more difficult. In such cases biliopancreatic diversion with duodenal switch as well as restriction procedures such as the addition of a silicon gastric band are possibilities.

RYGB is very effective in remission of Type 2 diabetes (see above) even before weight loss occurs whilst the metabolic improvement with LAGB is linked directly with weight loss. Evidence from a head to head comparison is lacking and dependent on severity and duration of diabetes [4].

Bariatric surgery improves overall mortality [7] and is cost-effective, especially at higher BMIs and is measured in cost-effectiveness ratios (£ per quality-adjusted life year (QALY)

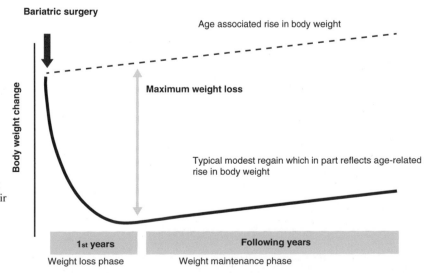

Fig. 22.2 General pattern of weight regain following bariatric surgery. The nadir of weight recordings is reached at 12–18 months postsurgery, after which subjects tend to start gaining weight

gained). It is greatest in people with BMI 40 kg/ m² or more followed by those with BMI 30 kg/ m² or more (and less than 40 kg/m²) with type 2 diabetes [8]. It is also an effective, safe and cost-effective treatment of Type 2 diabetes in obesity [9].

References

1. Scottish Intercollegiate Guidelines Network. Management of obesity. A national clinical guideline 115. 2010. http://www.sign.ac.uk/pdf/sign115.pdf.
2. Heber D, Greenway FL, Kaplan LM, Livingston E, Salvador J, Salvador J, Still C, Endocrine Society. Endocrine and nutritional management of the post-bariatric surgery patient: an Endocrine Society Clinical Practice Guideline. J Clin Endocrinol Metab. 2010;95(11):4823–43.
3. NICE (National Institute for Health and Clinical Excellence). Obesity guidance on the prevention, identification, assessment and management of overweight and obesity in adults and children. 2014. http://www.nice.org.uk/guidance/cg189.
4. Dirksen C, Jørgensen NB, Bojsen-Møller KN, Jacobsen SH, Hansen DL, Worm D, Holst JJ, Madsbad S. Mechanisms of improved glycaemic control after Roux-en-Y gastric bypass. Diabetologia. 2012;55(7): 1890–901.
5. Tack J, Arts J, Caenepeel P, De Wulf D, Bisschops R. Pathophysiology, diagnosis and management of postoperative dumping syndrome. Nat Rev Gastroenterol Hepatol. 2009;6(10):583–90.
6. Cui Y, Elahi D, Andersen DK. Advances in the etiology and management of hyperinsulinemic hypoglycemia after Roux-en-Y gastric bypass. J Gastrointest Surg. 2011;15(10):1879–88.
7. Sjöström L, Narbro K, Sjöström CD, Karason K, Larsson B, Wedel H, et al. Swedish Obese Subjects Study. Effects of bariatric surgery on mortality in Swedish obese subjects. N Engl J Med. 2007;357(8): 741–52.
8. Picot J, Jones J, Colquitt JL, Gospodarevskaya E, Loveman E, Baxter L, Clegg AJ. The clinical effectiveness and cost-effectiveness of bariatric (weight loss) surgery for obesity: a systematic review and economic evaluation. Health Technol Assess. 2009;13(41):1–190.
9. Dixon JB, le Roux CW, Rubino F, Zimmet P. Bariatric surgery for type 2 diabetes. Lancet. 2012;379(9833): 2300–11.

Medical Problems in Obesity

Case 23

Tolulope Shonibare,
Arelis Rodriguez-Farradas,
Mohan Ramasamy,
and Chinnadorai Rajeswaran

Abstract

The incidence of obesity and overweight is increasing worldwide. Obesity predisposes to the development of co-morbidities such as diabetes mellitus, hypertension, cardiovascular disease and malignancy. This chapter will focus on identifying and diagnosing common medical problems that obese patients encounter with an overview of managing these conditions.

Keywords

Obesity • Diabetes mellitus • Erectile dysfunction • Hypogonadotrophic hypogonadism • Obstructive sleep apnoea

Case

A 55-year-old heavy goods vehicle driver has been referred to the obesity clinic for further management of his weight. He has been recently made redundant and has a past medical history of

T. Shonibare, BSc, MBChB, MRCP
C. Rajeswaran, MBBS, FRCP(UK), MSc (✉)
Department of Diabetes, Endocrinology
and Obesity, Dewsbury District Hospital,
Halifax Road, Dewsbury, West Yorkshire
WF13 4HS, UK
e-mail: Chinnadorai.rajeswaran@midyorks.nhs.uk

A. Rodriguez-Farradas, BSc(Hons), RD
Diabetes Centre, Adult Weight Management
Services, Mid Yorkshire Hospitals NHS Trust,
Dewsbury, West Yorkshire, UK

M. Ramasamy, MScPT
Weight Management Service, The Mid Yorkshire
Hospitals NHS Trust, Dewsbury, West Yorkshire, UK

type 2 diabetes mellitus, hypertension, ischemic heart disease and hypercholesterolaemia. He is a smoker with a 35-pack-per-year history, and he does not drink alcohol. He is married with two biological children. His current medications include Metformin, Exanetide, Simvastatin, Atenolol and Ramipril. His glycaemic control is poor, and his most recent glycated haemoglobin (HbA1c) was 88 mmol/mol. On examination his weight was 135 kg; his height was 1.76 m with a body mass index of 43.58 kg/m^2. His waist circumference was 102 cm, and his blood pressure 146/89 mmHg.

He complains of feeling extremely tired during the day and admits to waking up in the middle of the night multiple times to pass urine. He always feels tired, and this has put a strain on his relationship with his wife recently. He has attempted to improve his personal life and intimacy with his wife, but he has been experiencing

R. Ajjan, S.M. Orme (eds.), *Endocrinology and Diabetes: Case Studies, Questions and Commentaries*,
DOI 10.1007/978-1-4471-2789-5_23, © Springer-Verlag London 2015

a low libido and has symptoms suggestive of erectile dysfunction. This has made him increasingly depressed, and his General Practitioner has recently prescribed amitriptyline.

What is the definition of obesity?

Obesity and overweight are defined as abnormal or excessive fat accumulation that may impair health [1]. This usually results from an imbalance between energy consumption and expenditure. According to the World Health Organisation (WHO), it is one of the leading causes of global deaths, with deaths of up to 3.4 million annually [1].

Body mass index (BMI) is used to classify these terms. The WHO definition is as follows: BMI >25-Overweight, BMI >30 –Obesity.

The use of BMI has great advantages in terms of ease of measurement and low cost, however there are drawbacks which exist with its use in ethnic populations. The WHO threshold was based largely on Caucasian populations, however it is now recognised that patients from Asian, black and other ethnic minority groups are at risk of obesity associated co-morbidities at lower BMI thresholds [2].

BMI alone is not a good reflection of the severity or extent of obesity related comorbidities. Figure 23.1 is a diagram of the Edmonton Obesity staging system, a clinical tool to compliment BMI. Both the National Institute of Clinical Excellence (NICE) and WHO have recommended the use of combined BMI and waist circumference categories for identifying an individual's risk of obesity-related ill health [1, 2].

What are the main points that should be considered when taking the medical history?

When assessing an obese patient, weight history is important and the following factors need to be considered [3].
- History from birth and life-changing events
- Previous strategies for weight loss and success
- Lifestyle habits, i.e., smoking, alcohol excess, eating and exercise
- Family history of obesity
- Comorbidities
- Symptoms suggestive of secondary causes of obesity such as Cushing's syndrome, acromegaly and hypothalamic disorders
- Psychological states and depression
- Medications

What are the main obesity-related comorbidities in this patient?

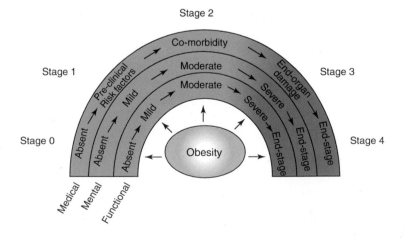

Fig. 23.1 Edmonton obesity staging system (Reprinted by permission from Macmillan Publishers Ltd.: Sharma and Kushner [27] copyright 2009)

Hypogonadotrophic Hypogonadism

The patient has a low libido and inability to maintain erections. Hypogonadotrophic hypogonadism (HH) is defined as subnormal free testosterone in the presence of inappropriately low gonadotrophins [4]. The clinical manifestations include low libido, erectile dysfunction, fatigue, loss of muscle mass, reduced bone density and depression [4].

About 25–40 % of men with type 2 diabetes mellitus (DM) have been found to have HH [5, 6]. The mechanism behind this is thought to be due to insulin resistance rather than hyperglycaemia itself [4]. Studies in mouse models have demonstrated that insulin facilitates secretion of gonadotrophin-releasing hormone (GnRH) from neuronal cells. Therefore insulin resistance would affect GnRH secretion, thus testosterone levels [7]. There have also been reports of raised inflammatory markers being associated with HH, suggesting an underlying inflammatory response [7].

Obesity is also associated with HH, with studies showing an inverse relationship between free testosterone and body mass index [8]. The proposed mechanism is related to an increase in adipose tissue which leads to increased oestradiol levels due to enhanced aromatase activity, thus leading to suppression of GnRH release [4]. Diabetes in conjunction contributes to low free testosterone levels, however studies have shown that low circulating testosterone levels are also observed in non-diabetic obese men [9].

Furthermore, low sex hormone binding globulin (SHBG) levels are observed in such patients [9]. Since a significant proportion of circulating testosterone is bound to SHBG, a low serum SHBG level will invariably result in lower total testosterone levels [9].

Another possible explanation for low free testosterone levels observed in obese diabetic and non-diabetic patients is an abnormal scrotal temperature [10]. Embryological descent of the testes outside the body aims to maintain scrotal temperatures at 2 °C less than core body temperature to facilitate adequate testosterone production [10]. In obese patients, an increase in abdominal fat envelopes the scrotum between the thighs and abdomen. This results in temperatures similar to that of core body temperature thus impeding testosterone production [10].

In summary, diabetes and obesity are independent factors for developing hypogonadotrophic hypogonadism. However, obesity in the presence of type 2 DM adds to that risk [4, 8]. This patient has two biological children so it is unlikely that he suffers from primary infertility.

What are the mechanisms for the erectile dysfunction in this patient?

Studies have shown a link between erectile dysfunction (ED), hypogonadotrophic hypogonadism, type 2 diabetes and obesity [11]. Both type 2 diabetes and obesity represent independent risk factors for development of ED [4]. The mechanisms involved are metabolic, neurogenic and vascular.

Hyperglycaemia, hyperlipidaemia and poor metabolic control give rise to biochemical perturbations that lead to microvascular changes [12].

In diabetic patients, there is impaired neurogenic and nitric oxide mediated endothelial relaxation of smooth muscle. As a result autonomic neuropathy and arterial disease lead to ED [12]. In obese patients, androgen deficiency due to increased aromatase action and microvascular changes are contributors [4].

In people with diabetes, it is also possible that use of beta-blockers might be contributing to ED. Furthermore an increase in nocturnal urinary frequency suggests benign prostatic hypertrophy.

Other than the metabolic/hormonal abnormalities, what else could be contributing to his tiredness?

This man is likely to have Obstructive sleep apnoea (OSA), which is usually underdiagnosed. OSA is defined as spectrum of breathing disorders which occur during sleep. This ranges from snoring to hypoapnoea and apnoea [13]. It results from collapse of the upper airways leading to upper airway resistance, airflow impedance and ultimately oxygen desaturation [13, 14].

The patient typically has interrupted sleep due to periods of apnoea and wakes up feeling unrefreshed in the morning; this leads to daytime somnolence [13, 14].

OSA has been linked to obesity, hypertension and diabetes. Risk factors for developing OSA include age, obesity and male sex. Also certain craniofacial characteristics such as changes associated with acromegaly increase the risk [13].

Other respiratory disorders that are associated with in obesity include obesity hypoventilation syndrome in which patients develop night time hypoxia and daytime hypercapnia [15].

It is likely that the patient has OSA, therefore a referral to the Respiratory physicians for further assessment and treatment will be necessary. Weight loss tends to alleviate symptoms.

> This man is feeling low in mood. How would this contribute to his clinical presentation?

This patient has been diagnosed with depression by his general practitioner which has resulted in a poor quality of life. Studies have shown that 55 % of obese patients have an increased risk of developing depression [16]. People who are depressed have a 58 % risk of becoming overweight [16]. Large epidemiological studies have found a relationship between socioeconomic factors, chronic disease and psychological stress [17]. Some alleviation might be achieved through management of each chronic disease; however in severe cases of depression management with pharmacological therapy might be necessary.

> What questions would you ask about lifestyle?

Diet and Eating Behaviour

It is important to identify potential eating behaviour contributing to the maintenance of obesity. It is also crucial to consider diabetes management which may be more relevant than aiming to quantify calorie intake or specific meal composition. Below is a list of eating behaviours that can contribute weight gain [18].

- Skipping meals
- Snacking/grazing
- Lack of structured eating patterns
- Night eating
- Inconsistent dieting behaviour
- Emotional eating

It is recommended that patients have contact with a dietitian to provide a detailed assessment of dieting history so as to identify problem areas or misconceptions that can be rectified [2].

Exercise

Evaluation of the amount of daily exercise and exercise tolerance is necessary. Some obese patients experience difficulty increasing physical activity level due to various co-morbidities such as the pain associated with osteoarthritis and fibromyalgia. They might also experience increased shortness of breath due to cardiac and respiratory disease.

Smoking

It would also be important to determine the history of pack years in smoking. Some observational studies have shown an increase in abdominal and visceral obesity in overweight smokers [19]. Combining smoking and obesity increases the risk of developing cancer as well as a tenfold increase in premature death [20]. However cessation of smoking can increase appetite and therefore cause weight gain which may be moderate and temporary if appropriate management is pre-empted [20].

How would you physically assess an obese patient?

General examination of an obese patient should include height and weight to determine BMI [1, 2]. Also it is useful to measure waist circumference to determine the waist to hip ratio. Body composition analyser helps to determine general distribution of fat [2]. It is however important to note that waist circumference determination becomes unreliable when BMI exceeds 35 kg/m^2 due to the effects of gravity on central adiposity creating folds of fat across the abdomen [2]. Neck circumference evaluation is necessary for those who are likely to suffer from OSA.

Assessment should include a skin examination for signs of insulin resistance such as acanthosis nigricans, skin tags and intertrigo. Also signs of dyslipidaemia such as xanthalesma and eruptive xanthoma should be sought [3]. Assessment of cardiovascular status is necessary with blood pressure and an electrocardiogram.

Examination of the abdomen might reveal hepatomegaly caused by fatty liver disease. Finally assessment of the musculoskeletal system is important to determine the presence of gout or osteoarthritis as this can affect future ability to exercise and attend rehabilitation programmes [3]. With regards to diabetes it is important to assess whether the patient has established microvascular and macrovascular complications.

What are the secondary causes of obesity?

During the assessment it is also important to rule out secondary causes of obesity as treatment of the underlying condition is also necessary [3]. Table 23.1 presents a summary of potential secondary causes.

Summary of possible medical conditions this patient has:
- Super-obesity
- Obstructive sleep apnoea

Table 23.1 Summary of potential secondary causes of obesity

Endocrine disorders	Cushing's syndrome
	Hypothyroidism
	Type 2 diabetes
	Acromegaly
Genetic	Prader-Willi syndrome
	Cohen syndrome
	Bardet-Biedel syndrome
Central nervous system	Hypothalamic disorders
Drugs	Atypical antipsychotics
	Tricyclic antidepressants
Other	Bulimia
	Binge-eating disorder

- Hypogonadotrophic hypogonadism
- Cardiovascular disease leading to impotence
- Benign prostatic hypertrophy
- Depression

What investigations would you consider to reach your diagnosis?

Anterior Pituitary Tests

Measurement of luteinising hormone (LH), follicular stimulating hormone (FSH), testosterone, Oestradiol, prolactin and cortisol is necessary to confirm hypogonadotrohic hypogonadism [3]. However if pituitary disease is suspected then a complete pituitary hormone profile will be required. Typically a subnormal testosterone level is observed with inappropriately normal levels of FSH and LH [3]. Oestradiol levels might also be raised due to increased aromatase activity from excessive adipose tissue [4].

To rule out a pituitary cause for HH, an insulin tolerance test (ITT) should be considered to assess cortisol and growth hormone reserve. Typically a dose of 0.15 U/kg of insulin is used, however due to insulin resistance patients with obesity, diabetes, acromegaly or Cushing's require a higher dose of 0.2–0.3 U/kg to induce adequate hypoglycaemia <2.2 mmol/l [3].

If there are any contraindications to an ITT such as epilepsy, ischaemic heart disease, hypothyroidism or hypocortisolism, then a glucagon stimulation test might be considered [3]. However the growth hormone response to glucagon stimulation tends to be attenuated in obese patients, therefore care will be needed in interpreting the results.

Imaging

Magnetic resonance imaging might be required to rule out pituitary lesions. In most cases of HH no abnormalities are found [21] but pituitary incidentalomas might be discovered, instigating a plethora of further investigations which can complicate the diagnosis.

Sleep Studies

Diagnosis of OSA is by use of polysomnography or sleep studies. To assess severity, the Epworth sleepiness scale is used. This entails a series of questions with a maximum score of 24. A score of 15 is classed as moderate and a score above 18 is classed as severe [14].

Prostate-Specific Antigen

This patient also describes urinary symptoms so it will be important to assess him with a detailed clinical history and a digital rectal examination. A baseline PSA is also required especially in the context of possible testosterone replacement. This will be discussed in detail later in the chapter.

Full Blood Count

Assessment of haemoglobin and haematocrit is necessary as polycythaemia can occur due to OSA. In the context of testosterone replacement therapy it is also necessary to determine the baseline haematocrit.

Annual Diabetes Screen

As part of the recommendation by NICE, patients with diabetes require at least an annual retinal screen, foot examination, urinary micro albumin as well as biochemical tests such as HbA1c, fasting lipid profile, liver function tests, estimated glomerular filtration rate (EGFR), urea and electrolytes [22].

Other Tests

24-h Urinary Cortisol
If clinical Cushing's syndrome is suspected then a 24 h urinary cortisol can be requested. It is important to note that the test has 98 % specificity and 95 % sensitivity. False positive results can occur due to pseudo-Cushing's which can be present in patients who are obese, consume alcohol in excess and suffer from depression [3].

> How will you aid this patient to reduce his weight?

Weight Management Services

Patients are more likely to have a successful outcome when referred to a structured weight management service. The availability of such services varies between regions and can either be available in the community or the hospital setting. This typically comprises of a multi-disciplinary team of dietitians, psychologists, physiotherapists and specialist weight management physicians [2].

Commercial programmes also exist with each attesting to varying degrees of success. The decision as to where to refer the patient to will depend on the patient's preference. However if significant co-morbidities exist, then it will be advisable to refer to a programme in the hospital setting.

The first step to weight control is the "willingness to change" in the patient. Once this has been established the intervention strategy has various components involving behavioural strategies and life style changes [2, 18].

Dietary advice should be individually tailored with a focus on the concept of healthy eating. The total energy intake should be less than energy expenditure. For sustainable weight loss, diet should have a 600Kcal/day deficit, ensuring that all other nutritional needs are met. Diets which involve more restriction of calories should be undertaken with clinical supervision [2].

With regards to exercise, the NICE recommendation is that of 30 min of moderate exercise 5 days a week. Due to increasing demands on time, the recommendation is to encourage that this physical activity is incorporated into daily life. To maintain weight loss exercise duration of 60–90 min might be needed with a combination of cardiovascular high intensity exercises and weight resistance exercise [2].

> What other management options are available?

Apart from lifestyle intervention, pharmacological and surgical management of obesity can be considered.

Drug therapy can be used in patients after dietary, exercise and behavioural approaches have been started and evaluated. It can also be considered in patients who have not reached their target weight loss or have plateaued on life style intervention [2].

The NICE criteria for prescribing drug therapy are
- BMI of 28.0 kg/m^2 or more with associated factors
- BMI of 30.0 kg/m^2 or more [2]

Currently, the only licensed product in the United Kingdom is Orlistat, which functions as a lipase inhibitor. It has also been shown to improve glycaemic control in patients with type 2 DM [23].

This patient is on a GLP-1 analogue for management of his diabetes, although it is not licensed for obesity management, systematic reviews and meta-analyses have shown that it can promote weight loss [24].

> When would you consider bariatric surgery as a management option?

Bariatric surgery is considered as second- or third-line therapy. It is usually recommended for patients who [2]:
- Have failed to achieve or maintain clinically beneficial weight loss despite appropriate non-surgical measures.
- Have a BMI of 40.0 kg/m^2 or more and as first line in those with a BMI of 50.0 kg/m^2
- BMI of between 35 and 40 kg/m^2 with significant co-morbidities
- Generally fit for surgery and anaesthesia
- Show commitment to the need for long-term follow-up

There are data to suggest that patients have a better outcome with bariatric surgery compared to lifestyle intervention alone, as patients are more likely to achieve a greater amount of weight loss with remission of type 2 DM. This will be discussed in greater detail in Chap. 25 in this book.

> How would you manage his other co-morbidities?

Diabetes Management

This patient is likely to need insulin however it is important to note that use of insulin can stimulate weight gain lead to a cycle of weight gain and increased doses of insulin. The approach should be a balance between aiming for reasonable glycaemic control as well as weight loss. He will need education on portion control as well as other lifestyle changes mentioned above.

Testosterone Replacement

This patient describes a constellation of symptoms consistent with ED, HH and benign prostatic hypertrophy (BPH). Management should include testosterone replacement therapy.

A baseline measurement of 9 am testosterone will be required using a reliable assay. Once treatment has been initiated, further evaluation of testosterone levels should be undertaken at 3 and 6 months [25]. The risks and benefits should be discussed with the patient as well as the various preparations available. In view of possible BPH further urological assessment is required prior to commencing therapy. This would include a baseline PSA and digital rectal examination. Patients who have known prostate cancer should not be offered testosterone replacement [25].

Annual monitoring of PSA is required with a PSA rise of no more than 1.4 ng/mL/year [25]. A greater increase than this should prompt urgent referral to urological services. There have been controversies regarding testosterone replacement in relation to prostate cancer. It is now accepted however that testosterone replacement does not result in the development of prostate cancer, but can accelerate pre-existing malignant prostatic lesions. In the context of BPH it can exacerbate prostatic symptoms.

Monitoring of haematocrit is also necessary with a haematocrit greater than 0.55 prompting either withdrawal of therapy or reduction of testosterone dose [25]. A rise in haematocrit above the recommended reference range can lead to an increased risk of thrombotic events [25].

Erectile Dysfunction

Phosphodiesterase inhibitor therapies such as sildenafil exist for management of ED. These promote penile smooth muscle relaxation, thereby helping to achieve erection. Careful consideration is needed in patients who have co-existing ischaemic heart disease particularly those on nitrate therapy [12].

Smoking Cessation

Smoking cessation advice and pharmacotherapy should be offered if necessary, to reduce the risk of both microvascular and macrovascular complications [19].

Obstructive Sleep Apnoea

Continuous positive air pressure (CPAP) is the most cost-effective treatment. However, surgical alternatives can be used with the aim of increasing pharyngeal calibre and reducing pharyngeal airflow obstruction during sleep [14, 26].

Summary

Management of obesity often requires individual management of associated co-morbidities as well as aiding weight loss. Patients who are managed under a structured weight management programme led by a multi-disciplinary team have been shown to achieve better overall outcomes. Obesity is a chronic illness that requires long-term follow-up. The frequency and duration may vary amongst individuals depending on parameters such as improvement of co-morbidities, degree of weight loss and evidence of permanent behavioural and lifestyle modification.

In this patient a 6-monthly review would be acceptable. Once all the medical, psychological and behavioural problems highlighted in the chapter have been adequately addressed, he can be subsequently discharged back to his primary care physician.

References

1. World Health Organization. Overweight and obesity. Fact sheet no. 311. WHO: Geneva; 2006.
2. National Institute for Clinical Excellence (NICE). Obesity: the prevention, identification, assessment and management of overweight and obesity in adults and children. 2006. http://www.nice.org.uk/guidance/CG43.
3. Wass J, Owen K. Oxford handbook of endocrinology and diabetes. 3rd ed. Oxford: Oxford University Press; 2014.
4. Dandona P, Dhindsa S. Update: hypogonadotropic hypogonadism in type 2 diabetes and obesity. J Clin Endocrinol Metab. 2011;96(9):2643–51.
5. Corona G, Mannucci E, Petrone L, Ricca V, Balercia G, Mansani R, et al. Association of hypogonadism and type II diabetes in men attending an outpatient erectile dysfunction clinic. Int J Impot Res. 2006;18(2):190–7.
6. Grossmann M, Thomas MC, Panagiotopoulos S, Sharpe K, Macisaac RJ, Jerums G, et al. Low testosterone levels are common and associated with insulin resistance in men with diabetes. J Clin Endocrinol Metab. 2008;93:1834–40.

7. Dandona P, Dhindsa S, Chaudhuri A, Bhatia V, Topiwala S, Mohanty P. Hypogonadotrophic hypogonadism in type 2 diabetes, obesity and the metabolic syndrome. Curr Mol Med. 2008;8:816–28.

8. Dhindsa S, Miller MG, McWhirter CL, Mager DE, Ghanim H, Chaudhuri A, et al. Testosterone concentrations in diabetic and nondiabetic obese men. Diabetes Care. 2010;33:1186–92.

9. Mulligan T, Frick MF, Zuraw QC, Stemhagen A, McWhirter C. Prevalence of hypogonadism in males aged at least 45 years: the HIM study. Int J Clin Pract. 2006;60(7):762–9.

10. Du Plessis SS, Cabler S, McAlister DA, Sabanegh E, Agarwal A. The effect of obesity on sperm disorders and male infertility. Nat Rev Urol. 2010;7(3): 153–61.

11. Chitaley K, Kupelian V, Subak L, Wessells H. Diabetes, obesity and erectile dysfunction: field overview and research priorities. J Urol. 2009;182 (6 Suppl):S45–50.

12. Basu A, Ryder RE. New treatment options for erectile dysfunction in patients with diabetes mellitus. Drugs. 2004;64(23):2667–88.

13. Hering R, Taheri S. Obstructive sleep apnoea and diabetes – an emerging link. J Diab Nurs. 2011;15(2): 46–8.

14. Scottish Intercollegiate/British Thoracic Society Guideline. Management of obstructive sleep apnoea/ hypopnoea syndrome in adults. Guideline No 73. 2003. http://www.sign.ac.uk/guidelines/fulltext/73/index. html.

15. Piper AJ, Grunstein RR. Obesity hypoventilation syndrome: mechanisms and management. Am J Respir Crit Care Med. 2011;183(3):292–8.

16. Luppino FS, de Wit LM, Bouvy PF, Stijnen T, Cuijpers P, Penninx BW, et al. Overweight, obesity, and depression: a systematic review and meta-analysis of longitudinal studies. Arch Gen Psychiatry. 2010;67(3):220–9.

17. Everson SA, Maty SC, Lynch JW, Kaplan GA. Epidemiologic evidence for the relation between socioeconomic status and depression, obesity, and diabetes. J Psychosom Res. 2002;53(4):891–5.

18. Brownell KD, Kramer FM. Behavioral management of obesity. Med Clin North Am. 1989;73(1): 185–201.

19. Kim JH, Shim KW, Yoon YS, Lee SY, Kim SS, Oh SW. Cigarette smoking increases abdominal and visceral obesity but not overall fatness: an observational study. PLoS One. 2012;7(9):e45815.

20. Sucharda P. Smoking and obesity. Vnitr Lek. 2010; 56(10):1053–7.

21. Silveira LF, Latronico AC. Approach to the patient with hypogonadotropic hypogonadism. J Clin Endocrinol Metab. 2013;98(5):1781–8.

22. Home P, Mant J, Diaz J, Turner C, Guideline Development Group. Guidelines: management of type 2 diabetes: summary of updated NICE guidance. BMJ. 2008;336(7656):1306.

23. Hollander PA, Elbein SC, Hirsch IB, Kelley D, McGill J, Taylor T, et al. Role of orlistat in the treatment of obese patients with type 2 diabetes: a 1-year randomized double-blind study. Diabetes Care. 1998;21(8):1288–94.

24. Vilsbøll T, Christensen M, Junker AE, Knop FK, Gluud LL. Effects of glucagon-like peptide-1 receptor agonists on weight loss: systematic review and meta-analyses of randomised controlled trials. BMJ. 2012;344:d7771.

25. Bhasin S, Cunningham GR, Hayes FJ, Matsumoto AM, Snyder PJ, Swerdloff RS, et al. Testosterone therapy in men with androgen deficiency syndromes: an Endocrine Society clinical practice guideline. J Clin Endocrinol Metab. 2010;95(6):2536–59.

26. NICE guidelines for Sleep Apnoea and CPAP use 2008 (UK). www.nice.org.uk/Guidance/TA139.

27. Sharma AM, Kushner RF. A proposed clinical staging system for obesity. Int J Obes (Lond). 2009;33(3):289–95.

A Case of Severe Hyponatraemia

Case 24

Deepa Narayanan and Julian H. Barth

Abstract

Hyponatraemia is the commonest electrolyte abnormality in hospitalised patients and is associated with increased mortality and inpatient stay. Evaluation and management of patients with hyponatraemia can be challenging as patients with hyponatraemia may be hypovolaemic, euvolaemic and even hypervolaemic.

Keywords

Hyponatraemia • Syndrome of inappropriate antidiuretic hormone secretion (SIADH) • Osmotic demyelination syndrome • Cerebral Pontine Myelinolysis • Euvolaemia • Hypovolaemia • Hypervolaemia • Vasopressin antagonists • Antidiuretic hormone • Renin angiotensin system • Aldosterone • Pseudohyponatraemia

Case

A previously well 52-year-old female was referred by her general practitioner with a 3-day history of confusion, and cough and vomiting of several days duration. She had recently returned from a holiday in Spain. She was known to be hypertensive and her blood pressure was relatively well controlled on Bendroflumethiazide 2.5 mg od. Her family history was insignificant and she was a non-smoker and drank very little alcohol.

> What are the differential diagnoses at this stage?

The common differential diagnoses of confusion are very wide and include:
1. Infection/inflammation – meningitis, encephalitis, sepsis, abscess
2. Vascular causes – intracerebral bleed, cerebral infarction, subarachnoid haemorrhage
3. Organ failure – renal failure, hepatic failure, respiratory failure (both type 1 and type 2)

D. Narayanan, MBBS, MRCP, FRCPath (✉)
J.H. Barth, FRCP, FRCPath, MD
Chemical Pathology/Metabolic Medicine,
Department of Blood Sciences, Leeds Teaching Hospitals NHS Trust, Great George Street, Leeds, West Yorkshire LS1 3EX, UK
e-mail: deepan@doctors.org.uk

R. Ajjan, S.M. Orme (eds.), *Endocrinology and Diabetes: Case Studies, Questions and Commentaries*,
DOI 10.1007/978-1-4471-2789-5_24, © Springer-Verlag London 2015

4. Biochemical causes – hypoglycaemia, electrolyte disturbances (hyponatraemia), vitamin deficiencies – Wernicke's Korsakoff psychosis
5. Intracranial space-occupying lesions – primary malignancy and secondaries
6. Toxins – alcohol
7. Drugs – hypnotics, tricyclic antidepressants
8. Endocrine causes – myxoedema, thyrotoxicosis, Addisonian crisis

On examination her heart rate was 90/min, regular in rhythm and blood pressure was 100/60 mmHg. The abbreviated mental test score was (AMTS) 4/10 and systemic examination was otherwise unremarkable.

What are the initial investigations needed to reach a diagnosis?
1. Urea and electrolyte profile
2. Liver function tests
3. Full blood count
4. Plasma glucose
5. C- reactive protein
6. Serum calcium
7. Mid-stream urine- culture and sensitivity
8. Blood culture and sensitivity
9. Chest x-ray
10. Arterial blood gases

The biochemistry laboratory contacted the acute medical team as serum sodium was < 100 mmol/L. The patient was noted to be clinically volume depleted and Bendroflumethiazide was stopped. A diagnosis of possible acute hyponatraemia was made in the absence of any previous available electrolyte results.

What further investigations are needed to investigate the aetiology of hyponatraemia?
1. Serum and urine osmolality
2. Urine sodium
3. Thyroid function tests
4. Total protein, albumin, albumin globulin gap
5. Plasma cortisol
6. CT brain
7. Lipids (Cholesterol, Triglycerides)

Table 24.1 Changes in serum sodium since admission

Days	Na mmol/L	Comments
On admission	<100	
Day 1	106	
Day 1	114	
Day 1	119	
Day 2	123	Confusion better
Day 3	128	
Day 4	129	
Day 6	129	IV fluids stopped
Day 8	131	

Further investigations showed serum osmolality of 211 mOsm/kg, urine osmolality of 444 mOsm/kg and urine sodium excretion was 77 mmol/L. A short synacthen test (SST) was performed and serum cortisol was 390 nmol/L on the basal sample peaking to 900 nmol/L at 30 minutes confirming adequate cortisol response. The serum thyroid stimulating hormone (TSH) was 1.3 m IU/L. The patient was commenced on 0.9 % saline 500 mLs 2 hourly initially and then 1.8 % saline 500 mL over 12 h. This intravenous fluid regimen of 2 litres over 24 hours was continued for 6 days. The change in serum sodium concentration over the subsequent days is tabulated in Table 24.1. On day 10, the patient was noted to be unresponsive and had developed a quadriparesis.

What complication has the patient developed?

Central pontine myelinolysis (CPM), also known as osmotic demyelination syndrome (ODS), is a potentially preventable complication of rapid sodium correction in hyponatraemic patients. ODS is associated with high mortality and morbidity and can be averted with early identification and management of patients with severe hyponatraemia.

An urgent magnetic resonance imaging (MRI) of the head confirmed the diagnosis of central pontine myelinolysis and the patient unfortunately died within a week of being diagnosed.

Introduction

Physiology

Sodium is an extracellular cation. The renin angiotensin system is the major regulator of sodium concentration in the body. Decreased renal blood flow can lead to increased renin with consequent conversion of angiotensinogen to angiotensin I and then to angiotensin II by angiotensin converting enzyme (ACE) in the lung. Angiotensin II stimulates aldosterone production from the adrenal cortex leading to increased sodium reabsorption from the distal convoluted tubule. Water homeostasis through stimulation of thirst and antidiuretic hormone (ADH) also plays a crucial role in the determination of sodium concentration in the body.

Hyponatraemia is defined as the presence of serum sodium of < 136 mmol/L [1]. Hyponatraemia is the commonest electrolyte abnormality in in-patients [1] (prevalence ranging from 5 to 15 %) and is more prevalent in some groups of patients including the elderly and postoperative patients [2]. Hyponatraemia has been linked with prolonged in-patient stay [3] particularly in patients with metastatic malignancy and heart failure [4]. Hyponatraemia has been shown to be an independent variable of increased mortality [5, 6] and the increased mortality may be secondary to the acute electrolyte disturbance and its management or the underlying aetiology of hyponatraemia [7]. Acute hyponatraemia is defined as onset of hyponatraemia of < 48 hours duration and chronic as the presence of hyponatraemia > 48 hours duration [5]. Hyponatraemia is further classified as mild (130–135 mmol/L), moderate (125–129 mmol/L) and severe (< 125 mmol/L). Patients with hyponatraemia are usually symptomatic when serum Na < 120 mmol/L.

The diagnosis of hyponatraemia is under reported [8] as its signs and symptoms are non-specific and require a high index of clinical suspicion. The signs and symptoms of hyponatraemia depend on the duration of onset and the degree of severity [1]. The clinical spectrum of hyponatraemia may range from nausea, vomiting, weakness and lethargy to symptoms like falls and increased fracture risk, impaired memory and cerebral

Table 24.2 Causes of hyponatraemia

Pseudohyponatraemia:
1. Hypertriglyceridaemia
2. Paraproteins- multiple myeloma
Hypertonic hyponatraemia:
1. Hyperglycaemia
2. Mannitol infusion
Hypotonic hyponatraemia:
Hypovolaemic hyponatraemia:
1. Diarrhoea and vomiting
2. Addison's disease
3. Cerebral salt wasting
4. Diuretics
5. Excess sweating, burns
Euvolaemic hyponatraemia:
1. SIADH- secondary to drugs (chlorpropamide, cytotoxics), malignancy (small cell lung carcinoma, intracranial causes (meningitis, cerebral or subarachnoid haemorrhage space occupying lesions), pulmonary causes (pneumonia, tuberculosis) and porphyria.
2. Stress – recent surgery
3. Endocrine causes – hypothyroidism, cortisol deficiency
4. Drugs- SSRI (selective seratonin reuptake inhibitors), diuretics, barbiturates, anticonvulsants and opiates.
5. Chronic renal failure
Hypervolaemic hyponatraemia:
1. Congestive cardiac failure
2. Decompensated chronic liver disease

oedema [9]. Hyponatraemia may be more than just a biochemical entity and may be a marker of sinister underlying pathology [2] (e.g., presence of congestive cardiac failure, chronic liver disease and malignancy).

Hyponatraemia may be secondary to excess water (secondary to excess infusion of hypotonic fluids or isotonic fluids like dextrose that are metabolised to water), low solute (salt losing conditions), artefactual (analytical or contaminated sample with intravenous fluids), high concentration of osmotically active substances (e.g., glucose and mannitol) and SIADH (syndrome of inappropriate ADH secretion). The common causes of hyponatraemia are tabulated in Table 24.2. Institution of appropriate therapy depends on the underlying aetiology and can be dramatically different ranging from restricting fluid intake to administering fluids.

Plasma osmolality = 2× (serum sodium + serum potassium) + urea + plasma glucose mOsm/Kg. Plasma osmolality is predominantly determined by plasma cations- sodium and potassium. In hyponatraemia, the fall in extracellular tonicity leads to an osmotic pressure gradient with movement of water into the intracellular compartment and consequent cerebral oedema if hyponatraemia is acute in onset [2]. The cerebral adaptation to the development of hyponatraemia involves movement of sodium, potassium and organic osmolytes from the intracellular to extracellular compartment to reduce intracellular tonicity [2]. This adaptation may take upto 48 h and hence the need for more cautious correction of sodium in patients with chronic symptomatic hyponatraemia [2]. However, hyponatraemia is also seen in hyperosmolar states (i.e., hyperglycaemia) where there is movement of water from the intracellular to the extracellular compartment with dilution of serum sodium concentration.

What is pseudohyponatraemia?

Hyponatraemia can be rarely secondary to the presence of paraproteins or elevated triglycerides causing analytical interference in the routine methodology used to measure serum sodium. Sodium is measured in plasma water (indirect ion selective electrode). Any condition associated with increased plasma solids like hypertriglyceridaemia or paraproteins lead to decreased plasma water. However, the effect of sample dilution prior to measurement and the assumption of constant proportion of plasma water and solids in the sample lead to artefactual hyponatraemia. The presence of normal plasma osmolality is a valuable clue to diagnose pseudohyponatraemia. When pseudohyponatraemia is suspected alternative methods to measure serum sodium may give an accurate measurement of sodium (direct ion selective electrode).

What is the commonest cause of dilutional hyponatraemia?

The most common cause of hyponatraemia is inappropriate hypotonic fluid replacement in postoperative patients (prevalence 1 %). Dextrose is essentially metabolised to free water leading to iatrogenic hyponatraemia [9]. There is sufficient literature on the need for judicious use of intravenous fluids in postoperative patients. Dilutional hyponatraemia is also seen in patients with excessive sweating and who drink plain water.

What is hypovolaemic hyponatraemia?

Hypovolaemic hyponatraemia is the loss of excess salt in relation to water. Loss of circulating volume leads to an increased plasma osmolality and accompanied with activation of renin angiotensin system (RAS) stimulates thirst and release of ADH. The net effect of RAS is increased sodium reabsorption from the distal convoluted tubule with sodium preservation and urine sodium excretion of < 10 mmol/L in extra-renal causes (e.g., diarrhoea and vomiting). However with diuretic therapy and salt losing kidney disease there is persistent natriuresis and hyponatraemia is further compounded by the stimulation of thirst mechanism leading to increased fluid intake.

What is cerebral salt wasting?

Cerebral salt wasting is characterised by massive natriuresis, dehydration and hyponatraemia and seen in patients with hypothalamic damage. It typically occurs after sub-arachnoid haemorrhage and is mediated by b-type natriuretic peptide. The patient's volume status, but not serum and urine electrolytes and osmolality, is crucial for making this diagnosis [10].

What is hypervolaemic hyponatraemia?

In congestive cardiac failure, the reduction in cardiac output leads to release of ADH and stimulation of RAS with aldosterone-mediated water and salt retention. In cirrhosis of liver, peripheral vasodilatation leads to a reduction in cardiac output and activation of mechanisms similar to congestive cardiac failure.

> What is the commonest cause of euvolaemic hyponatraemia?

Syndrome of inappropriate ADH is thought to be the most common cause of hyponatraemia and was first described by Bartter and Schwartz [11]. The diagnostic criteria for SIADH are tabulated in Table 24.3. SIADH is a diagnosis of exclusion. In SIADH the concentration of ADH is inappropriately high leading to water retention and consequent hyponatraemia. The main stimulants of ADH secretion are increased plasma osmolality and decreased intravascular volume. ADH binds to the V2 receptor in the collecting duct and leads to passive reabsorption of water from the collecting duct. In patients with SIADH, sodium handling by aldosterone and atrial natriuretic peptide (ANP) remains intact. Despite the reabsorption of water patients are not oedematous as the water is dispersed equally between the intra and extravascular compartments.

However, it has been debated that SIADH is a misnomer as not all patients have high concentrations of ADH and the term 'syndrome of inappropriate antidiuresis' is being proposed [12]. Fluid restriction (500–1000 mL) is the

Table 24.3 Diagnostic criteria for syndrome of inappropriate ADH secretion

1. Clinically euvolaemia
2. Low plasma osmolality (Plasma osmolality < 275 mOsm/kg)
3. High urine osmolality (> 100 mOsm/kg)
4. Natriuresis (urine Na > 40 mmol/L)
5. Normal renal, adrenal, thyroid and liver function

hallmark of SIADH treatment. Other treatment options include demeclocycline which produces an iatrogenic form of nephrogenic diabetes insipidus. Lithium is also used occasionally, although it is unlicensed for use. Vasopressin antagonists have been approved by NICE for oral use in adult patients with hyponatraemia secondary to SIADH. Their mode of action is to block binding of arginine-vasopressin to V2 receptors with resultant free water clearance without sodium depletion [13]. The vasopressin antagonists are expensive and need to be initiated with close monitoring of serum sodium and volume status [13].

> How to prevent osmotic demyelination syndrome?

Osmotic demyelination syndrome (ODS) is a serious complication associated with high mortality and morbidity and is seen with rapid sodium correction in chronic severe hyponatraemic patients [14]. It is a well-described phenomenon in particular groups of patients like chronic alcohol excess, malnutrition [14, 15], patients on diuretics and post liver transplant. The recent joint European guideline on the management of hyponatraemia recommends limiting the sodium increment to < 10 mmol/L in the first 24 hours and < 18 mmol/L in 48 hours [16]. However, determination of sodium increment completely free of risk may be improbable [15]. The rapid correction of chronic hyponatraemia leads to an increased osmolality with deficit of organic osmolytes and predisposes the oligodendrocytes to cell shrinkage and demyelination [15, 17]. The signs and symptoms of ODS are variable and influenced by the focus of demyelinating lesions [15, 17]. Treatment is conservative and the clinical outcome of patients with ODS is variable.

> What are the flaws in current clinical algorithms for the management of hyponatraemia?

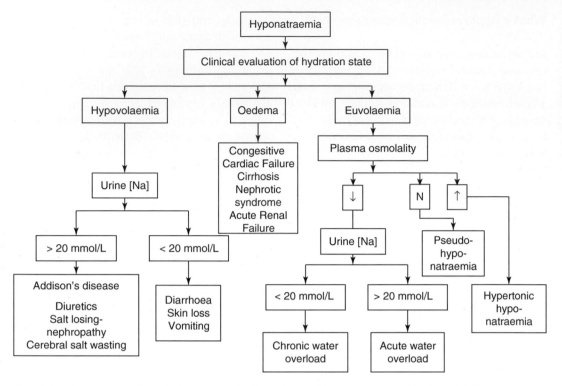

Fig. 24.1 Diagnostic algorithm for hyponatraemia (Reproduced with permission from Barth et al. [19])

There are different algorithms for diagnosis of hyponatraemia in review articles and medical textbooks [18]. The common parameters used in these algorithms clinical assessment of the extracellular fluid (ECF) volume and laboratory data [18]. The flaws in current algorithms include failure of inclusion of chronicity of low Na, reliance of correct estimation of volaemic state and the lack of consideration of underlying pathophysiology [18]. The commonly used equations for sodium correction fail to consider the effects of the added water and solutes and assume that there is no ongoing loss of fluid [18]. The European Society of Endocrinology, the European Society of Intensive Care Medicine (ESICM), and the European Renal Association – European Dialysis and Transplant Association have developed a new joint guideline on management of hyponatraemia [16]. The new joint clinical guideline suggests the use of urine osmolality and urine sodium initially and then assessment of volaemic status to categorise the various aetiologies of hyponatraemia [16]. Though the clinical assessment of fluid status is subjective, we however, propose an algorithm with fluid status as the key determinant to classify the different aetiologies (Fig. 24.1).

References

1. Adrogue HJ, Madias NE. Hyponatraemia. N Engl J Med. 2000;342:1581–9.
2. Anderson RJ, Chung HM, Kluge R, Schrier RW. Hyponatremia: a prospective analysis of its epidemiology and the pathogenesis. Ann Intern Med. 1985;102:164–8.
3. Waikar SS, Mount DB, Curhan GC. Mortality after hospitalization with mild, moderate, and severe hyponatremia. Am J Med. 2009;122:857–65.
4. Whelan B, Bennett K, O'Riordan D, Silke B. Serum sodium as a risk factor for in-hospital mortality in acute unselected general medical patients. QJM. 2009;102:175–82.
5. Arieff AI. Hyponatraemia, convulsions, respiratory arrest and permanent brain damage after elective surgery in healthy women. N Engl J Med. 1986;314:1529–34.
6. Gill G, Huda B, Boyd A, Skagen K, Wile D, Watson I et al. Characteristics and mortality of severe

hyponatraemia – a hospital-based study. Clin Endocrinol (Oxf). 2006;65:246–9.

7. Hoorn EJ, Lindemans J, Zietse R. Development of severe hyponatraemia in hospitalised patients: treatment-related risk factors and inadequate management. Nephrol Dial Transplant 2006;21:70–6.

8. Movig KL, Leufkens HG, Lenderink AW, Egberts AC. Validity of hospital discharge International Classification of Diseases (ICD) codes for identifying patients with hyponatremia. J Clin Epidemiol. 2003; 56:530–5.

9. Tambe AA, Hill R, Livesley PJ. Post-operative hyponatraemia in orthopaedic injury. Injury. 2003;34(4):253–5.

10. Yee AH, Burns JD, Wijdicks EF. Cerebral salt wasting: pathophysiology, diagnosis, and treatment. Neurosurg Clin N Am. 2010;21:339–52.

11. Schwartz WB, Bennett W, Curelop S, Bartter FC. A syndrome of renal sodium loss and hyponatremia probably resulting from inappropriate secretion of antidiuretic hormone. Am J Med. 1957;23:529–42.

12. Ellinson DH, Berl T. The syndrome of inappropriate antidiuresis. N Engl J Med. 2007;365:2064–72.

13. Decaux G, Soupart A, Vassart G. Non-peptide arginine-vasopressin antagonists: the vaptans. Lancet. 2008;371:1624–32.

14. Brown WD. Osmotic demyelination disorders: central pontine and extrapontine myelinolysis. Curr Opin Neurol. 2000;13:691–7.

15. Laureno R, Karp BI. Myelinolysis after correction of hyponatremia. Ann Intern Med. 1997;126:57–62.

16. Spasovski G, Vanholder R, Allolio B, Annane D, Ball S, Bichet D et al. Clinical practice guideline on diagnosis and treatment of hyponatraemia. Eur J Endocrinol. 2014;170:G1–47.

17. Ghosh N, DeLuca GC, Esiri MM. Evidence of axonal damage in human acute demyelinating diseases. J Neurol Sci. 2004;222:29–34.

18. Hoorn EJ, Halperin ML, Zietse R. Diagnostic approach to a patient with hyponatraemia: traditional versus physiology-based options. Q J Med. 2005; 98:529–40.

19. Barth JH, Butler GE, Hammond P. Biochemical investigations in laboratory medicine. London: ACB Venture Publications; 2001. p. 56.

Medical Problems Post Bariatric Surgery

Case 25

Chinnadorai Rajeswaran
and Tolulope Shonibare

Abstract

Bariatric surgery is a cost effective way of reducing weight and improving weight related complications. It also improves the quality of life to some extent. However it can precipitate a constellation of metabolic complications which can have serious consequences. This chapter will focus on the role and types of bariatric surgery and will discuss the advantages and complications of these surgical procedures.

Keywords

Obesity • Bariatric surgery • Nutrition complications • Metabolic complications • Depression • Eating disorder • Metabolic bone disease

Introduction

The rising incidence of worldwide obesity has resulted in an increase in the number of bariatric surgical procedures. The number of National Health Service (NHS)-commissioned bariatric procedures has increased by 530 % in the last 6 years with 5,407 procedures done in 2011, compared to 858 procedures in 2006 [1, 2]. The estimated annual cost for the NHS is £85 million [1].

C. Rajeswaran, MBBS, FRCP(UK), MSc (✉)
T. Shonibare, Bsc, MBchB, MRCP
Department of Diabetes, Endocrinology and Obesity,
Dewsbury District Hospital, Halifax Road, Dewsbury,
West Yorkshire WF13 4HS, UK
e-mail: Chinnadorai.rajeswaran@midyorks.nhs.uk;
tshons7@doctors.org.uk

There is emerging evidence to show that bariatric surgery is more effective in inducing and sustaining weight loss. In addition to this it improves weight-related metabolic conditions and quality of life [3].

Consideration of Bariatric Surgery

Lifestyle measures and pharmacotherapy are the current options which can be used to aid weight loss. However the National Institute of Clinical Excellence (NICE) have made recommendations for when to consider surgery [4]. The referral criteria are as follows:
- BMI of 40 kg/m^2 or more
- BMI 35–40 kg/m^2 with other significant co-morbidities which can be improved with weight loss

R. Ajjan, S.M. Orme (eds.), *Endocrinology and Diabetes: Case Studies, Questions and Commentaries*,
DOI 10.1007/978-1-4471-2789-5_25, © Springer-Verlag London 2015

- When appropriate non-surgical measures have failed to achieve or maintain clinically beneficial weight loss for 6 months
- Fit for general anaesthesia

Patients also need to show commitment to follow up and not have pre-existing psychiatric illness which can affect their outcome post-surgery.

Bariatric surgery and follow-up postoperatively should be undertaken by a specialist multi-disciplinary surgical team consisting of a bariatric surgeon, bariatric physicians (either an endocrinologist or gastroenterologist), physiotherapist and clinical psychologist [3].

Types of Bariatric Surgery

Surgery can be broadly divided into restrictive and malabsorptive procedures: In the United Kingdom, the three most common procedures carried out are laparoscopic adjustable gastric banding, gastric bypass and sleeve gastrectomy [2].

Restrictive Procedures

These rely on restricting the stomach capacity, thereby reducing oral intake and inducing early satiety. The anatomical continuity of the stomach and intestines are maintained, as a result the incidence of malabsorption and nutritional deficiencies are minimal [3].

Adjustable Gastric Band

This relies on restricting the stomach capacity by use of an adjustable gastric silicone band which is laparoscopically placed at the stomach fundus. The band contains saline, the volume of which can be altered via an external port which is tunnelled through the skin. Adjustment of the band width is made by injection or removal of the saline to alter the stomach capacity. This procedure is reversible [3].

Sleeve Gastrectomy

A vertical sleeve is created by removing 70–80 % of the stomach along the greater curvature and suturing the residual portion. This is a non-reversible procedure [3].

Intragastric Balloon

This reversible procedure is often as a bridge towards more complex bariatric surgery. A balloon is placed endoscopically in the stomach thereby restricting the stomach capacity [3].

Malabsorptive Procedures

These procedures employ a combination of malabsorptive and restrictive techniques to induce weight loss. Stomach capacity is reduced and intestinal reconstruction results in reduced food capacity and absorption. The incidence of nutritional deficiencies is much higher [3].

Roux-en-Y Gastric Bypass

This involves creating an anastomosis between the proximal segment of the stomach (gastric pouch) and the distal small bowel. As a result the proximal intestine (ileum and jejunum) are bypassed. This creates a blind end of proximal small bowel which is surgically re-attached at the distal small intestine. This is called the Roux limb, which acts as a secretory limb for digestive juices [3].

Bilio-Pancreatic Diversion with Duodenal Switch

A portion of the stomach is resected to create a small pouch which is anastomosed to the distal end of the small intestine, thereby bypassing the duodenum and jejunum [3].

Case

A 38-year-old married lawyer was referred to the medical bariatric clinic following a Roux-en-Y procedure. Her body mass index prior to surgery was 44.92 kg/m^2 with a weight of 134 kg and a height of 5 ft 8 in. She has a past medical history of type 2 diabetes mellitus, hypertension, menorrhagia and mild depression. Her blood pressure was 167/90 kg/m^2 and glycated haemoglobin

(HbA1c) was 77 mmol/mol. There were no immediate surgical complications post-operatively.

At her first follow up 6 months post surgery, her weight had reduced to 112 kg (BMI 37.54 kg/m^2). Her blood pressure was 149/88 and HbA1c 55 mmol/mol. She complained of hair falling out with brittle nails.

> What questions would you ask?

Medication History

Her blood pressure and glycaemic control have improved. A medication review is warranted to assess the need for insulin and oral metformin. It would be worthwhile enquiring about frequent hypoglycaemic events.

Several studies have shown that bariatric surgery improves glycaemic control in people with type 2 diabetes mellitus [5]. A meta-analyses cited a 78.1 % rate of remission and an 86.6 % rate of resolution in severely obese patients [6]. The rate of remission in patients who have undergone biliopancreatic diversion is highest followed by gastric bypass and banding [7, 8]. Remission is defined as a HbA1c less than 48 mmol/mol (6.5 %) when not on hypoglycaemic therapy [9].

A large observational study has however shown that 50 % of these patients suffer a relapse after 10 years apart from those who have had biliopancreatic diversion [7].

> What signs would you look for?

She describes symptoms of nutritional deficiency: thinning hair, brittle nails and lethargy all point to zinc and iron deficiency. It is important to specifically ask about these symptoms.

Screening for nutritional deficiencies in patients who have undergone malabsorptive surgery is necessary due to the anatomic changes that occur. The extent of nutritional evaluation is usually guided by the form of bariatric surgery

undertaken [10]. Frank deficiencies are less common in patients who have undergone restrictive surgery compared with malabsorptive procedures. Approximately 30 % of bariatric surgery patients will develop a nutritional deficiency following their operation [11, 12].

The types of nutritional deficiency can be broadly divided into macro-nutrient or micro-nutrient deficiencies. They can be further be classified into the following categories:
- Vitamin deficiency
- Mineral deficiency
- Trace element deficiency
- Protein deficiency
- Calorific deficiency

In practice patients are given dietary and multivitamin supplementation shortly after surgery [13]. Best practice guidelines recommend a lifelong daily multivitamin and calcium supplementation with added vitamin D [10]. A typical multivitamin preparation would consist of fat and water-soluble vitamins, alongside trace and minerals elements. It is also important to note that patients who have had Roux-en-Y surgery develop vitamin B12 deficiency due to bypass of the lower stomach thereby leading to impaired formation of intrinsic factor. Additional intramuscular preparations of vitamin B12 are usually needed in such patients. Iron deficiency is common in menstruating women [10].

Furthermore, studies have shown that daily multivitamin preparations are insufficient to prevent selective nutritional deficiencies. Therefore it is necessary to screen patients and tailor supplementation to the patient's requirements [12].

> What investigations do you need to reach a diagnosis?
> - Haemoglobin,
> - Ferritin
> - Mean cell volume
> - Zinc
> - Vitamin B12

Table 25.1 Nutrients and symptoms in deficiency

Nutrient	Biomarker(s)	Symptoms of deficiency
Vitamin A		Visual impairment reduced night vision
Vitamin B$_1$		Wernicke encephalopathy Nystagmus, ataxia Ophthalmoplegia
		Peripheral neuropathy
Vitamin B$_{12}$	Serum vitamin B$_{12}$	Anaemia
		Peripheral neuropathy
Vitamin D	Serum 25(OH) vitamin D, calcium,	Osteomalacia
	Parathyroid hormone	Secondary hyperparathyroidism
	Phosphate	
Vitamin E		Ataxia
		Neuropathy
Vitamin K	Clotting screen	Bleeding
		Bruising
Folate	Red blood cell folate	Anaemia
Iron	Serum ferritin, total iron binding capacity,	Microcytic anaemia
Zinc	Plasma zinc	Acrodermatitis
		Taste alterations
		Alopecia
		Glossitis
Copper	Serum copper	Anaemia
		Neuropathy
Selenium	Serum selenium	Cardiomyopathy
Protein	Serum albumin	Oedema
		Poor wound healing

Reprinted from Xanthakos [33], Copyright © 2009, with permission from Elsevier

Screening in Practice

Patients are routinely screened at 6-monthly intervals following surgery. Specific nutritional deficiencies can also be determined based on the patient's symptoms.

Table 25.1 presents nutrients and corresponding symptoms in deficiency.

At her second follow-up at 12 months following surgery, she revealed that she had recently split from her husband and had been drinking excessive amounts of alcohol. She had also received an official caution from work, pending a disciplinary hearing. Her depression had worsened and on examination she had a slight tremor. She admitted to not taking her vitamin supplements.

What are the main problems highlighted from this consultation?

This patient has developed an addiction to alcohol which has resulted in marital breakdown and problems at work. She is also non-compliant with her medication.

Premorbid Psychological Health

A range of psychological co-morbidities occur in obese individuals such as depression, anxiety and low self- esteem [14]. Also, obese patients tend to have psychosocial challenges that result in social isolation and tendency to belong to a lower socio-economic class [14, 15]. Furthermore, they are less likely to be in full time employment compared to non-obese counter parts [14].

Prior to bariatric surgery, a psychological evaluation is undertaken to assess readiness for surgery and manage patient's expectations following their operation. Also it is an opportunity to identify any potential contraindications such as active suicidal behaviour, hallucinations, delusions and severe cognitive impairment [16].

Post-operative Psychological Health

A prospective controlled study involving 4,047 obese patients showed a significant improvement in quality of life and a decrease in depression and anxiety in the first year following surgery compared to obese controls treated with diet and counselling [8, 17].

However, there are reports of patient's mental health returning to their pre-operative state or even deteriorating after 2–3 years [18].

Eating Disorders

There is also evidence to suggest that some patients do develop post-surgical eating disorders such as anorexia nervosa and bulimia. The suggested mechanism behind this is that patients either develop eating avoidance behaviours due to discomfort from early satiety induced by gastric restriction or patients fail to psychologically adjust to food portion sizes leading to bulimia [19, 20].

Addiction

There is some anecdotal evidence to suggest that patients develop a "transfer addiction," i.e., from food to alcohol after bariatric surgery. Alcohol has been recognised as a high risk substance of abuse in bariatric patients. Gastric bypass operations alter the metabolism of alcohol, which may enhance its effects [19, 21, 22].

The choice of alcohol is affected as patients prefer to abuse spirits as opposed to beer which require larger amounts to achieve the desired effects. It would be prudent in such patients to also screen for thiamine deficiency as there is a risk of developing Wernickes-Korsakoff syndrome from both the bariatric surgery and alcohol abuse [10]. A negative change in behaviour could potentially exacerbate psychosocial problems both at home and the work place.

Interpersonal Relationships

There have been reports of high divorce rates and relationship break downs following surgery. This can be attributable to the patient and their partner struggling with their new body image. Relationship dynamics can change if the patient gets more attention from other suitors thereby boosting their self-esteem, resulting in promiscuity. Finally, new-gained self- confidence can trigger patients to leave particularly abusive relationships in search of a better life [23].

At her third follow up her weight had increased to 170 kg. She was notably breathless during the consultation. She revealed that she has been experiencing dizziness and sweatiness following a meal. This was relieved by eating a snack. As a consequence her appetite had increased. She also complained of increased breathlessness on minimal exertion and had suffered from paroxysmal nocturnal dyspnoea for the last 2 months. On examination there was evidence of bilateral pitting oedema with a splint on her left wrist following a hairline fracture after a fainting episode.

What is the differential diagnosis?

Dumping Syndrome

This patient is describing features of dumping syndrome. This phenomenon arises as a result of food high in sugar and fat being delivered largely undigested to the small intestine causing osmotic overload. Fluid is drawn into the intestinal lumen by osmosis stimulating a vagal reaction [24]. Patients present with abdominal cramps, sweating, nausea, diarrhoea, flushing, tachycardia and syncope [10]. Dumping syndrome can occur in up to 70–76 % of patients who have had RYGB [5, 10, 25]. Symptoms tend to become less prominent with time, however if proven difficult, avoidance of energy dense foods can be effective [10]. Medical treatment includes Octreotide and Arcabose. Patients who suffer from frequent episodes of dumping syndrome should not be offered slow release preparation of tablets due to incomplete absorption by the digestive tract [3].

Cardiomyopathy

This patient appears to be developing symptomatic cardiac failure. She has admitted to not taking her vitamin supplements and it is likely that she has developed Selenium deficiency which can lead to cardiomyopathy. Selenium is a trace element which is a component of glutathione peroxidase, an enzyme that may help prevent oxidative damage to cells. There have been numerous case reports of congestive cardiomyopathy as a result of Selenium deficiency. This is fully reversible upon selenium supplementation [26, 27].

Metabolic Bone Disease

She has developed a fracture following a syncopal episode due to dumping syndrome. This fracture is as a result of metabolic bone disease secondary to bariatric surgery. Voluntary weight loss due to any cause in an obese person results in approximately 1–2 % bone loss in all sites [28]. This correlates with the speed of weight loss [29].

Metabolic bone disease in obese patients is due to a number of factors such as inadequate intake of calcium and vitamin D post-operatively [30]. Also malabsorptive bariatric surgery results in reduced absorption of calcium and vitamin D due to bypass of the duodenum and proximal jejunum [30]. This results in a rise in Parathyroid hormone (PTH), i.e., secondary hyperparathyroidism, leading to increased bone resorption [28].

It is a phenomenon which has been demonstrated in large studies with up to 70 % of patients who have had malabsorptive surgery being affected [28, 31]. Patients can present with bone and joint pain, muscle weakness and fatigue. In extreme cases they present with bone fractures [30].

Monitoring of patients can be carried out by measuring calcium, PTH and vitamin D levels every 6 months for the first 2 years then annually. Objective measurements of bone mass density can be carried out by using annual dual-energy x-ray absorptiometry (DEXA) scan to quantify the degree of bone loss pre and post operatively until bone mineral density is stable [10, 28].

Table 25.2 Causes and prevention of weight gain

Causes	Prevention
Non-compliance with dietary/lifestyle restrictions	Dietary and lifestyle compliance
Insulin use	Regular clinic follow-up
Surgical failure	Regular physical activity 150 min/week
Psychological factors	Surgical revision
Dumping syndrome	Avoid high sugar/fat containing food

Adapted from Heber et al. [10]

Management of this condition is mainly preventative by giving vitamin D and calcium supplements. There is a scarcity of data on the use of bisphosphonates in such patients who have had bariatric surgery [28].

Weight Regain

This patient has started to regain weight. The vast majority of weight loss occurs in the first year. At 18–24 months most patients reach a weight loss plateau and in some cases, suffer from weight regain [10, 24].

Patients need to be regularly reviewed by a dietitian to re-enforce changes in nutritional habits such as avoiding or minimising carbohydrate dense foods which can lead to dumping. One of the symptoms of dumping syndrome is hunger, as a result patients tend to continuously eat to alleviate symptoms leading to weight gain [10].

See Table 25.2 for the causes of and ways of preventing weight re-gain

> Do obesity-related complications resolve following bariatric surgery?

Obesity is associated with co-morbidities such as type 2 diabetes mellitus, hyperlipidaemia, hypertension, obstructive sleep apnoea, cerebrovascular accidents and cardiovascular disease, degenerative joint problems and malignancy [6]. These co-morbidities result in 2.5 million deaths per year worldwide [32].

Table 25.3 Co-morbidity outcomes

Co-morbidity	Outcome (meta-analysis mean)
Diabetes (resolution)	76.8 % (95 % C.I. 70.7–89.2 %)
Diabetes (resolution or improvement)	86.0 % (95 % C.I. 78.4–93.7 %)
Reduction in total cholesterol	33.20 mg/dL (95 % C.I. 23.17–43.63 mg/dL)
Hypertension (resolution)	61.7 % (95 % C.I. 55.6–67.8 %)
Hypertension (resolution or improvement)	78.5 % (95 % C.I. 70.8–86.1 %)
OSA (resolution)	85.7 % (95 % C.I. 79.2–92.2 %)
OSA (resolution or improvement)	83.6 % (95 % C.I. 71.8–95.4 %)

Adapted from Buchwald et al. [6]

In addition to weight loss, the added benefits of bariatric surgery include an improvement of life expectancy post-surgery. This is achieved by an improvement in the severity of some of the obesity-related complications [8].

A Swedish study which was a large prospective study of obese patients, followed 4,047 obese subjects for an average of 10 years. These subjects were control matched to obese patients who were treated conventionally. This study showed an 80 % decrease in the annual mortality of diabetic patients who had surgery. After 9 years, the surgical group had a 9 % mortality compared to the control group which had a 28 % mortality [6, 8]. Improvements in glycaemic control have been observed with some patients discontinuing insulin [10]. It is however important to note that the longer the duration of diabetes, the less likely the patient would respond to surgically induced weight loss due to poor beta cell reserve.

A Meta-analysis has shown the percentage of patients who experience an improvement in hyperlipidaemia is 70 %. The maximum improvements were noted in patients who have had biliopancreatic diversion or duodenal switch [6]. The total amount of patients with resolution or improvement of hypertension was 78.5 %, and those with obstructive sleep apnoea were 83.6 % [6].

Table 25.3 summarises the co-morbidity outcomes post-surgery.

What are the complications of bariatric surgery?

The operative risk needs to be balanced against the benefits that occur following surgery. A meta-analysis has shown that the operative mortality at 30 days or less was 0.1 % for purely restrictive procedures, 0.5 % in patients undergoing a gastric bypass procedure and 1.1 % in those undergoing biliopancreatic diversion or duodenal switch procedures [6]. Finally, there is emerging evidence to suggest a link between bariatric surgery and colorectal carcinoma. A retrospective register-based cohort study on post bariatric surgery patients has demonstrated an increased risk of developing colorectal carcinoma [32].

Table 25.4 summarises complications that can occur following bariatric surgery.

Table 25.4 Complications of bariatric surgery

Immediate
Bleeding
Wound infection
Anaesthetic complications
Early
Leakage from staple lines
Thromboembolism
Infection
Bleeding
Late
Gall stones
Ulcers at anastomotic sites
Anastomotic strictures
Intestinal adhesions/obstructions
Dumping syndrome
Diarrhoea
Band erosion or slippage after gastric band surgery
Nutritional deficiencies
Weight regain
Excess skin following weight loss
Psychological or psychiatric issues

Reprinted from Rajeswaran et al. [3]. Copyright © 2013, MA Healthcare Limited

Summary

As the incidence of obesity increases, more patients will begin to fit the criteria for bariatric surgery. The increasing popularity stems from the evidence which shows that it is indeed a viable option for weight loss, with the added benefit of ameliorating the severity of the associated co-morbidities. However, clinicians should also be mindful of the potential post-operative complications and their respective management. To ensure long-term success, patients should be managed by a specialist multi-disciplinary team prior to surgery and thereafter. Finally patients should be reminded of the need for life-long supplementation.

References

1. Gastric Bypass up 530 % in 6 years, NHS choices, Health News; Aug 2012. http://www.nhs.uk/news/2012/08august/Pages/gastric-bypass-surgery-up-fivefold-in-six-years.aspx.
2. Bariatric surgery for obesity, national obesity observatory. Aug 2010. http://www.noo.org.uk/uploads/doc/vid_8774_NOO%20Bariatric%20Surgery%20for%20Obesity%20FINAL%20MG%2011210.pdf.
3. Rajeswaran C, Shaikh R, Mohammad M. Bariatric surgery: a long-term solution to managing diabesity. Pract Nurs. 2013;24(12):608–15.
4. Obesity. Guidance on the prevention of overweight and obesity is adults and children. https://www.nice.org.uk/guidance/cg43.
5. Pories WJ, Swanson MS, MacDonald KG, Long SB, Morris PG, Brown BM, Barakat HA, et al. Who would have thought it? An operation proves to be the most effective therapy for adult-onset diabetes mellitus. Ann Surg. 1995;222(3):339.
6. Buchwald H, et al. Bariatric surgery: a systematic review and meta-analysis. JAMA. 2004;292(14):1724–37.
7. Sjöström L. Review of the key results from the Swedish Obese Subjects (SOS) trial–a prospective controlled intervention study of bariatric surgery. J Intern Med. 2013;273(3):219–34.
8. Sjöström L, Lindroos AK, Peltonen M, Torgerson J, Bouchard C, Carlsson B, Dahlgren S, et al. Lifestyle, diabetes, and cardiovascular risk factors 10 years after bariatric surgery. N Engl J Med. 2004;351(26):2683–93.
9. Spanou M, Tziomalos K. Bariatric surgery as a treatment option in patients with type 2 diabetes mellitus. World J Diabetes. 2013;4(2):14.
10. Heber D, Greenway FL, Kaplan LM, Livingston E, Salvador J, Still C, Endocrine Society. Endocrine and nutritional management of the post-bariatric surgery patient: an Endocrine Society Clinical Practice Guideline. J Clin Endocrinol Metab. 2010;95(11):4823–43.
11. National Institute of Diabetes and Digestive and Kidney Diseases. www.niddk.nih.gov/health/nutrit/pubs/gastsurg.htm. Accessed November 2014.
12. Fujioka K, DiBaise JK, Martindale RG. Nutrition and metabolic complications after bariatric surgery and their treatment. JPEN J Parenter Enteral Nutr. 2011;35(5 Suppl):52S–9.
13. John S, Hoegerl C. Nutritional deficiencies after gastric bypass surgery. J Am Osteopath Assoc. 2009;109(11):601–4.
14. Kubik JF, Gill RS, Laffin M, Karmali S. The impact of bariatric surgery on psychological health. J Obes. 2013;2013:837989.
15. Stunkard AJ, Wadden TA. Psychological aspects of severe obesity. Am J Clin Nutr. 1992;55(2):524S–32.
16. Snyder AG. Psychological assessment of the patient undergoing bariatric surgery. Ochsner J. 2009;9(3):144–8.
17. Karlsson J, Sjöström L, Sullivan M. Swedish obese subjects (SOS)–an intervention study of obesity. Two-year follow-up of health-related quality of life (HRQL) and eating behavior after gastric surgery for severe obesity. Int J Obes Relat Metab Disord. 1998;22(2):113–26.
18. Van Hout G. Psychosocial effects of bariatric surgery. Acta Chir Belg. 2005;105(1):40–3.
19. Marcus M, Kalarchian M, Courcoulas A. Psychiatric evaluation and follow-up of bariatric surgery patients. Am J Psychiatry. 2009;166(3):285–91.
20. Deitel M. Anorexia nervosa following bariatric surgery. Obes Surg. 2002;12(6):729–30.
21. Sogg S. Alcohol misuse after bariatric surgery: epiphenomenon or "Oprah" phenomenon? Surg Obes Relat Dis. 2007;3(3):366–8.
22. Hagedorn JC, Encarnacion B, Brat GA, Morton JM. Does gastric bypass alter alcohol metabolism? Surg Obes Relat Dis. 2007;3(5):543–8.
23. Orzech D. Counselling bariatric surgery patients. Social Work Today. 5(6):24.
24. Fujioka K. Follow-up of nutritional and metabolic problems after bariatric surgery. Diabetes Care. 2005;28(2):481–4.
25. Monteforte MJ, Turkelson CM. Bariatric surgery for morbid obesity. Obes Surg. 2000;10(5):391–401.
26. Cheng TO. Selenium deficiency and cardiomyopathy. J R Soc Med. 2002;95(4):219–20.
27. Bergqvist AG, Chee CM, Lutchka L, Rychik J, Stallings VA. Selenium deficiency associated with cardiomyopathy: a complication of the ketogenic diet. Epilepsia. 2003;44(4):618–20.
28. Williams SE. Metabolic bone disease in the bariatric surgery patient. J Obes. 2011;2011:634614.

29. Shapses SA, Riedt CS. Bone, body weight, and weight reduction: what are the concerns? J Nutr. 2006;136(6): 1453–6.

30. Sanghera TS, Kang SN, Hamdan K. Metabolic bone disease and bariatric surgery. Rheumatol Curr Res. 2012;S5:001.

31. Collazo-Clavell ML, Jimenez A, Hodgson SF, Sarr MG. Osteomalacia after Roux-en-Y gastric bypass. Endocr Pract. 2004;10(3):195–8.

32. Derogar M, Hull MA, Kant P, Östlund M, Lu Y, Lagergren J. Increased risk of colorectal cancer after obesity surgery. Ann Surg. 2013;258(6):983–8.

33. Xanthakos SA. Nutritional deficiencies in obesity and after bariatric surgery. Pediatr Clin North Am. 2009;56(5):1105–21.

Index

R. Ajjan, S.M. Orme (eds.), *Endocrinology and Diabetes: Case Studies, Questions and Commentaries*,
DOI 10.1007/978-1-4471-2789-5, © Springer-Verlag London 2015

Printed by Printforce, the Netherlands